Springer Wien New York

Jeremy C. Ganz

Gamma Knife Neurosurgery

SpringerWienNewYork

Dr. Jeremy C. Ganz
Oysteinsgate 16
5007 Bergen
Norway
jcganz@gmail.com

© Springer-Verlag/Wien 2011
Printed in Germany

SpringerWienNewYork is a part of Springer Science+Business Media
springer.at

Typesetting: SPI, Pondicherry, India

Printed on acid-free and chlorine-free bleached paper
SPIN: 12791149

With 73 Figures

Library of Congress Control Number: 2010935853

ISBN 978-3-7091-0342-5   e-ISBN 978-3-7091-0343-2
DOI 10.1007/978-3-7091-0343-2
SpringerWienNewYork

This book is dedicated to my wife "Annie" Gao Nan Ping. Only the wives of authors can truly understand the domestic upheaval that results from an author's pre-occupation and obsession over his writing. Without her constant and unceasing support this book would never have been written.

Foreword

This new addition to the plethora of literature on radiosurgery in general and Gamma Knife surgery in particular, is a massive and phenomenal accomplishment.

In 1993 Doctor Ganz wrote the book "**Gamma Knife Surgery – A Guide for referring physicians**". A revised edition was published again by Springer in 1997. As indicated by its title, this book was intended for the general practitioner who needed to get a fleeting understanding of Gamma Knife surgery in order to be able to make informed recommendations to his or her patients. While the book accomplished this objective it was too sketchy to become a true work of reference, for a novice in the field or even for an established practitioner of Gamma Knife surgery.

All the limitations of the previous book(s) have been addressed in detail in this tome. As you read this work you will be led through every relevant aspect of the field in a most didactic and enjoyable way. Doctor Ganz, never known to be shy, doesn't steer away from controversial issues but rather, and admirably, addresses them head on!

Part I of "**Gamma Knife Neurosurgery**" starts with a look at the definition of radiosurgery and how this has evolved recently. The original definition of radiosurgery called for a high dose of ionizing radiation being delivered in a single session. This is how radiosurgery is administered to intracerebral targets, mostly using a stereotactic frame anchored to the skull. As the use of radiosurgery has become increasingly widespread it has also been attractive to apply it to various extracerebral targets. As a consequence fixation principles also have changed. Face masks are used in place of bony frame fixation and various methods of body immobilization have been developed. Since none of these are as accurate as bony fixation, a need for fractionation has emerged. The "surgical" properties of single session high dose radiation are lost when fractionating. Nevertheless, the two principles now coexist, hopefully to the benefit of a larger number of patients.

In reading the manuscript I enjoyed the proposed new name of **Gamma Knife Neurosurgery (GKNS)**. Neurosurgeons have often not been particularly good at protecting the interests of their own specialty. The proposed name change would clarify who the gatekeeper is!

Several additional chapters in Part I will help the reader grasp many of the finer points of radiosurgery, including the use of stereotaxy as well as the radiophysics and radiobiology of radiosurgery. Dose planning and the importance of good quality neuroimaging are highlighted and well explained.

Part II highlights numerous factors relevant to the patient. Some of the things brought up in this chapter are mandatory reading for any doctor, in his face to face encounter with patients deeply worried about their disease, its treatment and its prognosis.

In Part III the reader will gain innumerable insights into each and every indication to which the Gamma Knife has been applied, historically and currently, as well as indications for which its use is being currently researched. The author has also diligently included sections on movement disorders, epilepsy and pain. Movement disorder surgery fell out of favor with advent of L-Dopa in the early 1970s, for which Swedish pharmacologist Arvid Carlsson was awarded the Nobel Prize in 2000. However, since a decade or so we have seen a remarkable resurgence of interventional therapies for these disorders. One such remedy has become DBS which by some has been promoted as the "final solution" for many functional disorders. On this I beg to differ. I do not believe DBS to be the panacea it is described as by some. It is invasive, it is expensive and it is definitely not free of complications. If non-invasive radiosurgery can be suspected of accomplishing the same results as DBS, without the morbidity associated with DBS and without adding new morbidity, then it would be unethical not to explore its utility further.

The only section I tend to disagree with, largely for the same reasons as above, is the small section on so-called psychosurgery. Firstly I disagree with the use of the term itself. We do surgery for vestibular schwannomas, for AVM's and for pain. By the same token we should say that we do surgery for OCD and depression. The stigma associated with the term psychosurgery needs to be relegated to the past. Secondly, I disagree with Doctor Ganz's conclusion that DBS "is likely to become the preferred treatment". The disadvantages of DBS are possibly even more pronounced in cases of OCD than they are in some of the other disorders it is being used for. More research is needed in this area before drawing any definitive conclusions about the future.

Nonetheless, in summary, this is a very comprehensive and well written book on Gamma Knife Neurosurgery. It is extremely well illustrated and a lot of work has gone into providing us with relevant references.

Every neurosurgical department should have at least one copy of this book in its library. It should be mandatory reading for neurosurgery residents and it is mandatory reading for anyone involved with, or planning to get involved with Gamma Knife Neurosurgery.

GP's who want to refer patients to be considered for radiosurgery would be greatly helped by the knowledge and guidance provided by this excellent addition to the existing literature on radiosurgery in general and Gamma Knife Neurosurgery in particular.

It has been a pleasure to be one of the first readers and I will cherish my copy once it's printed.

Stockholm, Sweden   Dan Leksell

Preface

In 1993 the author of this book published a short work on Gamma Knife surgery. At the time less than 20,000 patients had been treated world wide and there were only a handful of centres equipped with Gamma Knives. Since that time radiosurgery has exploded so that there are now over 250 machines installed world wide and over 500,000 patients have been treated with the Gamma Knife. Moreover, the machine itself has developed through several generations to its current model "Perfexion".

The use of focused radiation to improve the sparing of normal tissue is now used outside the head. This means that there has also been a development of other methods for delivering stereotactic radiation than the Gamma Knife. The extent of this development was demonstrated in 2008 with the publication the first exhaustive text on radiosurgery embracing all its aspects. This was "Principles and Practice of Stereotactic Radiosurgery", edited by Lawrence S. Chin and William F. Regine and published by Springer Verlag. This book marks a new departure, signalling as it does that radiosurgery is today truly a whole body concern.

Despite the publication of such a comprehensive text there remain several reasons for writing a book limited to just the Gamma Knife. These reasons are based less on the technology and more on the development of the modern medical milieu over the past 20 years.

Firstly, it is no longer possible for an individual hospital physician/surgeon to manage patients alone. The complexity of modern knowledge requires management with teams. This is mentioned in a little more detail in the final chapter. Nonetheless, the ultimate responsibility for the management of a disease should be in the hands of a specialist trained in the understanding of the disease and not by the method of treatment. Thus, neurosurgical diseases should be managed by neurosurgeons and neurosurgeons should all be familiar with radiosurgery. Even so the neurosurgeon will require the advice and guidance of radiologists, pathologists, oncologists, neurologists, nurses and in the case of the Gamma Knife physicists. This notion will be mentioned repeatedly in different contexts throughout the book as it is considered to be of prime importance.

Secondly, there is a vast literature on the management of different diseases using the Gamma Knife. This is by no means uniform in its opinions of indications for treatment and the technique of radiosurgery when that is deemed the treatment of choice. This book aims to provide a guide through the maze of varying opinions. It is not for the author to say which opinion is correct, though it is possible for him to state a personal preference. However, it is hoped that the differing opinions and their underlying reasoning are fairly presented so that the reader may make a balanced judgment.

This book is intended primarily for neurosurgeons in training and referring physicians including neurosurgeons. It is emphasized it is a book limited to intracranial disease and has thus been given the title *Gamma Knife Neurosurgery*. The relevant basic science aspects of intracranial radiosurgery are described.

To simplify access to information of interest for any given reader, the book is divided into three main parts. Firstly there is an outline of the scientific principles underlying radiosurgery. This part is concluded with an account of how the Leksell Gamma Knife has developed. Secondly, there is a short part, containing information directly related to the patients and how they experience the treatment. This part also contains comments on the impact of computer networks on clinical practice and the patient's experience. In the third part there is an account of current thinking on the commonest diseases treated in the Gamma Knife. At the end of the book there is a short concluding chapter indicating desirable directions of future interest and expansion.

In conclusion, the author would like to emphasise two points. Firstly, the reader's attention is drawn once again to the importance of radiation dose in the Gamma Knife treatment of diseases. The first question that must be asked when comparing results from one centre with those of another is – *what was the dose*? If this simple information is not available then assessment of the results is impossible. There are of course other variables which may be considered but dose is essential. The second point concerns choices of the best method for treatment. It is regrettable that different methods of treatment are viewed all too often as competitors. On reflection it seems that in reality different methods complement rather than compete with each other. Once again the allocation of patient management to teams of experts instead of individual physicians should help to make such competition and debate unnecessary.

Bergen, Norway   Jeremy G. Ganz
30 June 2010

Acknowledgements

Nobody can write a book without help from other people. The first step is to obtain relevant background literature and the University Library in Bergen with its easy electronic access to research literature has been absolutely vital.

The contents of this work cover amongst other fields the mathematical labyrinth which is medical and nuclear physics. Jan Heggdal in Haukeland Hospital has been of great assistance especially with regard to matters related to the α/β ratio and the significance of the linear quadratic equation. He is the latest in a long line of physicists who have pointed the author in the direction of accuracy of concept and expression. They include his predecessor at the Gamma Knife in Bergen, Frits Thorsen. However, the physicist who has had the greatest influence on the author's albeit limited understanding of the behaviour of ionizing radiation is of course Jürgen Arndt, friend and mentor and one of the pioneers of radiosurgery. Discussing science with Jürgen is one of life's real pleasures. I should also like to thank Professor Herbert van der Kogel of Niejmegen in Holland. He is a leading authority on radiobiology, especially the radiobiology of the CNS. His recently published volume on radiobiology has proved invaluable.

Much of the clinical material on which this book and the author's experience is based was acquired during 6 years working with the new Gamma Knife Center in Cairo. Firstly on the administrative level, the managing team of Moustafa El Asmar and Amr Rifaat ensured that the necessary facilities were always available, which was no easy task. Importing wooden crates to carry necessary equipment provided unforeseen and unforgettable difficulties. Of course thanks are also due to the Nasser Institute which proved creatively positive for the stranger which had been constructed within their grounds. Without their help the Centre would have had insurmountable difficulties. On the clinical level I should like say thank you to the various nurses who were with us during the 6 years. They were ever pleasant and helpful and skilful with the patients. Then, I should like to thank Mr. Magdy the physicist for his unfailing good humour and willingness to solve problems. However, my major thanks go the team of young physicians with whom I had the pleasure to co-operate and teach. It has been truly said that the best way to learn a subject is to teach it and this proved to be the case. So thanks go to Drs. Wael Reda,

Khalid Abdelkarim and Amr El Shehaby who kept the author constantly on his toes; asking sensible questions that were by no means always easy to answer. They also provided invaluable assistance in enabling communication with the patients. It is a great pleasure to see how their careers are developing and to know that they are achieving the increasing respect and recognition they deserve.

Having returned to Bergen, in the daily work with the Gamma Knife if there were no patients there would be no basis for this book. In this respect I should like to mention the group of nurses who are responsible for all the work involved in arranging appointments and admissions and who are never less than helpful. They are led by Sidsel Bragstad and including Marianne Flatebø, Håvard Teksle, Kjersti Klett and Eirik Johansen, Elisabeth Larsen who looks after all the paper work generated by the activity with speed and efficiency has been great to work with.

Many colleagues have contributed to the establishment of Gamma Knife treatment in Bergen. Professor Backlund acquired the machine and was the author's mentor in its use. However, since 1993 to the present day the Bergen Gamma Knife has been run with skill, knowledge and expertise by Professor Paal-Henning Pedersen. He is also the co-author of the chapter on intrinsic brain tumours. One of the sadder parts of retiring from work is to have to wish him goodbye. The head of neurosurgery in Bergen, Erling Myrseth also deserves my thanks for offering me the possibility to rejoin the old team and continue to work in the hospital where I have spent most of my professional career. It has also been a pleasure to work with Dr. Bente Skeie who is a willing and enthusiastic student of radiosurgery; definitely a quick study. Gamma Knife treatment is impossible without images and it is a pleasure to thank Jostein Kråkenes, Alf Inge Smievoll, Gunnar Moen and Jonas Lind, who have devoted much time and patience to the pre- and post-treatment assessment of patients and of course in helping to ensure that the targets are defined with maximum accuracy. Also I should like to thank the large number of radiographers who were always helpful and sometimes challenging. They truly contributed to the author's somewhat uncertain belief that maybe he understands something of MRI; though clearly never enough.

This author also owes a permanent debt to Gerhard Pendl of Karl-Franzens-University in Graz, Austria who welcomed the author as an academic colleague and placed all the resources of his department at his disposal. Today, I should also like to thank Drs. Michael Mokry and Frank Unger for their assistance and help in the use of images from their department.

The author is also indebted to Elekta Instruments AB, the manufacturer of the Gamma Knife for permission to use parts of their presentation material in the design of Figs. 6.9 and 6.11.

Finally, I should like to express my gratitude to the Gamma Knife itself and to its inventor Professor Lars Leksell. This machine is a constant source of satisfaction, with its elegant simplicity of concept and its equally elegant simplicity in daily use.

Contents

Part III   The Gamma Knife and Specific Diseases: Tumours

Part I
Background Principles and Technical Development

Chapter 1
Introduction and the Nature of Radiosurgery

The impulse to perform surgery antedates literacy by some thousands of years, as demonstrated by the large number of prehistoric trephined skulls that have been discovered. These earliest operations were based at best on superficial empirical experience and not on knowledge, in any way in which that term could be understood today. Thus it is remarkable that they were performed at all. What is even more remarkable is that the "patients" allowed themselves to be subjected to such surgery. All this suggests that the need to operate or to suffer surgery is primitive and not entirely rational. In fairness to the Stone Age surgeons, many of these prehistoric trephine openings show signs of healing. Thus their operations were in fact often successful, measured by the yardstick of technical success.

The next stage in neurosurgical development following prehistoric trepanation came with Hippocrates. This remarkable man told us "First do no harm". Even so, the same Hippocrates, with very little if any neuroanatomical knowledge described in detail the indications and procedures to be followed in the treatment of skull injuries. His practical advice, for example on cooling the trephine was excellent. His indications for surgery were often, by any rational modern standard, bizarre.

These few examples could be multiplied ad infinitum. The point is that even wise people can be tempted to perform surgery in situations where the indications are dubious. And it must be admitted; there is something theatrical and attractive about the whole concept of a surgical operation. There is the exciting setting, in an operating room, with all its attendant technology, ritual and regalia. There is the dramatic procedure, with its attendant risks and rewards. However, it is an undeniable fact that all surgery is potentially dangerous. There cannot be a surgeon alive who has not, when re-operating a patient, witnessed the scar tissue resulting from previous surgery, itself a witness to the fact that all surgery exacts a price. Happily, such scar tissue usually does no apparent harm but its presence is a reminder that the body resents mechanical interference. In addition, all operations carry with them local risks of bleeding and infection in the operating field and more systemic risks related to immobilization.

J.C. Ganz, *Gamma Knife Neurosurgery*,
DOI 10.1007/978-3-7091-0343-2_1, © Springer-Verlag/Wien 2011

Thus, it is perhaps wise to consider the advice of earlier generations and accept surgery as a treatment, which is appropriate when all else has failed. "Desperate diseases require desperate remedies".

None of the foregoing is meant in any way to minimise the achievements of modern surgery. The author has been an active neurosurgeon, who has enjoyed and been convinced of the value of his profession. Nonetheless, while good surgery is always acceptable and where used, most often unavoidable, it is a brave person who would describe it as desirable. It is more in the nature of an elegant necessary evil. This notion gains support from the knowledge that while people have allowed themselves to be subjected to strange surgical procedures, from prehistoric times, there is nonetheless a tradition in literature, indicating a yearning for more painless methods of treatment. Thus, Homer describes the miraculous effects of ointments on wounds in the Iliad and Christ heals by strength of spirit in the New Testament. And while such treatments are still, in the main, unattainable, it must be sensible to long for them. Anyone can understand a patient's reluctance to undergo surgery, with the resulting pain and possibly disfiguring scar. Concern about disfigurement is particularly worrying for the neurosurgical patient. The consequences of even successful neurosurgical procedures can be very distressing for a particular reason. Anyone with a dent in the forehead, or with epilepsy or a paralysis is viewed by many people as having a changed, disturbed or indeed deranged personality. This is an onerous burden to be avoided if at all possible.

Bearing the above in mind, the surgeon takes precautions against the dreaded complications of wound haemorrhage and wound sepsis, by applying meticulous asepsis in the operating theatre and by operating with a gentle technique which respects the living tissue under the knife. He also relies heavily on the body's ability to compensate for the surgical invasion. For neurosurgeons it is particularly important to gain as much space as possible within the crowded intracranial cavity, thus reducing the force necessary to retract the brain. The brain may react badly to prolonged retraction, particularly if too great a force is applied. To this end, the neurosurgeon releases CSF before applying the retractor and the neuro-anaesthetist manipulates the intracranial circulation to minimise blood volume, without prejudicing tissue perfusion. Moreover, the neurosurgeon knows just how surprisingly large quantities of the brain may be removed, without causing social embarrassment to the patient.

The principles of gentle sterile surgery based on knowledge of and respect for the body's compensation mechanisms is part of the mainstream tradition of medical development in this century. As medical men tend to be conservative, it would take a powerful and courageous intellect to break with such a tradition. Lars Leksell, for many years Professor of Neurosurgery, at the Karolinska Hospital in Stockholm was possessed of such an intellect. He was certainly one of the most creative neurosurgeons of the twentieth century. Over a period from the 1940s to the 1980s, he devoted his time to methods of treatment, which were not confined to taking advantage of the compensation mechanisms that make open surgery possible. On the contrary, his work seems to have had a central aim to reduce operation trauma to an absolute minimum. In his monograph, *Stereotaxis and Radiosurgery*, he states: "The tools used by the surgeon must be adapted to the task, and where the human brain is concerned they cannot be too refined".

One of Leksell's first clinical contributions was to devise a stereotactic frame for routine use in humans. Prior to this, stereotaxy had been primarily an experimental tool, though a stereotactic technique had been used in the treatment of trigeminal neuralgia and for intracerebral targets. The advantage of the Leksell system was that it was relatively simple and versatile in operation, when compared with other contemporary stereotactic systems. As a result stereotactic surgery gained an impetus, which has been maintained to the present day. With Leksell's system, access could be gained to any intracranial region with minimal trauma. However, Leksell's attempt to minimise operative trauma did not stop with the design and further development of a clinical stereotactic system. He went further and with a small group of associates devised an apparatus for treating intracranial pathological processes, without opening the cranium. This instrument, the Leksell Gamma Unit, was designed for use with the Leksell stereotactic system.

The terms radiosurgery and Gamma Knife have been the source of some controversy. Those who use radiosurgical techniques would justify the use of the term as follows. When ionising radiation is employed to damage or destroy a pathological process, it is vital that normal tissue in the neighbourhood of the lesion remains undamaged. This is achieved in conventional radiotherapy by fractionating the dose and by directing the radiations first from one side and then from the other. The beams are few, broad and seldom more than 8 different beam directions are used. With the Gamma Knife technique, there are around 200 beams of radiation and they are individually very narrow. This arrangement enables the construction of a very precise radiation field, limited to the pathological lesion. Normal tissue is excluded from dangerous levels of irradiation, because in radiosurgery a correlate of the very precise radiation field is a rapid fall in radiation levels just beyond the edge of the lesion. It is the surgical precision of the radiation field, administered at a single session that has led to the term radiosurgery.

Definitions of Radiosurgery

1. Leksell's Definition
   Leksell's definition was "... **Stereotactic radiosurgery is a technique for the non-invasive destruction of intracranial tissues or lesions that may be inaccessible to or unsuitable for open surgery [1]**".
2. Börje Larsson's Definition
   Leksell's physicist co-inventor of the Gamma Knife expanded the definition culminating in "**Radiosurgery signifies any kind of application of ionizing radiation energy, in experimental biology or clinical medicine, aiming at the precise and complete destruction of chosen target structures containing healthy and/or pathological cells without significant concomitant or late radiation damage to adjacent tissues [2]**". The Larsson definition specifies

radiation as the agent of tissue damage. It also states overtly what is implicit to surgeons in the Leksell definition. Like Leksell, Larsson states that the aim of the method is the destruction of the intended target. However, his definition also specifies openly that the avoidance of damage to adjacent tissue is part of the technique. He went on to state an important corollary that "Multiple fraction radiotherapy" is in principle excluded [2].

3. The Official Current USA Definition

A modern definition has been approved in the USA. "The AANS Board of Directors, the Executive Committee of the Congress of Neurological Surgeons and the Board of Directors of the American Society for Therapeutic Radiology and Oncology agreed on a contemporary definition of stereotactic radiosurgery. This position statement follows and also is published online at www.AANS.org, article ID 38198." It is a little prolix compared with its predecessors but admirably covers the elements that require covering.

(a) "**Stereotactic radiosurgery is a distinct discipline that utilizes externally generated ionizing radiation in certain cases to inactivate or eradicate (a) defined target(s) in the head and spine without the need to make an incision. The target is defined by high-resolution stereotactic imaging. To assure quality of patient care the procedure involves a multidisciplinary team consisting of a neurosurgeon, radiation oncologist, and medical physicist.**"

(b) **Stereotactic radiosurgery typically is performed in a single session, using a rigidly attached stereotactic guiding device, other immobilization technology and/or a stereotactic image-guidance system, but can be performed in a limited number of sessions, _up to a maximum of five_.**

(c) **Technologies that are used to perform stereotactic radiosurgery include linear accelerators, particle beam accelerators, and multisource Cobalt 60 units. In order to enhance precision, various devices may incorporate robotics and real time imaging**.

The first comprehensive text on radiosurgery was published in 2008. It is a careful extensive text, filling a substantial need but it is clearly written in the light of the AANS definition quoted above [3].

Consequences of Changing Definitions of Radiosurgery

Non-neurosurgical Treatments and Fractionation

It would seem therefore that there is a contradiction of understanding between Leksell and Larsson who favoured single session treatment and the modern definition which permits limited fractionation. This is a not unexpected direction in view of how changing practice uses stereotactically guided focused radiation therapy. Increasingly the method is applied to treat malignant lesions not only inside but outside the cranium. This in effect is directing the methodology more in the direction of radiation oncology than neurosurgery; the speciality of origin. Such a development is both natural, unavoidable and has the advantage it makes the benefits of stereotactic radiation therapies available to a greater number of needy patients. Indeed, the Gamma Knife itself, in its latest edition (Perfexion) is designed to apply fractionated treatments to the skull base and the neck. Thus, for extracranial disease, irrespective of the treatment machine, the evolution is moving in the direction of various forms of sophisticated stereotactically guided radiotherapy. This also means that it is moving in the direction of treatment with fractionation. This is an area which lies outside the expertise of the neurosurgeon.

Microsurgery, Gamma Knife Surgery and Their Relationship to Each Other

Leaving aside extracranial diseases, it is no exaggeration to say that within the neurosurgical milieu itself, Gamma Knife surgery (GKS) has had its opponents and no doubt will continue to do so. This is part of the healthy development of evidence based medicine and is a positive sign. However, the author would like to suggest that a clarification directed at co-operation would simplify the management of patients, save money and improve the methods available to clinicians.

It seems unavoidable that the term **radiosurgery** is likely to expand and develop along the lines outlined above. Yet the Gamma Knife was originally intended to treat intracranial lesions. This will remain the major part of its work for the foreseeable future. This being so, perhaps the time has come to adjust the classification.

GKS as applied intracranially might be re-christened **Gamma Knife Neurosurgery (GKNS)**. This term will be used throughout this book. GKNS will most probably continue along the successful patterns of treatment laid down by the pioneers and practised over two and a half decades, specialising for the most in non fractionated single session treatment of intracranial lesions. It will be a treatment in which neurosurgeons will continue to have a dominant role in the team involved in the use of the machine. However, there is a caveat. There can be little disagreement that modern neurosurgical department members should be involved in multi-speciality teams, to optimise treatment by using the competence of experts from diverse converging fields to the benefit of the patients. If GKNS is to develop its full potential there is an absolute need for Gamma Knife users to be involved with their microsurgery colleagues in such teams. Indeed the optimal situation would be that all neurosurgeons in a department with a Gamma Knife should be competent in its use. **The time has surely come for systematically planned multi-stage treatments in which the sequence of treatments are determined prior to their implementation; for example sometimes microsurgery alone, sometimes GKNS alone and sometimes both in sequence. This will replace the common current practice where GKNS is requested only when**

safe radical microsurgery has proved impossible. Such planning must surely offer patients safer and more effective management.

Aims of This Book

Today there are many specialist texts published covering every aspect of radiosurgery with every available method. There are however few books covering the hands-on detailed daily use of the various radiosurgery techniques. To write such a book to cover the field of GKNS is relatively easier than for other technologies since the technique is so uniform. The current volume is designed firstly as a manual for those beginning a career in Gamma Knife treatment, specifically aimed at users of Gamma Knife Perfexion. It is also intended as a guide for those who wish to be involved in **multi-treatment teams** as mentioned above. It should be also helpful to anyone who wishes to refer a patient to Gamma Knife treatment. Finally, for those who wish to deepen their knowledge in respect of the subject, extensive References are attached to every chapter.

References

1. Leksell L. Stereotactic Radiosurgery. J Neurol Neurosurg Psychiat 46: 797–803; 1983
2. Larsson B. Radiobiological Fundamentals in Radiosurgery. In Radiosurgery: Baselines and Trends. Ed Steiner L et al. Raven Press Ltd., New York: pp 3–14; 1992
3. Chin LS, Regine WF eds. Principles and Practice of Stereotactic Radiosurgery. Springer Verlag, New York; 2008

Chapter 2
Principles of Stereotaxy

Introduction

There are few parts of the body, which may not be approached by means of a surgical operation. An exception to this rule is the deep parts of the brain. The reasons are easy to understand. The head is a rigid cavity and about 90% by volume of its contents is cerebral tissue. This tissue tolerates retraction and displacement badly. Moreover, access to, for example, the basal ganglia involves an unavoidable and unacceptable risk of damage to eloquent areas lying superficial to or adjacent to these ganglia. Thus, conventional open surgical techniques are an essentially inappropriate method to use for operations in the depths of the brain, irrespective of the sophistication of modern microsurgical techniques. These problems have been appreciated for a long time. A solution, at least in principle, has also been around for a long time, in fact since before the First World War.

The famous British neurosurgeon and neurophysiologist, Victor Horsley, wished to gain access to deep cerebellar structures in animal experiments. He sought the help of an Oxford mathematician and physician, Robert Clarke and together they published an account of the first stereotactic instrument in 1908 [1]. However, neither this instrument, nor any modification of it was ever used in clinical work, though one was designed but abandoned for lack of interest. Approximately 40 years were to pass before two Americans, Spiegel and Wycis in 1947 published the results of their operations with a "stereoencephalatome", as they called it; designed for use for pain and psychiatric disorders [2].

The term stereotaxy derives from two Greek roots "stereos" meaning solid and "takse" meaning arrangement. However, in the past there has been an at times passionate debate, as to whether the correct adjective from stereotaxy should be stereotaxic or stereotactic. The former is etymologically correct. However, the latter was felt to be somehow more in keeping with a surgical procedure, in that "tactic is derived from touch. But! It is derived from the *Latin* word for touch, so that etymologically speaking stereotactic is a chimera. Nonetheless, in 1973 the international body responsible for furthering the interests of those involved in this

J.C. Ganz, *Gamma Knife Neurosurgery*,
DOI 10.1007/978-3-7091-0343-2_2, © Springer-Verlag/Wien 2011

form of surgery changed its previously rather cumbersome name to "World Society for Stereotactic and Functional Neurosurgery". Thus, this is the form, which will be used throughout this book.

Principles

While knowing what the word stereotaxy means may indicate the area of interest, it does not tell us any more about the principles of the method. The aim of the technique is to relate the location of deep and inaccessible intracerebral structures to a three-dimensional Cartesian axis system. The first step in this process is to enclose the head in such a system. This is done by fixing a rigid metal frame to the head. The borders of the frame then constitute the Cartesian axes, while the cranium serves as a platform to support the frame and the cerebrum is enclosed both physically and conceptually within a microcosm, where every point can be precisely defined in space. The zero for the three axes lies above and behind the right ear. Thus the "X" axis increases from right to left, the "Y" axis from back to front and the "Z" axis from above downwards. The way in which a point within the frame is defined in terms of the three Cartesian axes is depicted in Fig. 2.1.

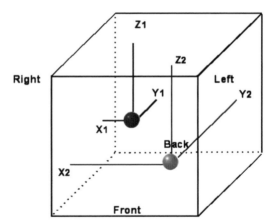

Fig. 2.1 Stereotactic technique relates the position of targets within the body to a system of appropriately designed markers or "fiducials". The system employed for GKNS uses a Cartesian axis system as illustrated in this figure. The system consists of a notional rectangular hexahedron (or cuboid with some definitions). Any point can be connected to the sides of the cube by a line meeting that side at a right angle. If a line is dropped from the top back and right side the length of the lines are characteristic for that particular location which is thus defined by these lengths, or in other words by three numbers. As shown the two locations in the illustration each have sets of lines with different lengths characterising the two locations with two sets of three numbers. It is to be remembered that stereotaxy is performed in relation to the axis system and markers. Any structure within a stereotactically defined space can be characterised in the way shown. Thus if a frame, substituting for the notional box is fitted to the skull, any intracranial location can be defined in relation to that frame

Thus, it is possible to define any intracranial target in respect of the frame. However, to be of any use the frame must itself be a platform for a device, which will hold an instrument or electrode, to be introduced into the brain, to reach the target. The small diameter of the instruments used and the mechanical stability with which they are held and introduced, by means of a rigid holder and guide, and the extreme accuracy of the localization implicit in the method are the basis of the exceptionally atraumatic nature of stereotactic procedures.

The Leksell System

A great variety of different stereotactic systems have been designed over the last 40 years. Each system has its protagonists and its special fields of application. For a description of the essential technical principles of stereotactic surgery reference will be made only to the Leksell system, because it is the system used in GKNS. These principles are on the whole independent of the system used, though the ways in which technical problems are solved differ from system to system. As indicated in Chap.1, while the Leksell stereotactic system was not the first, it was the first to be constructed with a view to ease of application and frequent use [3]. The sides of the cuboid frame constitute the axes of the instrument. An arc is mounted on the instrument in an adjustable holder, which is regulated in respect of the desired values in the three axes. The arc may be rotated backwards and forwards, with respect to the frame. The instrument holder is mounted on the arc and may be moved transversely across the whole circumference of the arc. When the axis values for the target point have been determined, the centre of the arc will always coincide with this target point. This arrangement allows a needle to be pointed at its target from an almost infinite number of directions. Thus, it is simple to design an optimal trajectory for the instrument to be introduced into the depths of the brain, avoiding especially sensitive structures, for example eloquent brain or important blood vessels. An important point of the design is that, for a given target setting, the point of the instrument introduced to the centre of the arc does not move. It does not move irrespective of how the direction of the shaft of the instrument is varied, by moving the arc backwards and forwards or by moving the needle holder transversely across the arc. This effect is quite uncanny and is illustrated in Fig. 2.2.

Target Identification

The features of a stereotactic system, which have been outlined so far, describe how a point in space, a so-called target point may be defined in terms of the reference axis system, built into the stereotactic frame that is fixed to the head. If the target is "visible", for example a space occupying lesion, then a general knowledge of cerebral anatomy together with adequate imaging techniques will suffice. However,

Fig. 2.2 This is an illustration of the Leksell stereotactic frame with the arc attached for use in open surgery. A needle is fixed to the ark and is moved across its circumference in 5° movements. The picture is taken repeatedly and as can be seen, while the direction of approach of the needle varies, there is an uncanny stability of its tip located at a stereotactically defined point. The Gamma Knife is built on the same principle with a single needle on an arc being replaced by multiple fine radiation beams mounted on a 3 dimensional array

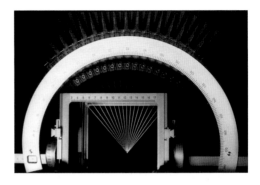

in the early days, stereotactic technique was almost exclusively used for the treatment of functional disorders. The targets in this situation are "invisible", consisting of discrete nuclei or tracts within larger anatomical entities, such as the thalamus or the basal ganglia. To locate such targets, a map of the region is required or rather a collection of maps in an atlas. An atlas of the internal cerebral anatomy of a variety of laboratory animals had already been produced by Horsley and Clarke, in the first decade of this century [1]. The production of a human stereotactic atlas in 1962 was one of the major contributions of the pioneers Spiegel and Wycis, mentioned above [4].

While an atlas will show where a given nucleus or tract should be it will not show its precise location in an individual patient. It is necessary to have some visible structure with a constant relationship to intracerebral structures. In Horsley and Clarke's experimental work, skull landmarks were used. They had no choice in this, because contrast materials, which could outline soft tissues on X-ray, were not available, at the time they performed their studies. They were aware of the limitations of this method of localization and checked the location of the lesions they made at post-mortem. Their physiological studies included only those animals where the lesion was correctly placed. This sort of inaccuracy would clearly be inappropriate for operations performed in human patients, so some other means of localization was necessary. To accomplish this, an internal cerebral reference system had to be defined. Air ventriculography had been first described by Harvey Cushing's pupil, Walter Dandy, in 1918 [5]. This technique was thus well established at the time when Spiegel and Wycis performed the first stereotactic operations, in humans. They outlined the third ventricle and used a line drawn between the posterior border of the Foramen of Monro and the anterior border of the pineal body, as a reference. They could then relate the anatomical structures, as depicted in their atlas, to this line.

Moreover, they used the technique to demonstrate just how great the variability of the relationship between intracerebral structures and skull landmarks really is. Subsequently, Tailairach in France used a line joining the anterior and posterior commissures, visualized on an air ventriculogram of the third ventricle, as a reference in his atlas. This reference line is more constant than that based on the Foramen of Monro and the Pineal Body. This is because the borders of the former can be difficult to see and the latter varies a lot, in terms of size and ease of definition. Since that time the intercommissural line has been a standard reference in functional stereotactic surgery. The adequate definition of the posterior commissure required a somewhat refined air ventriculography technique. The subsequent introduction of iodinated positive contrast substances, in particular the discovery of water-soluble contrast media greatly improved the quality of the anatomical definition of the boundaries of the third ventricle. This technique is still used in many centres during treatment, because it is still unusual to find a CT scanner in the operating room. Moreover, repeated ventriculograms can be used not only to identify a target location but also to check that the instruments are placed correctly at the target. Thus, with adequate X-ray definition and using the intercommissural line and an appropriate stereotactic atlas, the location of "invisible" targets became reliable enough for systematic clinical use. The "invisible" targets had been made "visible".

Newer Localization Methods

The treatment of pain, Parkinsonism and psychiatric disturbance, which required the localization of invisible targets, remained the dominating indication for stereotactic neurosurgery for approximately 20 years. However, stereotactic technique could also enable completely accurate placement of instruments into deep-sitting space occupying lesions, where this is appropriate. And it is clearly desirable to obtain a biopsy from those deep-sitting lesions that are tumours and puncture those that are cysts, haematomas or abscesses. Prior to the stereotactic era, these procedures were performed free hand, with a considerable margin of error. It is interesting, in this context, that Leksell's first stereotactic operation on a patient, using his own instrument, was to instil radioactive isotopes into a craniopharyngioma cyst. The problem in the early days, with using stereotaxy in the investigation and treatment of space-occupying lesions was that the X-rays available were inadequate for localization in many cases. Angiography could help with those lesions, which show pathological vessels, but often distortion or displacement of blood vessels is all that can be seen and this is too imprecise. Even so, with the advent of radiosurgery, the angiogram became the examination of choice in the treatment of arteriovenous malformations. The various techniques for displaying the CSF spaces were really only adequate for the stereotactic localization of lesions which distort these spaces. Thus, identification of smaller lesions, deep in the cerebral parenchyma was difficult. However, the development of computer assisted tomography (CT) and more recently magnetic resonance imaging (MRI) has greatly facilitated stereotactic procedures. These techniques render space-occupying lesions truly visible and thus simple to localize. The stereotactic CT or MRI is performed with an adapter [6], to fit and fix the patient's frame to the table of the imaging machine. Then an indicator box is affixed to the frame to enable definition of the stereotactic space. This is described in detail in more Chap. 8. However, the principles of this system are illustrated in Fig. 2.3.

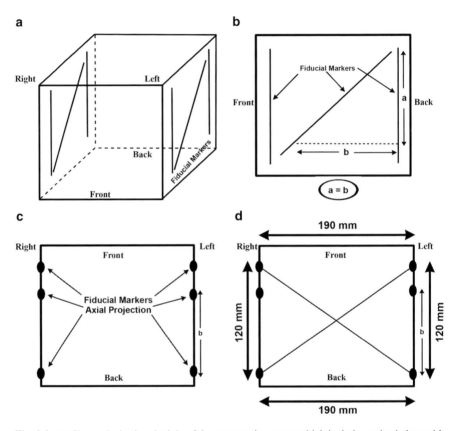

Fig. 2.3 (**a**) Shows the basic principle of the stereotaxic system which includes a plastic box with fiducial markers in the walls. The vertical markers at the front and back are at fixed positions in the stereotactic space and define positions in the XY (axial) plane. The oblique marker permits estimation of the position in the "Z" direction. (**b**) Shows how the distance from the posterior vertical fiducial to the oblique fiducial is the same as the distance from the top of the fiducial to the level of the slice. This is because the oblique fiducial forms part of an isosceles right angled triangle. (**c**) shows how this arrangement appears in axial slice on a computerised image, be it CT or more commonly MRI. (**d**) Shows the distances between the vertical fiducial markers from back to front (120 mm) and side to side (190 mm). These distances MUST be checked at every MR examination to ensure geometric accuracy. It is permissible for the measurement to deviate 1 mm from the true distance because of the size of the pixels. However, the two opposite measurements must not differ by more than 1 mm. The presence of such a difference indicates that the MR machine must be shimmed

Modern Indications for Stereotaxy

Stereotactic technique, following the advent of CT imaging has a large number of indications, most of which have been mentioned. There has however been a tendency for its use to be restricted to a relatively small number of enthusiasts. It is not, even today, used routinely by all neurosurgeons. This is partly because, in the majority of centres, it has been used for functional work, which requires a specialised neurophysiological knowledge that is not a part of all general neurosurgical training programs. Furthermore, the basis of the technique is not technical surgical virtuosity but rather the avoidance of the need for such virtuosity. The Karolinska Hospital Neurosurgery Department, under Leksell's aegis taught that stereotaxy was not to be considered an alternative to other forms of treatment but to be used in addition. This teaching has spread. Moreover, the spread of radiosurgery has encouraged the concomitant spread of intracranial stereotaxy as well. Another result is that stereotactic technique is today no longer limited to the cranium. There are a variety of instruments, both linear accelerators and particle accelerators which can be adapted or specifically designed to deliver focussed radiation using stereotactic methods to any place in the body. This does not of course apply to the Gamma Knife which is and always will be mainly used on intracranial illnesses. It is true, that the latest model, "Perfexion" has the capability to treat lesions in the neck but this method is still in its infancy. Moreover, it would be inappropriate to make machines for use outside the head with the extreme sub-millimetre accuracy of the Gamma Knife. The body movements due to heart beat and respiration prevent the application of focussed radiation with the same accuracy as applies intracranially. These matters are mentioned as they represent a modern trend which has grown up in the last 15 years and which clearly is here to stay. Focussed radiation has many advantages. However, extracranial radiosurgery lies outside the scope of this book so no further mention will be made. Moreover, this is a book exclusively about GKNS. Thus, other methods of delivering stereotactically guided focused radiation such as linear accelerators or particle accelerators are considered outside the range of this text and will not be described or discussed. This is not a comment on the value of alternative techniques. There are plenty of texts which describe their value and use in detail. They simply lie outside the context of this particular book.

Conclusion

Thus after a slow start in the 1950s, stereotaxy is now a commonly used technique both in neurosurgery and radiation oncology. In view of the relative frequency of appropriate extracranial disease this is a trend which is likely to expand. However, it is emphasised that the current book is concerned with Gamma Knife Neurosurgery and discussion of other techniques, except in very special situations is considered outside the range of the topic.

References

1. Horsley V, Clarke RH. The structure and functions of the cerebellum examined by a new method. Brain **31**: 45–124; 1908
2. Spiegel EA, Wycis HT. Stereotaxic apparatus for operations on the human brain. Science **106**: 349–350; 1947
3. Leksell LA. Stereotaxic apparatus for intracerebral surgery. Acta Chir Scand **99**: 229–233; 1949
4. Spiegel EA, Wycis HT. Stereoencephalatomy. Part II. Clincal and Physiological Applications. Gruve, New York; 1962
5. Dandy WE. Ventriculography following the injection of air into the cerebral ventricles. Ann Surg **68**: 5–11; 1918
6. Leksell L, Jernberg B. Stereotaxis and tomography. A technical note. Acta Neurochir 52(1–2): 1–7; 1980

Chapter 3
Ionising Radiation and Its Effects on Living Tissue

Introduction

Some knowledge of the effects of ionising radiation on living tissue is necessary, for those who wish to understand the nature of any treatment using radiation and who also wish to inform patients about such treatment. Correct information is particularly important in this regard, because of the associations that the word radiation has for most people. Most powerful therapeutic methods arouse concern or anxiety amongst those who will be subjected to them. However, medicine or the surgeon's knife may also be viewed with some degree of relief. This is not the case for treatment involving ionising radiation. There are several reasons for this. Firstly, everyone has seen films of the agonising effects of radiation fall-out from nuclear bombs. Secondly, there is something particularly horrid about the idea of an invisible entity, creeping into the body, producing no apparent initial effect but followed by untold harm, at a later date. The unpleasantness is compounded by the nature of the harm that may develop: in that sterility and cancer are amongst the commonest consequences of exposure to excess irradiation. Thirdly the concept of radiotherapy is indissolubly linked in the public mind with cancer. This last provides particular difficulties for the patient with an intracranial tumour, where radiation treatment may be advisable because of a tumour's inaccessibility, rather than its malignancy. What follows is simple and qualitative. Those seeking a more definitive account of these matters should refer to the excellent "Basic Clinical Radiobiology" [1].

Radiophysics

Basic Concepts

The basic mechanisms, underlying the effect of radiation on matter occur at the atomic and subatomic level. Thus, understanding of these effects is necessarily

J.C. Ganz, *Gamma Knife Neurosurgery*,
DOI 10.1007/978-3-7091-0343-2_3, © Springer-Verlag/Wien 2011

predicated on some elementary knowledge of atomic theory. The concept of an atom, consisting of a nucleus containing a specific number of positively charged protons and non-charged neutrons, surrounded by orbits of electrons is familiar.

Another important set of concepts in the study of atoms and subatomic particles are embodied in a theory; Quantum Theory. Quantum theory was developed to explain findings which indicated that electromagnetic radiation (see below) sometimes appeared to behave as a wave and sometimes appeared to behave as a stream of particles or quanta, each carrying a certain specific amount of energy, defined by the Planck Radiation Formula:

$$E = h\nu$$

Where E is energy, h is Planck's constant and ν is the frequency of the radiation. Moreover, it is also true that subatomic particles may be considered to have wave like properties. Another important concept, for the understanding of radiation's interaction with matter, is that energy and matter are interconvertable, according to Einstein's famous equation:

$$E = mc^2$$

Where E is energy, m is the mass of the particle being converted into or arising from energy and c is the velocity of light. This dual nature of radiation and subatomic particles is not intuitive and has been considered difficult to understand. However, it is not really so. Many familiar objects have different properties depending on how they are observed. For example, a meadow will be viewed by a farmer in terms of what he can grow on it. A geologist, looking at the vegetation and terrain may try to deduce if there is oil below. The archaeologist will use other observations to deduce what artefacts may lie buried. It is the same meadow showing different properties depending on how it is observed. Another analogy is to consider looking at a cone. When viewed from, the side it can appear as a triangle. When viewed from the top it can seem to be a circle. Obviously, it is both and neither. Moreover, in keeping with the Quantum conception of waves and particles, the two views of the cylinder are mutually exclusive. In the same way, a wave may seem to be a wave or a particle, but never both at the same time. This notion is illustrated in Fig. 3.1

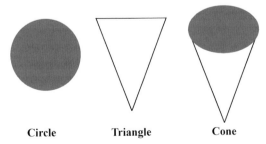

Fig. 3.1 Point of view. Affects appearance and understanding

Circle   **Triangle**   **Cone**

Now we must return to quantum mechanics. Irrespective of whether waves or particles are considered, an atom can only emit or absorb energy in discrete, discontinuous quanta. The quanta so emitted or absorbed will have a particular energy and by the same token a particular wavelength; in accordance with Planck's equation.

The term **ionising radiation** refers to radiation, which has a sufficiently high energy to be able to dislodge electrons from atoms, or disrupt the bonds between atoms and molecules. Examples of this sort of radiation are ultraviolet light, X-rays and gamma rays. An atom deprived of an electron will have a net positive charge and thus will have become an ion hence the term ionising radiation.

There are two sorts of radiation **source** used in radiation treatment; artificially generated irradiation from man-made machines and spontaneously generated radiation from radionuclides. (A nuclide is a variety of an atom. It may be used as an alternative to the word isotope. Some atoms exist in several forms with the same number of protons and electrons but varying numbers of neutrons. They have the same atomic number but differing atomic weights. They are all the same element. Some elements exist in only a single form making the term isotope inappropriate. Examples are sodium or fluorine. A nuclide is an alternative term to an isotope and includes the atoms which exist only in a single form. It is thus a more general term. A radionuclide is an unstable atomic variety exhibiting spontaneous radioactive breakdown).

There are two basic kinds of radiation in current use. *Electro-magnetic radiation* has no mass and travels at the velocity of light ($c = 3 \times 10^8$ m/s). *Particle radiation* consisting of for example protons, neutrons or electrons, has mass and travels at a lesser velocity. Both particles and electromagnetic radiation lose energy to matter by interacting with it. If a radiation passes through matter without striking an atom no ionisation will occur.

Units

A variety of units are used to quantify the phenomena associated with ionising radiation. The units relate to the expenditure of energy and common to a number of them is the SI unit for energy, the joule. A **joule** is the energy expended when a force of one newton works through one metre. A **newton** is a force, which will accelerate a mass of 1 kg by 1 m/s^2. The following are among the more useful units used in relation to radiation therapy.

1. In the measurement of the energy of photons and particle beams electron volts are used.
   The **volt** is the difference in potential between two points within an electric field which requires one joule of energy to move one coulomb of electric charge between the two points. A **coulomb** is the quantity of electricity transported by a one ampere of current in 1 s.

1 **electron volt** (eV) is the energy acquired by an electron passing through a potential difference of 1 V and is equal to 1.60219×10^{-19} J.

Kilo electron volts (keV) and mega electron volts (MeV) are the customary units used in radiation therapy.

$$1 \, \text{KeV} = 10^3 \, \text{eV} \quad \text{and} \quad 1 \, \text{MeV} = 10^6 \, \text{eV}$$

2. An older out-dated set of units is **Kilovolts** (kV) and **Megavolts** are used. These are descriptive terms related to the quality and not the energy of the radiation. They are only mentioned because they occur commonly in older texts.

3. The **Activity** of an amount of a radioactive nuclide is the number of spontaneous nuclear transitions (dV) in the time interval.

The unit of activity is the **Becquerel** (Bq)

An older unit of activity is the Curie (Ci)

In the measurement of nuclear disintegration of a radionuclide:

$$1 \, \text{Curie(Ci)} = 3.7 \times 10^{10} \text{ disintegrations per second.}$$

$$1 \, \text{Becquerel} = 1 \, \text{disintegration/s}$$

4. In the measurement of the tissue absorption of radiation: The absorbed dose, D, is the mean energy imparted, dE, by ionising radiation to matter, in a volume element with mass dm.

$$D = dE/d_m$$

The unit of absorbed dose is the gray (Gy)

$$1 \, \text{Gy} = 1 \, \text{joule/kg}$$

1 Radiation Absorbed Dose (rad) is a familiar and older radiation absorption dose, using CGS units so that

$$1 \, \text{rad} = 1 \, \text{erg}/100 \, \text{g}$$

It should no longer be used.

The relation of rads to Gy is described by the equation

$$1 \, \text{Gy} = 100 \, \text{rads}$$

In the U.S.A. and the U.K. the cGy is popular.

$$100 \, \text{cGy} = 1 \, \text{Gy} = 100 \, \text{rad.}$$

Electromagnetic Radiation

There is of course a vast range of electromagnetic radiations from the lowest frequency radio waves (frequency 10 kHz, wavelength 30 km) up to cosmic rays (frequency 10^{24} kHz, wavelength 1/1,000 millionth of an Angstrom unit). In low frequency, long wavelength radiation the wave-like properties dominate. In high frequency, short wavelength radiation, the particle-like properties dominate. For the present purpose, the range of interest is X-rays (approx. 10^{15}–10^{21} Hz) and gamma rays (approx. 10^{18}–10^{24} Hz).

The essential difference between X-rays and gamma rays is their manner of production. X-rays are the product of deceleration of a stream of electrons. According to electromagnetic theory, acceleration or deceleration of electrically charged particles results in the emission of radiation. This radiation produced by this sudden deceleration is called "bremsstrahlung"; from the German "bremsen" meaning to brake and "Strahlung" meaning radiation. This phenomenon is used in the production of X-rays from a machine, in which negatively charged electrons are accelerated in a vacuum and strike a target with a high atomic weight, usually tungsten. The X-rays produced by the deceleration of the electrons may diffuse in many directions and are directed where desired through a device called a **collimator**. The X-rays produced by different machines can have different energies. **Linear Accelerators**, much used in conventional radiotherapy, and which may be adapted to perform radiosurgery, produce X-ray beams with energies between 4 and 30 MeV.

It is important not to confuse the **energy** of a radiation beam with its *intensity* (see the Planck Radiation Formula). The energy of the beam is proportional to the frequency of the radiation. It will be seen later that this is in turn related to the penetration of the beam and the sort of effects it has on the atoms, which it strikes. The intensity of the beam is related to the number of photons the machine is delivering; in other words to the dose. This may become clearer by considering the same characteristics in respect of a beam of light. Increasing the energy, or frequency of a beam of light will change its colour from red through the spectrum up to violet. For a particular colour, increasing the intensity will make the light brighter. It will not change the colour.

Gamma rays, which are also electromagnetic radiations, differ from X-rays in that they are produced in a different way (Fig. 3.2). When the nucleus of an atom is in an excited state it can decay to a stable state by the emission of one or more photons, (quanta of electromagnetic radiation energy) called in this case gamma rays or gamma photons. The other products of radioactive breakdown are alpha particles (helium nuclei with two protons and two neutrons) and beta particles (electrons) and neutrons. Alpha particles produced by radioactive transformation have too low a penetration to be of much use in clinical practice. Beta radiation also has a low penetration but it may be used following implantation of isotopes in tissue. One example, in the field of neurosurgery is in the treatment of the thin walls of craniopharyngioma cysts with the instillation of radioactive Yttrium, which

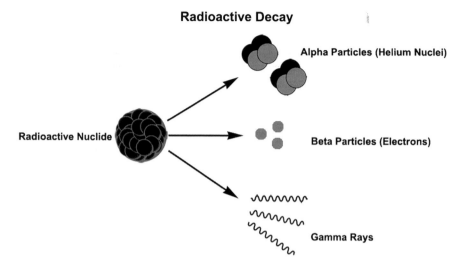

Fig. 3.2 Radioactive decay. There are three main types of radioactive breakdown, producing three main products are indicated here. However, not all radioactive breakdowns produce all products. Thus alpha particles are mostly produced by isotopes of high atomic weight, for example Uranium. Cobalt-60 produces gamma waves, but also loses electrons

emits pure beta radiation into the cyst cavity. This is not unusual. Many nuclides emit a greater proportion of one of the products of radioactive breakdown than of the others. Thus Uranium-235 is primarily an alpha emitter, just as Cobalt-60 is mainly a gamma emitter but also emits beta particles.

Particle Radiation

The most commonly used particles in current therapy are electrons and protons. Electron beams can be produced by an adapted linear accelerator or a special sort of accelerator called a betatron. High-energy electrons have a definite limited range in tissues, with a rapid fall of dose over distance. This makes this form of radiation advantageous in the treatment of cutaneous and subcutaneous lesions, such as lymph nodes or the parotid gland. The commonest energies of electron beams are 7–18 MeV, for the linear accelerator and 12.4–124 MeV for a betatron.

Proton particles are produced in particle accelerators, such as the synchrocyclotron. These are rare and costly and are found in only a few centres, for example Boston, and Loma Linda in the USA and Uppsala in Sweden. Particle beams have special characteristics, enabling the delivery of a sharply defined dose deep in the tissues, with relative sparing of the tissues on the way in to the high dose volume. The energies of those in current use ranges from 72 to 1,000 MeV.

The Effect of Electromagnetic Radiation on Matter at the Atomic Level

Ionisation is a chemical change. Electromagnetic radiations can react with matter in a variety of ways; for example reflection, refraction interference that is different forms of scattering. They can induce chemical change only by *absorption*. When ionising radiation is absorbed it interacts with atoms to detach electrons from their orbits. The energy of these electrons is part of the energy of the incoming photons. There are three main ways in which such interactions between radiation and matter occur, depending on the energy of the radiation. Finally, it should be repeated that some radiation will go through whatever matter is being irradiated without interacting with it.

The Photoelectric Effect

This is the major energy absorption mechanism for low energy X-ray beams up to 50 keV, though it also occurs at higher energy levels. All the energy of a given photon is absorbed in detaching an electron from one of the inmost shell of an atom. An outer electron will then hop into the insufficiently filled inner shell, resulting in a change in energy level and the emission of a photon of X-rays (Fig. 3.3). The kinetic energy of the originally ejected inner electron will be equal to the energy of the incident photon minus the energy required to detach it from its orbit. It is *not* related to the *intensity* of the photon beam, which will determine the *number* of detached electrons. These liberated electrons will then cause the ejection of further electrons from other atoms, until their kinetic energy is no longer great enough to change an atomic energy state. At this stage they can produce vibrations within atoms but not ionisation. The discovery of the mechanism underlying the photoelectric effect was what won Albert Einstein his Nobel Prize in physics, not his theories of relativity.

Compton Scattering

With higher energy X-ray beams and gamma rays, with an energy between approximately 90 keV and 5 MeV, a different effect occurs; involving the interaction of the radiation photon with electrons in the outer shell of the atom. Some of the photon's energy will be dissipated in detaching the electron from its path and in giving it kinetic energy. The rest of the energy will continue as a new photon with an energy equal to the energy of the incident photon less the energy required to detach the electron and the kinetic energy delivered to that electron (Fig. 3.4). This new photon with a lower energy will naturally have a longer wavelength. Quantitative analysis of the effects of radiation in water has shown that the vast majority of the energy absorbed is related to the detached electrons and not to the ongoing lower energy photons.

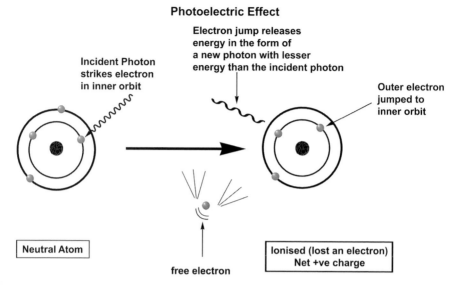

Fig. 3.3 Photoelectric effect. The photoelectric effect was discovered following the observation that when a spark appears at a gap between two electrodes its appearance could be facilitated by shining light at the gap. The photoelectric effect is due to the incoming photon from the light loosening an electron and thus facilitating the generation of a spark. The electron released is from the inner shell. The energy of the ongoing photon is discharged when an electron jumps from an outer to the inner electron shell. The energy of this photon is equal to the energy of the incoming photon less the energy imparted to the free electron. Note that the frequency of the incoming photon is higher than that of the outgoing photon. This reflects the relationship between the energy and frequency of a photon. See text

Pair Production

When a photon passes close to the nucleus of an atom it is exposed to the powerful energy field around that nucleus and may thus be converted from a photon of energy into matter, in the form of a pair of electrons. Since the mass of an electron is equivalent to 0.511 MeV the energy of the incident photon must be at least 0.511 × 2 or 1.022 MeV. One of the pair of electrons has a positive charge (positron) and the other a negative charge (electron). Both these electrons pass through the absorbing matter exciting and ionising atoms as described earlier (see Fig. 3.5).

The different mechanisms of energy absorption are not mutually exclusive: though the coexistence of the photoelectric effect and pair production is not thought to occur. However, the radiation energy range, associated with Compton scattering will at its lower end also be associated with the photoelectric effect, while at its upper range it will be associated with pair production.

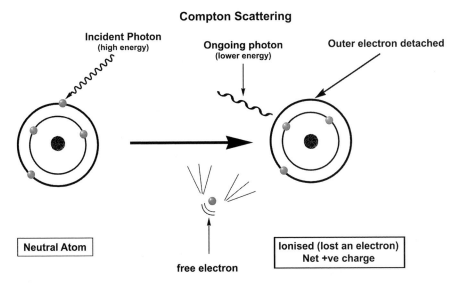

Fig. 3.4 Compton scattering. Compton found that when X-rays are dispersed in a crystal. There was a change in the frequency of the X-rays, indicating a loss of energy. At the same time an outer electron is freed. The lower frequency of the ongoing X-rays reflects the energy of the incoming X-ray photon less the energy imparted to the ongoing electron. Note that, as in the photoelectric effect, there is a net gain of one positive charge and the atom is ionised. This time the energy liberated comes directly from the incoming photon. It is not mediated by means of an electron hopping from one orbit to another. It s the most likely process to be responsible for ionisation during Gamma Knife Neurosurgery

The Effect of Charged Particles on Matter

A crucial difference in the pattern of energy absorption between particles and electromagnetic radiation is related to this characteristic of particles: that they can decelerate while radiations are bound to travel at the speed of light.

The absorption of energy associated with the passage of particles or radiation through matter is described by the Linear Energy Transfer (LET), described by the formula – dE/dX where dE is energy loss and dX is unit distance travelled.

The units of LET are KeV/mμ: where $1\,\text{m}\mu = 10^{-6}\,\text{m}$.

The energy loss of a particle is reflected by ionisations along the course of its passage. How far the particles will travel in a medium – such as living tissue – is a function of the density of the medium and its atomic weight on the one hand, and the mass and velocity of the particle on the other. Protons as an example of "charged heavy particles", with their greater mass can penetrate more deeply. There is relatively little energy loss along the track of a proton beam, so long as

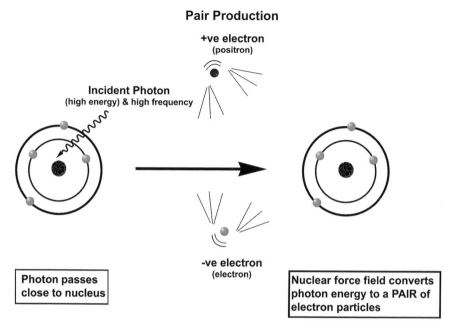

Fig. 3.5 Pair production. In this case, the incoming photon has enough energy to reach close to the nucleus. Here it is affected by the powerful field and is converted into particles. Two electrons are formed in accordance with the law of Conservation of Electric Charge. Thus, the minimum number of electrons that can be formed in this way is 2; one with a positive and one with a negative charge. In this way the law is obeyed and neutrality is maintained

the particle is moving quickly. Thus, such heavy particles have a low LET in the part of their tracks where they are moving fast. However, more and more of their energy is absorbed as they decelerate, so that this part of the track has a high LET. Since most energy absorption occurs at the distal end of the track, most of the ionisations also occur in this region. A consequence of this phenomenon is that particles like protons, with an appropriate delivery system can be used to produce very precisely defined radiation fields at specific distances from the particle source. The precisely defined area of intense irradiation at the end of a low LET track following the passage of protons is called a "Bragg Peak". However, taking advantage of the Bragg Peak phenomenon is not the only way in which a proton beam may be used to produce a well-localized volume of high radiation energy delivery. **Cross firing** of a number of *narrow* proton beams will also produce a region of high dose where the beams cross, while the amount of dose delivered along the beam outside the cross firing region will be low because of proton radiation's low LET. To avoid the development of a Bragg Peak a proton source is used with a high energy and therefore a high penetration, so that the deceleration of protons, necessary for a Bragg Peak will occur after the protons have passed through the living tissue and emerged on the far side (Fig. 3.6). This principle for

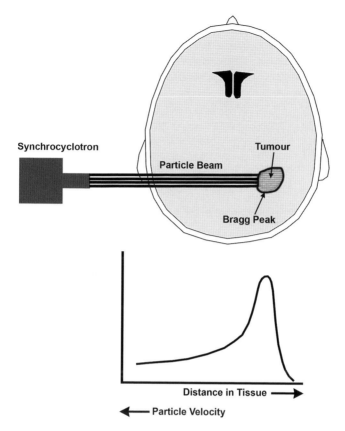

Fig. 3.6 Focal radiation (Bragg Peak). Most radiation energy delivered from particle radiation is lost when the particles decelerate. This deceleration of particles enables the concentration of the radiation dose over a tightly controlled sharply defined volume, called the Bragg Peak. This is one of the best known techniques for delivering focused radiation. For the sake of presenting the picture of the radiation and the graph of the particle deceleration concordantly, the source in this diagram is placed on the opposite side from the lesion. This would not really happen in the clinic

producing focused ionisation is mentioned again in the chapters dealing with the development of the Gamma Knife. Obtaining a sharply defined radiation dose, by using cross firing of a number of narrow radiation beams is a central principle of Gamma Knife radiosurgery.

The principles of particle radiation applying to protons apply also to electrons, but because of their lower mass they penetrate less well into tissues, at comparable energies and are most useful for the discrete irradiation of superficial structures.

In conclusion, it is important to emphasise that irrespective of the kind or dose of radiation energy delivered to a substance, the majority of the energy absorbed by the cell is mediated through the free electrons, produced by the radiation.

Consequences of Radiation Induced Damage on Biological Tissue

Early Effects

The events described in the previous section relate to the effects of radiation energy on atoms – the so-called direct effect of radiation. These events take place within *fractions of a microsecond*. As stated above, a common feature of all forms of radiation is the production of free electrons moving that speed through an absorbent medium. These can combine with ions of the same sort as those from which they were derived. They can also combine with atoms of other molecules, producing energised unstable products. This is the basis of the **indirect effect** of radiation. In living tissues, among the available molecules which can thus react with electrons is the water molecule, which is present in abundance. In a *matter of microseconds* free radicals can form according to, for example, the following equations.

$$H_2O \leftrightarrow H_2O^+ + e^-_{aq}$$

$$H_2O+ \leftrightarrow H^+ + OH^-$$

$$H_2O + e^- \leftrightarrow H^+ + OH^-$$

Other possible products of this kind of reaction are H_2, H_2O_2. Which radicals are formed and in which direction the equations are predominantly balanced will depend on the nature of the absorbent medium, including its physical state and also the energy of the radiation. These free radicals can then react with other molecules, within the cell to do damage. These chemical reactions are enhanced by the presence of oxygen. Or perhaps it is more precise to say, that if hypoxia induces a tissue pO_2 of less than 30 mmHg, then these reactions are inhibited and the damaging effect of the radiation is reduced. Because the half-life of the free radicals is so short, they cannot travel great distances and the damage they induce is effectively limited close to the path of the radiation and does not spread to any great extent through the tissues.

Everything that has been described so far in this chapter would be of little interest, if the effects of radiation were consistently reversible. However, they are not, because the energy that is deposited within living cells proceeds, also within *microseconds* to damage the macromolecules, which are the substrate of living processes. Chemical bonds may be broken, polymers may depolymerise or new unphysiological polymerization may occur. These processes may be reversible and be subsequently repaired, but they may be permanent leading to biochemical injury. The biochemical changes occur over the *seconds to hours* following irradiation and will be considered in the next chapter. It is generally thought that the most important target for biochemical injury is the hereditary molecule DNA.

Radiation Injuries to Nucleic Acid Molecules

The question then arises as to why DNA is considered to be the most likely target for radiation injury. There are a number of reasons. Firstly, while ionising radiation is absorbed in random locations, there are multiple copies of most molecules. DNA is present however in only two copies, has limited turnover and is the biggest molecule and hence the easiest target to hit. Also experimental evidence, using needles placing α particles in either cytoplasm or the nucleus, cell death only occurred if the radiation damaged the DNA. There are three major sorts of DNA injuries, which are considered to be the most common caused by radiation. These are base excision (BE), cross links with nuclear proteins, single DNA strand breaks – SSB – or double DNA strand breaks – DSB (Fig. 3.7). It is relevant in this context to mention that BEs and SSBs occur frequently without radiation in every cell in the body every day. For this reason effective mechanisms exist to repair such common processes. The evidence suggests that it is the DSBs, which do not repair after several hours, which are responsible for the sterilization of the cell. It would seem that 1 Gy of radiation may produce about 1,000 initial single strand breaks and about 20–40 double strand breaks. However, the lesion that counts is as stated the DSB, which is not repaired. However, the repair is so efficient that it is reckoned that 1 Gy will only kill about 30% of a typical mammalian cell line [1]. This reflects the comprehensive and effective DNA damage response.

Response to Radiation Damage of DNA Molecules

It is outside the scope of this book to go into too much detail about the biochemistry of DNA repair. The interested reader is again referred to "Basic Clinical

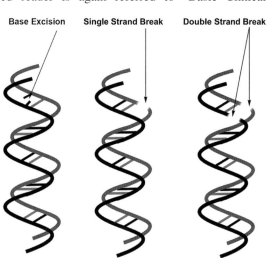

Base Excision   **Single Strand Break**   **Double Strand Break**

Fig. 3.7 Types of radiation damage. About 1,000 SSBs occur for 1 Gy and 20–40 DSBs. The SSBS and the BE excisions are easily repaired. The DSBs are the danger and it is reckoned that 1 Gy of absorbed radiation kills around 30% of the cells involved, indicating the efficiency of the repair processes

Radiobiology" [1]. However, there exist specialized repair systems for the repair of BEs and SSBs. These injuries not only follow irradiation injury but are a common component of normal cellular function. In consequence they are not that important because means of repair are to hand, since they are commonly occurring phenomena. To understand the outline of the repair of DSBs it must be remembered that the DNA is associated with a group of proteins with various functions. The DNA plus associated proteins constitute chromatin. Many of the proteins have enzymatic functions related to metabolism, transcription, replication and repair. The DNA damage response consists of three main steps involving the synthesis, movement and activation of various necessary proteins. The first step is damage detection and there exist DNA damage sensors for this. When these are activated a signal process is established which sends signals to one of three effector pathways. The end result of these processes is one of three possibilities. These are cell death, DNA repair or an effect on the checkpoints. This last possibility requires a brief digression.

Checkpoints in the Cell Cycle

The movement of dividing cells through the cell cycle (see Chap. 5) is controlled by enzymes which in essence constitute a checkpoint for permitting the cell to proceed from one stage in the cycle to the next. These checkpoints may be affected by DNB damage and may delay the passage of the cell through the cell cycle. While this in theory could provide a protective mechanism for stopping cells with dangerous mutations from dividing, there is little evidence to suggest at present that this is an important role. All that can be said is that the all the checkpoints are affected following radiation damage with concomitant delays in the process of cell division. The specifics of these processes is not at present better understood [1]. No further consideration will be given to the details of checkpoint control as this is considered to be outside the range of this book.

Cell Death

Cell death is associated with an increase in p53 and MDM2 in the cells. These two substances normally interact in such a way that their secretion and destruction result in limited levels in normal cells. In radiation damaged cells the substances are phosphorylated and this inhibits p53 breakdown so that it accumulates. The substance p53 is a tumour suppressor which regulates genes that control cell cycle check points and also apoptosis. The thought is that these processes exclude cells whose continued survival would be more of a threat than a benefit to the organism as a whole.

Cell death is a normal function occurring all the time in a healthy body. There are a variety of genetically programmed regulated mechanisms necessary for tissue homeostasis. They include, apoptosis, senescence, autophagy and necrosis. A detailed account may be found in "Basic Clinical Radiobiology" [1]. The cause of cell death after radiation damage is quite different. Early cell death following radiation damage (pre-mitotic cell death) is unusual but can occur within a few hours of the radiation. It affects a minority of tissues all of which have in common rapid cell division. Examples include hair follicles, the small intestine, developing embryos and spermatogenesis. It may also affect some tumours for example lymphomas [1].

The great majority of cells killed by radiation die after a latent interval after attempting mitosis one or more times. This is called post-mitotic cell death. For some reason the cells are no longer capable of the proper completion of mitosis so that mitotic catastrophe occurs. This is the commonest cause of cell death following radiation damage to living tissue.

DNA Repair

The third possibility is that the DNA is repaired. There are thought to be two possible mechanisms for this. In outline there is homologous recombination and non-homologous end joining. More detail will be found in "Basic Clinical Radiobiology" [1]. Homologous recombination requires the presence of lengths of DNA identical to the section with the break. This process can only occur in the S and G_2 stages of cell division. Non-homologous end joining can occur at any stage whether the cell is dividing or not. It is more rapid than homologous recombination but less accurate. There is a tiny risk this form or repair could increase the chance of harmful mutation. However, since only a tiny proportion of the DNA is concerned with gene coding and regulation, this risk is considered minimal and this notion would indicate why this mechanism has been able to survive.

This chapter has consisted of an outline of how ionising radiation can damage living tissue at the subatomic and molecular level. It has been shown that much of the damage may be repaired. When repair fails there are a variety of possible biological expressions of this failure. The membranes, enzymes and protein factory of the affected cells may cease to function or function in a deranged fashion. The reproductive functions of the cell may be damaged with destruction or damage to chromosomes, delay in mitosis, mutation and changes in the cell cycle. Moreover, even if the above changes are not lethal in the short term, over a time scale of months to years late effects may be seen in the form of premature aging, carcinogenesis or growth disturbances in the young.

References

1. Basic Clinical Radiobiology eds. Joiner M, van der Kogel A. Hodder Arnold an Hachette London UK company. 2009

Chapter 4
Biological Effects of Ionising Radiation

Introduction

The effects of radiation at atomic and molecular levels have been discussed in the previous chapter: events that occur over a time frame of nanoseconds to milliseconds. The present chapter relates to the effects of radiation on visible structures, in other words cells and tissues: events that occur within a time range of seconds to months or even years. To begin with, the theories relating to the infliction of radiation damage at the cellular level must be mentioned. It is considered that this may occur in one of two main ways. There is the *Direct Action* theory, whereby the ionisation of and lesion to the target, most probably DNA, is the primary event. The *Indirect Action* theory refers to the formation of DNA lesions produced by free radicals, which have in this instance been the primary target for ionisation by the radiation. Experimental work shows that the effect of oxygen on radiosensitivity is mediated by indirect action, since the tissue pO_2 affects the formation of the free radicals, which damage the DNA. Today, both modes of action are considered to be important in producing cell death. It may be mentioned that while there is, as stated above, broad agreement that the most important site of damage is the DNA of the cell nucleus, it may not be the only one. Some radiation effects, for example radiation oedema, indicate that cell membranes may also be important targets. As stated in the previous chapter, the majority of cell deaths are delayed and the result of mitotic catastrophe.

Cell Survival Studies [1]

Scientific analysis of any phenomenon requires quantitation, as an aid to improving understanding of that phenomenon and radiobiology is no exception. This involves the selection of variables to be observed and the registration of end-points. One of the most useful of radiobiological variables to study has been cell survival.

Cell survival studies are for the most part based on the effects of radiation on cells in culture, in other words in vitro. It must also be emphasised that cell death in

J.C. Ganz, *Gamma Knife Neurosurgery*,
DOI 10.1007/978-3-7091-0343-2_4, © Springer-Verlag/Wien 2011

the present context has a particular precise definition. Cell death is the loss of the capacity for <u>indefinite</u> proliferation usually due to mitotic catastrophe. The methods for studying cell survival, following a dose of radiation are designed with this definition in mind. Various models are used, including commonly cell culture where cells are plated out and the colonies of dividing and thereby surviving cells are counted. Such surviving cells are termed *Clonogenic Cells*. The proportion of surviving cells is called the *Survival Fraction* and is a much-used quantitative indicator of the effect of the radiation.

To appreciate the significance of these survival studies, it must be understood that the chance of radiation producing a cell kill is a random event. Thus, if a group of cells receive a dose, which is just big enough to provide one lethal event per cell, not all cells will be killed. Some will receive no lethal dose and some will receive several. The type of statistics used in calculating the chance of a cell kill is called Poisson statistics. This statistical technique is employed when the chance of a specific given change being produced is very small, in relation to the number of events taking place. This method is obviously relevant in the present context, since it is estimated that the absorption of 1 Gy of radiation will give rise to 10^5 ionisations per cell. On the other hand this amount of radiation produces only about 40 double strand breaks in the cell's DNA. Using Poisson statistics it is calculated that the percentage of cells which survive, when a radiation dose, sufficient to produce an average one lethal lesion per cell is delivered, is e^{-1} or 37%. This is called the *Survival Fraction*. The relationship between the survival fraction and the dose can be expressed as an equation. The form of such an equation should reflect the underlying pathophysiological mechanisms involved in cell death. The dose producing a survival fraction of e^{-1} used to be called D_0. However that assumes that a survival curve has a flat portion which it doesn't, so that D_o is not used today. Over the years a number of equations have been derived which have all been more or less complex exponential functions. They have been derived on the basis of the concept of *Target Theory*. This theory proposes that there exist a specific number of targets in the DNA which must be damaged if cell death is to occur. In the last 10 years the linear quadratic equation, has been increasingly used as having the best fit with what is observed in survival fraction experiments. A further mechanism of cell death is called bystander cell death. It affects cells adjacent to irradiated cells but not struck by radiation themselves. The underlying mechanisms and significance of this phenomenon is not currently clear.

The Linear Quadratic Equation [2–4]

The linear quadratic equation has the form

$$p = e^{-(\alpha D + \beta D)}$$

where p is the survival fraction. α and β are constants, descriptive of the linear and quadratic components of the equation respectively. Various experimental models have been used, from which the cells are plated out and the colonies of dividing – thereby surviving – cells are counted. Such surviving cells are termed *Clonogenic Cells*. The proportion of surviving cells is called the *Survival Fraction* and is a much-used quantitative indicator of the effect of the radiation. The applicability of the linear quadratic formula carries with it certain implications.

The linear part of the curve reflects direct lethal DNA damage from a single hit without repair. The logarithmic part reflects multiple sub-lethal hits which together become lethal.

Firstly, it is necessary to consider possible pathophysiological mechanisms, which are both consistent with the formula and at the same time, are consistent with the observed data of cell killing by radiation. The formula is presumed to reflect cell death produced by lesions, which are not related to any notional number of predetermined targets. The shape of any cell survival curve will be determined by the α/β ratio. This defines the dose at which the linear and quadratic contributions to cell killing are equal. The units of the α/β ratio are Gy. The linear quadratic equation has over the last 10 years not only been used for assessment of in vitro studies but has been widely applied in vivo, in the clinic. It is depicted in Fig. 4.1.

The vertical axis is logarithmic and Régisters the survival fraction. Thus the higher the value on this scale the less successful the treatment. The scale is logarithmic to reflect the logarithmic equation on which it is based. Low α/β ratios like 2–3 are associated with slowly dividing tissues which show late reactions to radiation (see Chap. 5) like brain. High values like 10 or more apply to rapidly dividing tissues like malignant tumours. Intermediate values can apply to rapidly dividing normal tissues like skin. However, the relationship is not a simple one. Thus skin and oral mucosa have an α/β ratio over 8 while melanomas have an α/β ratio of less than one. The benefit for the purpose or radiosurgery is to illustrate the two basic mechanisms of cell damage, direct and cumulative. The equation is mainly based on in vitro experiments but has been a useful clinical tool. If the α/β ratios for given normal or pathological tissues are known then this information can be used to guide the radiotherapy dosimetry. The applicability of the equation is supported by its similarity to the equations underlying the two most commonly accepted methods of cell repair after radiation.

Mechanisms of Cellular Repair [1]

There are two main conceptual models which, it is postulated produce survival curves consistent with the linear quadratic curve.

Lethal–Potentially-Lethal model

In this model, attention is focused on patterns of lesion production. There are two types of lesion reflected by different parts of the linear quadratic curve. The linear part of the equation reflects lesions, which are in themselves lethal. The quadratic

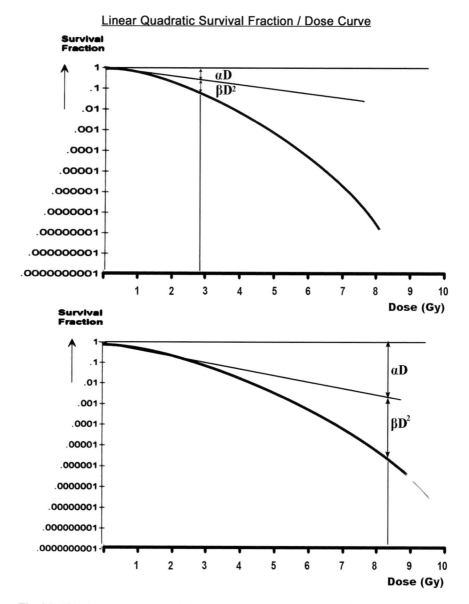

Fig. 4.1 This shows two linear quadratic survival curves, one where the α/β ratio is low (<3) and one where it is high (>8). For an explanation of the curve please see the text

part of the equation reflects lesions which of themselves maybe reparable, or potentially lethal. While such lesions may repair, they can combine to produce lethal lesions. Thus, with increasing the dose, it is conceived that a lethal outcome of such lesions will increase according to a quadratic function. Moreover, with

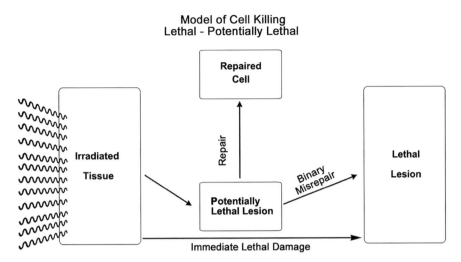

Fig. 4.2 Lethal–Potentially Lethal Model of Cell Killing. For details see text

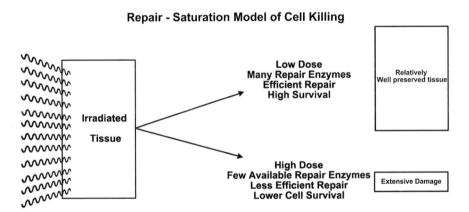

Fig. 4.3 Repair Saturation Model of Cell Killing. For details see text

increasing dose the direct lethal damage will increase. Thus the lesion has two possibilities, to become lethal or to repair (Fig. 4.2).

Saturation Repair Model

This is illustrated in Fig. 4.3. In this model there is only one kind of lesion produced by a single "hit", but it may be repaired if there is sufficient repair enzyme around. It is suggested that the main biological substrate of the linear quadratic equation relates exclusively to the processes of repair. Thus, with increasing doses an increasing number of potentially lethal lesions will be produced. With a greater number of lesions to repair, the repair enzymes and processes may be saturated by the number of repairs to be performed. Thus, a greater number of lesions end up lethal. It is conceivable that both models may contribute to the outcome, following radiation.

It is necessary to specify that *repair* and *recovery* do not mean the same thing when applied to the processes within a tissue, following a dose of ionising radiation. Repair refers to the intracellular restitution of damaged structures, in particular DNA. *Recovery* refers to the way in which the repair processes express themselves in the tissue; for example in terms of increased cell survival or reduction in the extent of radiation damage.

There are other factors to consider, in addition to the basic interaction between radiation and cells that has been discussed so far. These factors relate both to the tissue and to the radiation.

Different Factors Affecting the Effects of Radiation

Biological Factors

The Cell Cycle [5]

Under the microscope, the only time that the DNA is visible is during mitosis. However, using autoradiography techniques, the DNA can be shown to pass through a cycle of changes (Fig. 4.4).

The M phase is mitosis. This is followed by an inactive phase or gap, the G_1 phase which is turn is followed by the S phase or phase of active synthesis. The S

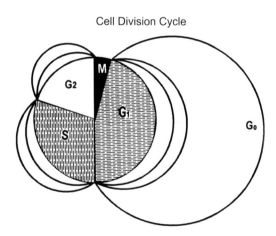

Fig. 4.4 Diagram of Cell Cycle. For details see text

phase is in turn followed by a second gap, the G_2 phase which ends with the next mitosis. Figure 4.4 depicts a variety of cell cycles. A variety is shown to indicate the variability between cells. There is also a G_o phase, which is a state of apparent suspended animation, when the cell cycle is either resting or changing so slowly as to be undetectable. As indicated by the diagram the G_o can vary in duration in different situations. During this phase, the rest of the cell's activities, that are not related to cell division continue unabated. Since normal adult tissues do not grow, the process of synthesis described by the cell cycle must also be accompanied by a process of cell loss, to provide the steady state of unchanged tissue size. In tumours, this steady state is disrupted. Also as mentioned in Chap. 3 the passage from one phase to the next in the cell cycle is under the control of checkpoints where different enzymes control the processes. These checkpoints can be affected during the processes damaging DNA after radiation.

Oxygenation [1]

This has already been mentioned a number of times. Hypoxia, at levels of pO_2 below 30 mmHg reduces the development of damaging free radicals and thus the degree of radiation damage (Fig. 4.5). Moreover, there is experimental evidence, which suggests that hypoxic areas of a tumour may reoxygenate, during fractionated radiotherapy, due to a variety of factors. These include reduction in oxygen consumption by dead cells, reduction in the number of cells in relation to area of the capillary bed and reduction of the intratumoural pressure, permitting reopening of the microcirculation. Since normal tissues are well oxygenated in relation to tumour tissue, reoxygenation of tumour tissue theoretically improves the therapeutic index (see Fig. 4.5).

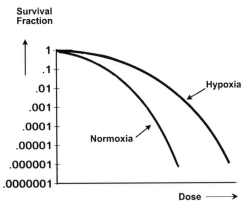

Fig. 4.5 Effect of Hypoxia on Dose Response. Radioresponsiveness is dependent on adequate oxygenation. If the tissue oxygen tension falls below 30 mmHg, the radiation is noticeably less effective as indicated in this diagram

Radiation Factors

Fractionation and Fraction Size [2, 4]

In conventional radiotherapy, it is customary to deliver the dose in fractions. This permits a higher target dose while keeping the normal tissue damage down to acceptable levels. It was originally based on the presumption that normal cells repair sublethal damage more quickly than tumour cells. It also has some other theoretical advantages In principle, it increases the chance of catching a tumour cell at a radiosensitive stage of the cell cycle (see above), by killing sensitive cells early and establishing cell cycle synchronisation; thus facilitating synchronisation of the cells at a sensitive phase, later in the treatment. This process is called reassortment. However, it may be seen that increasing the number of fractions increases the tumour cell survival, or decreases the proportion of cells killed. Figure 4.6 depicts the effect of fractionation on the total dose required to produce the same degree of cell death as shown using survival fraction studies. Thus, it is a general principle that to produce the same dose effect, using fractionation, a greater total dose is required than would be needed if all the radiation were given at one time. This is because of the capacity for repair of DNA and repopulation by undamaged cells that occurs between the individual fractions, which make up the total dose. The phenomena described in this paragraph have been summarized as the 4 "Rs" of radiotherapy, Repair, Reassortment, Repopulation, and Reoxygenation. To these a fifth "R" may be added, Radiosensitivity, indicating the intrinsic sensitivity of individual tissues to radiation. **This** term must be distinguished from *radiorespon-siveness*, which does **not** refer to a fundamental biological characteristic but to the clinical responsiveness to a given radiation treatment. It may be noted that of the 4 "Rs", repair and repopulation should reduce the effectiveness of the radiation with fractionation, while reoxygenation and reassortment should increase it. Finally, the

Fig. 4.6 Fractionation and Dose response. In general, the biological effect of a given dose of radiation is less if it is divided between several fractions. A corollary of this is that with an increasing number of fractions an equivalent increasing dose will be required to achieve the same amount of cell killing. This is illustrated diagrammatically here

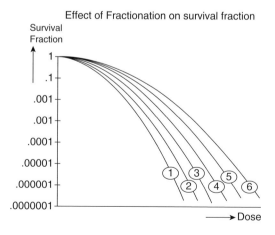

Effect of Fractionation on survival fraction

linear quadratic equation has proven to be useful in determining appropriate fractionation strategies for different clinical situations and a little more on this will be mentioned in the next chapter.

There is another matter relating to fractionation. Tissues with a low α/β ratio tend to show a reduced biological effect with increased fractionation more than those with a high α/β ratio. Thus fractionating the dose for tissues with a low α/β ratio will require a proportionally higher total dose to achieve the same cell killing effect. This applies to both the brain and to the majority of benign intracranial tumours treated by GKNS. In situations with high α/β ratios and particularly if the value is high for the tumour and low for the surrounding tissue, there is a possibility of using these differences to optimise the design of fractionation schedules.

Time Between Fractions

This is another radiation therapeutic variable that must be taken into account when fractionated doses are given. It must be obvious that two fractions given with one hour's interval and two fractions given with a month's interval are not equivalent. This becomes even more apparent when it is remembered that single band DNA damage repair is for the most part completed in 2–4 h. Thus, in general, the first 5–6 h are important: thereafter the time interval is not so significant.

Dose

Dose, as stated earlier, equals energy absorbed per unit mass of absorber, (dE/dM). Yet the term dose is, if unqualified, unacceptably imprecise. According to Webster's Collegiate Dictionary, the noun "*dose*" derives from Middle English, which derives from Old French which in turn derives from a Greek noun "*dosis*", a giving: this noun being a derivative of the verb "*didonai*", to give. However, there are a variety of different types of dose definition as outlined below, lending greater precision to our understanding.

The Surface Dose is the dose absorbed in the superficial layers of the skin.

The Maximum Dose is the maximum dose absorbed.

The Target Dose is, in general, the minimum dose delivered to the target volume.

The Prescription Dose is, in general the same as the Target dose but is the dose chosen to treat the target margin.

The Margin Dose is a much used term to be avoided. It is in effect used as a synonym for the prescription dose. However, the term implies that the dose at the margin is the same at all points of the surface of the target whereas in reality there are always some small portions of a target which have a lesser or greater dose. Because of this, the term should probably be abandoned in favour of prescription dose.

The Integral Dose is the total absorbed dose in a specified volume (of tissue) and is comprised of Gy and cm^3 and its units are units of work that is, joules or millijoules

Isodoses are volumes containing is the same dose. In a tissue volume, seen in computerised image slices the isodoses appear as lines in each slice, but in reality they comprise a volume. They are commonly referred to as isodose lines, but this is an imprecise usage to be avoided. They are not unlike other lines of equal value such as isobars on a weather map or height contour lines on a survey map. Isodoses express relative dose distribution as a percentage of the maximum dose. Moreover, they reflect dose homogeneity.

The dose to the tumour is designed to be adequate for its destruction without producing unacceptable damage to the surrounding normal tissues. For fractionated radiotherapy total doses to brain tumours, vary between 30 and about 50 Gy. There is no absolute consistency of practice but it is common for example to give patients with glial tumours 50 Gy in roughly 2 Gy fractions. On the other hand it has been more and more usual to give whole brain radiotherapy for metastases with doses of 30 Gy in ten 3 Gy fractions.

Dose Homogeneity

In conventional radiotherapy, radiant energy is delivered in one of two ways. With teletherapy, radiation is beamed into the patient from a distance. This technique enables the construction of radiation fields with a high degree of homogeneity over the target. This should be highly desirable, because the radiation effect cannot be greater than that due to the lowest dose delivered. There will be more on this in Chap. 7. Brachytherapy is the other principle radiotherapy technique and here a radiation source is implanted within the target. Lack of homogeneity is an intrinsic weakness of brachytherapy for solid tumours, though the degree of inhomogeneity can be reduced by using multiple radiation sources. Nonetheless, intracystic instillation of an isotope with limited penetration provides an excellent way of delivering an adequate dose to the walls of a thin walled neoplastic cyst. The cyst fluid diffuses the isotope, evens out the dose and is radioinsensitive, so that the dose at the wall is the only factor, which needs consideration.

Dose Volume

It has long been appreciated that the volume of a tumour is an important determinant of the success of radiotherapy on that tumour. In general, larger tumours do less well than smaller. On the other hand, it is known that for the same dose, the larger the area of skin receiving the dose the greater the chance of skin complications from that dose. Dose volume may be defined, for convenience, as the volume within a given isodose. Its significance may be demonstrated as follows. While 5 Gy to the whole human body is usually lethal, 5 Gy to a tumour volume is wholly inadequate. Indeed doses of up to 50 Gy can be tolerated with gastrointestinal cancer, while it is the gastrointestinal tract, which is one of the main victims of whole body radiation. Moreover, considerations of volume must be made within the bounds of a single species. Some insects and bacteria can survive radiation doses vastly in excess of those tolerated by mammals. Within the brain, the volume of normal brain receiving a high dose of radiation is crucial to the development of adverse radiation effects. This is the factor which limits the volume of target which may be safely treated by radiosurgery. However, the permissible volume that may be treated has been on the increase over the years with the use of repeated partial treatments on the one hand and the reduction of the prescription dose on the other. While a target diameter of 2.5–3 cm remains a reasonable guideline there are ways of treating larger lesions, provided the dose to sensitive adjacent tissues is kept within acceptable bounds.

Dose Rate

Dose rate is the dose per unit time. Within certain limits dose rate appears to affect the biological effectiveness of a given dose. Between 1 Gy/min and 0.1 cGy/min there is a gradual fall off in dose effectiveness. Increasing or decreasing the dose rate beyond these limits has little extra effect [6]. The mechanism behind the dose rate effect is attributed to the speed of repair processes within the affected cell. Radiation damage occurs in micro-seconds. Repair processes take several hours. With lower dose rates, there is a bigger chance for repair for a given dose. Dose rate calculations become important when the radiation source is an isotope, where the age of the isotope has reduced the dose rate below 1 Gy/min.

Clinical Radiobiological Correlates

The Fate of the Normal Tissue

The fate of normal tissue, subjected to ionising radiation is closely related to the cellular architecture and internal organization of the tissue. In general, tissues are considered to have two main kinds of organization.

Hierarchical Tissues (H-Type)

In these tissues, the cell division is carried out by a minority of pluripotential cells, stem cells, while the functions of the tissue are performed by differentiated cells. These tissues usually show rapid renewal; such as skin, mucosae and the haemo-poietic system. The rate of cell production is determined by the lifetime of the mature cells.

Flexible Tissues (F-Type)

These are the tissues, which do not have a clear-cut hierarchical organization. In these tissues there is thought to be less of a clear-cut division into primitive dividing and mature non-dividing cells. It is considered that even mature cells maintain some capacity for division. These tissues are generally slowly self-renewing, for example, liver, kidney, lung and the CNS. However, it seems likely that purely F tissues may not exist and that, for example, the CNS is a mixed H-F tissue.

However, the different types of cellular organization imply different responses to radiation. Thus, if H-tissues are considered, while the intensity of response to radiation and the duration of recovery is dose related, the latency time between delivery of radiation and the appearance of the response is not dose related. It is dependent on the survival time of the mature cells. On the other hand the latency from dose to response in F-tissues is dose dependent. This is significant for the user of the Gamma Knife.

Tissue Architecture

Another tissue factor, beyond cellular organization is tissue architecture. The H-type tissues have a largely serial architecture, but so does the CNS. This means that function is so organized that removal of one segment can affect the whole tissue. The kidney or lung are examples of parallel organization. Thus, the destruction of many nephrons may have little effect on total kidney function, at least not until so many are destroyed, that the organ's reserve capacity is used up. This is an important concept, in that the relatively radiosensitive kidney can compensate well for radiation damage, so that it is less radioresponsive than would be expected. On the other hand, the relatively radioinsensitive CNS is radioresponsive, because damage to even a small part can produce damage to the function of the whole organ.

Cell Cycle Time (Tc) and Tumour Doubling Time (Td)

The Tc for most tumours, where it has been measured is of the order of 1–4 days. This is in contrast with the time it takes the tumour to double in volume; the tumour doubling time (Td). The Td for most tumours is between 1 and 2 months. This implies a considerable loss of cells during the tumour growth. Even so, in most tumours the growth rate approximates to a simple exponential function, emphasising the need for early detection and treatment.

The Fate of Irradiated Tumour Cells

Cells may be lethally injured. Lethal Injury, as stated above, is defined as a loss of capacity for indefinite proliferation. The expression of lethal injury may not be seen immediately. Usually, cell lysis occurs at the time of a subsequent mitosis, though not necessarily the first, following the radiation. In extreme cases, interphase lysis without a subsequent mitosis can occur. The timing of the observed damage may well be delayed by two additional factors. Firstly, the cells of a slowly growing tumour will take longer to die than those of a quickly dividing one. Secondly, the sensitivity of irradiated tumour cells varies with their position in the cell cycle. M phase and G_2 phase cells are more sensitive while S phase cells are more resistant. When G_1 is long cells in the early G_1 are also relatively resistant. Thus, radiation during an insensitive portion of the cycle may be associated with division delay. This division delay appears to be a linear function of dose. At all events, it is important to emphasise that the aim of conventional radiotherapy of malignant neoplasms is to destroy all neoplastic cells. Nonetheless, this may be impossible of achievement because certain tumours may require a tumour control dose, which will give unacceptable normal tissue damage. Thus, tumour growth delay is a much used clinical/radiological endpoint: used to indicate that radiation gives benefit even if the tumour is not killed. The following tumour factors can influence the outcome of treatment.

The Radiosensitivity of the Tumour

Radiosensitivity of a given tumour appears to be closely related to the slope of the linear component of the linear quadratic curve of cell survival, for the cells of the individual tumour.

The Volume of the Tumour

It is obvious that with a larger tumour there will be a greater number of clonogenic cells to destroy, and for a given tolerated dose of radiation, the chance of therapeutic success must be less. Moreover, there is some evidence that the clonogenic cells of larger tumours may be less radiosensitive.

Accelerated Repopulation

There is evidence that clonogenic cells that survive a dose of radiation may repopulate the tumour at a faster rate than before. This effect may be independent of tumour growth and indeed may be seen when a tumour is in fact shrinking.

The Tumour Bed Effect

This effect relates to a reduction in tumour growth or regrowth in an irradiated region and is considered to relate to damage to the surrounding tissue stroma, including the blood vessels. It is considered to contribute to retarded growth.

The Hypoxic Reaction

Those clonogenic cells that are hypoxic at the time of radiation will have a better chance of survival. This means that in the immediate period following a dose of radiation, the proportion of hypoxic cells will be greater than before the treatment.

Reoxygenation

This process, described above will contribute to increased radio-responsiveness during a course of fractionated radiotherapy. The speed of reoxygenation varies greatly from a few hours to several days.

References

1. Horsman MR, Wouters BG, Joiner MC, Overgaard J. The oxygen effect and fractionated radiotherapy. in Clinical Radiobiology eds. Joiner M, van der Kogel A. Hodder Arnold and Hachette UK company, London: pp 207–216; 2009.
2. Bentzen SM, Joiner MC. The Linear Quadratic Equation in Clinical Practice. in Clinical Radiobiology eds. Joiner M, van der Kogel A. Hodder Arnold and Hachette UK company, London: pp 120–34; 2009.
3. Joiner MC, Bentzen SM. Fractionation: the linear-quadratic approach. in Clinical Radiobiology eds. Joiner M, van der Kogel A. Hodder Arnold and Hachette UK company, London: pp 102–119; 2009.
4. Joiner MC. Quantifying cell kill and cell survival. in Clinical Radiobiology eds. Joiner M, van der Kogel A. Hodder Arnold and Hachette UK company, London: pp 41–55; 2009.
5. Ganz JC. Gamma Knife Surgery, Second Revised Edition. Springer, Vienna: pp 40–41; 1997.
6. Van der Kogel A. The dose rate effect. in Clinical Radiobiology eds. Joiner M, van der Kogel A. Hodder Arnold and Hachette UK company, London: pp 41–55; 2009.

Chapter 5
Ionising Radiation and Clinical Practice

Introduction

This chapter will consider some of the information, outlined in the previous chapter, in relation to clinical practice in general. The concept of radioresponsiveness has been mentioned already, in relation to both tumours and normal tissues. The aim of the doctor using ionising radiation in the treatment of tumours is to kill the tumour and not damage the normal tissues. While this is desirable in theory, it is difficult to achieve in practice. In this context, the concept of the therapeutic index has been much used.

General Clinico/Pathological Principles

The Therapeutic Index

The therapeutic index describes the relationship between tumour damage and normal tissue damage. The tumour response curve and the normal tissue response curve are both sigmoid. This is illustrated by Fig. 5.1. The limiting factor is the appearance of unacceptable, normal tissue damage. Thus, the normal tissue damage will limit the dose. The ideal tumour is so radioresponsive that it may be destroyed without inducing significant normal tissue damage. However, the ideal tumour does not exist and in terms of the CNS, many of the tumours are markedly radioresistant. It will be noticed from Fig. 5.1 that only the lower part of the normal tissue complication frequency is charted, because to treat to higher doses would be unethical. It was at one time thought that the difference in response between normal tissues and tumours was a result of a difference in radiosensitivity between a radiosensitive tissue, the tumour, with a high rate of cell division, and a relatively less sensitive normal tissue, with a low rate of cell division. This notion was based on the concept that radiosensitivity correlated with the rate of cell division. Today,

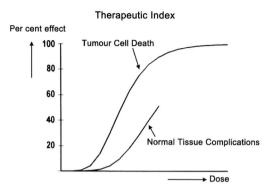

Fig. 5.1 The Therapeutic Index. The therapeutic index is a measure of the difference between an effective treatment and associated complications. In this instance it is the difference between killing a tumour and damaging the surrounding normal tissue. The dose to normal tissue is the limiting factor because if too high the clinical consequences of the damaged tissue can be unacceptable. It may be noted that only the lower part of the tissue complications curve is shown since a higher complication rate would be unacceptable. In any given case the acceptable complication rate has to be assessed in relation to the danger of the disease being treated. It is however, true to say that the risk of damage to normal tissues can be big enough to prevent a radiation dose which will have a 100% chance of killing the tumour. This is the major factor limiting the effect of clinical radiotherapy

it is more conventional to consider the therapeutic index in terms of radiorespon-siveness, which reflects a clinical response rather than an intrinsic biological characteristic. Other factors are thought to be more significant than the 5th "R" of radiotherapy – radiosensitivity. Amongst these are tumour volume and the effect of fractionation in respect of the 4 "Rs".

The significance of volume on successful radiotherapy was mentioned in the previous chapter. It is a commonplace of clinical management that all attempts should be made to reduce the volume of a tumour surgically, prior to radiotherapy, in order to improve the chances of Success. There is, of course, no tumour related reason why the dose should not be increased to a level, which is uniformly lethal. But as stated above, the unwanted effects of radiation on normal tissues will limit the acceptable radiation dose, which may be given. Thus, the rest of this chapter will consider, in a little more detail than hitherto, the effects of radiation on normal tissue, in particular in relation to clinical practice.

Time Dose Relationships

It has long been known that the biological effect of a dose is less if given in a protracted, fractionated course, instead of in one session. One of the earliest attempts to quantify this phenomenon was undertaken by Strandqvist, who tried to assess the duration of treatment on the biologically equivalent dose. Nowadays, this is called the iso-effect dose. This work, while seminal can be criticised for a number of important weaknesses. Amongst these is that it did not separate the effects of duration of dose, number of fractions and fraction dose. An even more important weakness is that the mathematical formalism used in the study, and other related formalisms derived on the same principle have subsequently been shown to be inherently incorrect. Today, the linear quadratic formula is more often used in the assessment of the effect of fractionation and duration of treatment on iso-effect doses. The effect of fractionation in sparing normal tissue was described in the previous chapter. However, it is necessary to mention another factor, if the effect of fractionation on normal tissue is to be understood. Tissue damage may be early or late and these two categories may be distinguished as follows. There is an arbitrary cut-off between early and late complication set at 90 days. Another way of looking at this notion is to consider early complications as arising during treatment while late complications occur after treatment is over.

The effect of the duration of treatment is now considered to be complex and, at least in terms of late complications, of little relevance. Treatment duration will of course be of importance in relation to tumour response and acute reactions occurring during the course of treatment. The importance of duration of treatment is of current interest in relation to hyperfractionation and accelerated radiotherapy, but is of little more interest here. It is of limited interest in Gamma Knife treatment, for reasons, which are outlined later.

Early and Late Reactions

The Linear Quadratic Equation and Early and Late Complications

It has been stated in Chap. 4 that the α/β ratio characterised the cell survival response, for a given tissue/tumour type. A characteristic of tissues which show early complications is that they have a high α/β ratio. On the other hand tissues with late complications have a low α/β ratio. Moreover, late complications and the tissues, which develop them, are more sensitive to fractionation, while early complications and the tissues, which develop them, are less sensitive to fractionation. In general, the α/β ratio for tissues showing early reactions is 7–20 Gy and for tissues showing late reactions it is 0.5–6 Gy.

Early Reactions

As stated above, these reactions occur while radiation treatment is still going on and/or before 90 days after the start of treatment. They are characterised by a high α/β ratio [3]. They occur chiefly in H-tissues, are due to an effect on parenchymal stem cells and are largely reversible. Their intensity is dose dependant and the time taken to resolve is dose dependent, but the latency from start of treatment to appearance of complication is not dose dependent. It is related instead to the life span of the mature cells in the tissue concerned. These complications are not fractionation sensitive and for a given dose, on the whole, the shorter the duration of treatment, the greater the injury. Typical early reactions are the erythema and desquamation seen in the skin.

As stated the early reactions usually are reversible. However, they can be a great risk to the organism in situations of whole body radiation, as after a nuclear explosion, where they can be the major causes of death. However, for the focal low volume focal irradiation arising during therapy they are in the main reversible and not a threat to life.

Late Reactions

These reactions have a low α/β ratio [6]. They occur in all sorts of tissues and are thought to be related to effects on connective tissue rather than parenchyma. They occur after 60 days and often after many months or even years. At all events they occur after the cessation of treatment [1, 2, 4]. The intensity of response and the shortness of the latency to the complications' inception are dose dependant. They are in general irreversible. They are fractionation sensitive but not sensitive to the duration of treatment. Subcutaneous fibrosis, skin telangiectasia or radiation damage to the CNS are all late reactions.

Adverse Radiation Effects in the Brain

These are the complications which are of relevance to the Gamma Knife user. They are of the late reaction type since the brain is an F type tissue and the cells do not have the high turn over necessary for early reactions. The components of the late reaction are as elsewhere with the complications of irradiation both somatic and genetic. The complications may be acute sub-acute or chronic. These terms apply to the kind of lesion irrespective of when the lesion arises. The complications may also be immediate, early, intermediate or delayed. These terms apply to the latency between the irradiation and onset of the complication. This topic will be pursued further in Chap. 7, in relation to GKNS.

Severe Somatic Adverse Radiation Effects in the Brain

As stated earlier the acute reactions tend to apply in the brain only in those patients who have been exposed to total body radiation. However, one of the reasons it is not seen in clinical practice is that the correct radiation dosimetry to the brain is now widely known. Thus early complications may occur following whole brain radiotherapy if the fraction dose exceeds 2 Gy or the total dose is more than 50–60 Gy.

The patient will suffer from headache, nausea, vomiting and maybe fever and even unsteadiness. All signs of raised intracranial pressure. They are however at these doses usually reversible and indeed are seldom seen if doses are kept within the limits mentioned. It should however be emphasised that children are far more at risk for these complications and at lower doses.

The components of delayed radiation damage are epithelial (parenchymal) stromal and vascular. Like all radiation injuries an inflammatory response is not a major component of the reaction. The stromal reaction consists in the deposition of fibrosis which is not seen in the brain. Gliosis, the cerebral equivalent of fibrosis is a minor and inconsistent component of brain damage after radiation. Radiation damage is known to be commonly associated with oedema. Moreover demyelination is seen. Thus, the radiation is damaging the astrocytes and endothelial cells which are the anatomical basis of the blood brain barrier, allowing the development of oedema. The damage to the oligodendroglia results in demyelination. The extent and severity of the damage is dose and volume dependent. Perivascular lymphocytic cuffing is seen and a major pathogenetic mechanism is thought to be small vessel damage. This is consistent with the finding that the damage is most severe in the relatively less vascular white matter. Large infarcts due to the occlusion of larger vessels are less common. While the pathogenesis of the radiation damage is thought to be due to microvascular injury how this is converted into clumps of coagulation necrosis is currently less clear.

Less Severe Somatic Adverse Radiation Effects in the Brain After Gamma Knife Treatment

It is known that after Gamma Knife surgery, that perilesional oedema may be seen on follow up MR imaging. This is mostly temporary. Sometimes it is expansive sometimes not. It does not correlate well with the appearance of symptoms. It seems probable that the source of this oedema may in many cases not be direct brain damage by radiation but by blood brain barrier damage due to peptides originating in the pathological process being treated. Its presence does mean that interpreting the MR findings may be difficult and the determination that radiation necrosis has occurred in association with Gamma Knife treatment is by no means simple.

Genetic Adverse Effects Following Brain Irradiation

It is of interest that no survivor of the Japanese atomic explosions has been recorded to develop a primary glial tumour. A number of meningiomas have been reported. On the other hand in over 10,000 children treated with scalp radiation for tinea capitis there was a relative risk of developing a gliomas of 2.6% a meningioma of 9.5%, a schwannoma of 18.8% and other neural tumours of 3.4%. The mean latency from tumour to secondary neoplasm was 17.6 years [2]. The ideal characteristics for the development of a radiation induced neoplasm are a susceptible recipient, a fairly low dose over a large volume and a long latency period. The Gamma Knife delivers high doses to small volumes. The machine has been in use for over 25 years with over 500,000 patients treated. The risk of Gamma Knife induced neoplasia is unknown. With the passage of time this incidence will become clearer. Currently estimates vary between 1 and 2% at 20 years to 1 per 1,000 to 1 per 20,000 patients.

References

1. Yang I, Sneed PK, Larson DA, McDermott MW. Complications and Management in Radio-surgery. In Chin LS & Regine WR (eds) Principles and Practice of Stereotactic Radiosurgery. Springer Verlag, Vienna New York, pp 649–662, 2008
2. Fajaro LF, Berthrong M, Anderson RE. Radiation Pathology. Nervous System. Oxford University Press, Oxford, pp 351–361, 2001
3. Ganz JC, Gamma Knife Surgery, Second Revised Edition. Springer Verlag Vienna New York, pp 40–54, 1997
4. Dörr W. Pathogenesis of normal tissue side-effects. In Joiner M, van der Kogel A (eds) Basic Clinical Radiobiology. Hodder Arnold an Hachette UK company London, pp 169–190, 2009
5. McNally MJ. (ed) The Scientific Basis of Modern Radiotherapy. British Institute of Radiology, London. 1989
6. Withers HR, Peters LJ. Biological aspects of radiation therapy. In: Fletcher GH. (ed) Textbook of Radiotherapy. Lea & Febiger, Philadelphia: pp 103–180, 1981

Chapter 6
Gamma Knife Development from 1967 to 2010

General Information

Introduction

The *first* Gamma Unit was constructed after more than two decades of research, in both the laboratory and the clinic. The primary intention, at the start of this research was the non-invasive treatment of functional disease, rather than a commitment to a particular technology. Ultrasound was considered and rejected, because at that time it could not be used with precision without opening the skull. Leksell's first paper with the word radiosurgery in the title was published in 1951. Thus, the concept of a non-invasive surgical procedure and the development of a simple usable stereotactic system seem to have been contemporary. Moreover, it is easy to forget today, when the major indications for Gamma Knife surgery are tumours and malformations that the limits of imaging techniques applying to open stereotaxy also apply to radiosurgery. In the nineteen fifties and sixties radiological tumour delineation was approximate, seen in relation to the precision of stereotactic treatment. Thus, the early experimental work was performed and the first clinical instruments were designed with a view to making cerebral lesions, for treating functional disorders. It seems likely that it was considered particularly important to avoid the potential dangers of surgery when treating conditions, which did not present a short-term threat to life.

Preparatory Basic Research

The first steps in the basic research were taken in association with the distinguished radiobiologist, Börje Larsson, at the University of Uppsala, at that time a very young man. The first matter to be decided was the choice of a suitable type of radiation. The radiation should be able to penetrate to the desired depth, without delivering potentially damaging energy to the tissues along its path, in other words

J.C. Ganz, *Gamma Knife Neurosurgery*,
DOI 10.1007/978-3-7091-0343-2_6, © Springer-Verlag/Wien 2011

radiation with a low Linear Energy Transfer or LET (see Chap. 3). Furthermore, the method of delivery of the radiation had to fulfil certain criteria. It must be possible to localize the radiation target accurately. Moreover, it should enable the design of a radiation field with a high dose where it was needed, at the target and a very sharp dose fall at the edge of the target, enabling protection of tissue around the target from damaging radiation. High energy protons from the 185 MeV synchrocyclotron, at the University of Uppsala, close to Stockholm provided such a source of radiation. The localization was achieved by fitting a Leksell stereotactic frame to the head and directing the beam in accordance with the frame's axes. The desired dose distribution could be achieved by cross firing a number (20–22) of small diameter beams. It should be noted that with this cross firing technique, deceleration of the protons, producing a Bragg Peak was not the aim. Using high energy proton beams, with the low LET characteristic of protons, which have not yet begun to decelerate, cross firing produced a very low radiation-tissue interaction along the individual beams, with a concentration of radiation activity in the volume where the beams crossed (Fig. 6.1).

A consequence of this design is that the effects of the technique cannot be compared with the effects of Bragg Peak radiation (see Fig. 3.6), since the two types of lesion are radiobiologically dissimilar. It must be emphasised that it is the narrow diameter of the beams, which enables the great precision of the radiation field (Fig. 6.2). Since the intended clinical application was a lesion in the brain parenchyma, the early experiments studied the characteristics of lesions in the cerebrum of the goat. Goats were used because their skulls are large and rigid enough to allow the application of a human stereotactic frame. Moreover, their

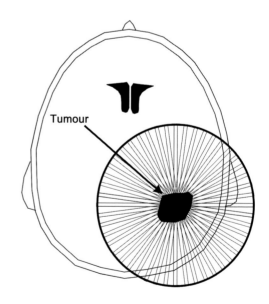

Fig. 6.1 Focal radiation – cross firing cross firing individually weak beams of low LET through a focal point leads to a focused concentration of radiation energy by a different method from the Bragg Peak described in Chap. 3. This is the method used with nearly all other radiosurgery methods including the Gamma Knife

Tumour

Collimator Width & Dose Precision

**40 mm diameter
Collimator**

**8 mm diameter
Collimator**

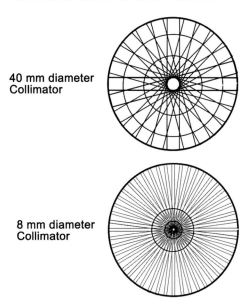

Fig. 6.2 Effect of collimation on dose precision this illustration shows the distribution of the lines joining equivalent points of intersection, between the beams of radiation arranged around a central target. In the *upper* diagram the beams are broad while in the lower picture they are much narrower. It is obvious that with narrow beams, in the *lower* picture, the radiation is much more concentrated at the centre of the irradiated volume with a sharp fall in dose away from the high dose central region. In the upper diagram the fall off is more diffuse and spread. This diagram emphasises the requirement for multiple narrow beams for precise focal radiation as used in the Gamma Knife

brains are large enough, in proportion to the lesion to avoid such complications as generalised radiation oedema.

Disk shaped lesions were produced, because the disk shape would be most appropriate when performing a thalamotomy, in patients. 200 Gy was used and a somewhat stereotyped lesion was produced. After 4 weeks, necrosis, degeneration and inflammatory reactions could be observed. Over the subsequent weeks there was intense cellular activity, characterised by phagocytosis and the beginning of scar formation. After a year, a stable glial scar had developed. Like the radiation volume, the lesions were disk shaped. The lesions were also characterised by a sharply defined edge lying at the region of maximum dose fall, roughly equivalent to the 50% isodose. Moreover, there was very little increase in lesion volume over time. If the dose was doubled to 400 Gy a much more marked and diffuse lesion was seen, with even a risk of oedema in the entire cerebral hemisphere. These lesions were chronically inflammatory and did not result in stable avascular scars. Thus, there was clearly an upper acceptable target dose that should not be exceeded. Another finding was that above a certain threshold, of about 150 Gy, the time to the development of a lesion was within limits a function of dose. The existence of the threshold indicated that there was also a lower dose limit, below which no adequate lesion would develop. All these findings indicated that in radiosurgery, the dose would be critical. Moreover, below 130 Gy in most cases lesions did not develop.

The First Patients

The above is only the merest outline of the detailed research, which was performed before the first patients were treated radiosurgically. However, it indicated that sharply defined small radiosurgical lesions, appropriate for the treatment of functional disorders could be relatively easily obtained. The next step was a clinical trial. It was still too early to build a new dedicated machine for the first patients so they were treated using already existing machines. The first patient reported following radiosurgery in 1955 suffered from long lasting, severe chronic schizophrenia. She was treated with 280 kV X-rays from an industrial X-ray tube. A dose of 40 Gy was delivered first to the right rostral internal capsule, followed 33 days later by the same dose to the left. The result was indeterminate but the following conclusions could be drawn. After 2 years follow-up, the patient had suffered no harmful effects of the treatment. She responded to ECT and chlorpromazine afterwards, something she had not done before. She was eventually able to return home a year later, after a 4-year stay in a mental institution. In retrospect, the dose today seems rather low, but the result was sufficiently encouraging to stimulate Leksell and his colleagues to continue with the method.

The next patients to be treated, suffering from Parkinsonism or chronic pain, were treated using the Uppsala synchrocyclotron. The results of this series were also promising enough to suggest that radiosurgery had a definite future, as a clinical technique. However, Leksell felt that the synchrocyclotron, using the cross firing technique, was too inconvenient for routine clinical use, so an alternative technology was required. A number of options were considered, including accelerated ions or electrons, supervoltage X-rays, neutrons and gamma emitting nuclides. The final choice fell on gamma nuclides, because the radiobiological characteristics of this form of radiation were so similar to those of the protons that had been used hitherto. Of available nuclides, ^{60}Co was finally chosen, not least because its half-life of 5.27 years was seen to be the most practical.

The First Gamma Unit

Requirements

The requirements of the instrument, the main application of which was to be functional neurosurgery, were as follows:

1. Adequate precision. This requires both accuracy of localization, accuracy of the radiation field and immobility of the patient, in respect of the radiation. The accuracy of *localization* was achieved with the stereotactic frame and high quality X-rays taken with the central beam at right angles to the frame. This requirement of a central beam at right angle to the stereotactic system remained a requirement into the late 1990s. The accurate *radiation field* was achieved by beaming 179 cobalt beams, mounted on a hemisphere towards a sharply defined focus at the centre of the hemisphere. The beams were directed through collimators with a rectangular cross section in order to obtain the desired disc shaped lesion. Two collimator sizes were available, 3 × 5 mm and 3 × 7 mm. The collimators were held in a helmet. Immobility of the patient was achieved by rigid fixation of the stereotactic frame attached to the patient's head, to axis rods attached to this helmet. The machine incorporated a hydraulic system to move the target to the focus of the machine. The use of the same frame for X-rays and treatment resulted in concordance of the stereotactic target on the X-rays and in the machine. The extreme rigidity of the head fixation and the lack of moving parts during radiation are central to the high degree of accuracy of the technique.

2. Bringing the patient's head to the correct position. The machine must be able to move the patients head into the machine in such a way the region to be irradiated will lie at the immovable focal point of the machine.

3. Acceptable treatment time. It was clearly desirable that the treatment should be carried out as quickly as possible. It is not easy for often elderly patients, with severe pain or paralysis agitans to remain in one position for long periods. The major determinant of the treatment time is the energy of the radiation source. The ^{60}Co used provided a beam of 1.17 or 1.33 MeV. Leksell commented in his description of the first cases that the treatment time was on the long side and discussed the possibility of using isotopes with a higher energy in future.

4. The brain integral dose should not be greater than that commonly accepted for a single radiation of malignant brain tumours. With the tiny lesions produced with the small collimators used, the geometry of the machine ensured that the spread of radiation dose was very restricted, even with a maximum dose of 250 Gy.

5. Adequate radiation protection for the patient's body and the treatment personnel. The patient's protection is related to a single exposure and was guaranteed by the geometry of the machine, which precluded the spread of any unacceptable amount of radiation away from the focus. For the personnel who would be repeatedly exposed to the machine, their absence from the treatment room during treatment and the massive casings and doors of the device were the major factors. Of course, the usual routines for any department using radioactive material, of repeated measurements of radiation in the locale, radiation absorption badges and the like were employed.

The machine which was developed to achieve all these aims was the first Gamma Unit shown in Fig. 6.3. This is now of mainly historical interest, so that only a brief description is given of the principles in the legend of the figure.

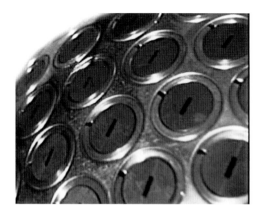

Fig. 6.3 The superficial ends of the collimators are the round visible in this picture. Note that the opening is rectangular. This shape was optimal for the thalamotomies which a major indication for which the Gamma Unit was designed. This indication became much reduced following the introduction of L-Dopa at about the same time. Thus, the Gamma unit's major use was against tumours and AVMs and subsequent collimators would have circular openings

Early Experience

The first patients were treated after installation of the prototype machine, in the Sofiahemmet hospital in Stockholm early in 1968. This prototype was called a Gamma Unit and the first patients were treated with gamma thalamotomy for intractable cancer pain. Doses of 160 to 250 Gy were used. This was a clinical material, which inevitably allowed post-mortem examination of the lesion produced, only a relatively short time after the treatment. The lesions and the dose time relationships of the lesions were similar to those seen in the experimental work on animals, using the synchrocyclotron. However, the very first patient treated was a tumour case, a small craniopharyngioma. This patient was treated in the autumn of 1967 before the machine had left the nuclear power facility where the radiation sources had been inserted. Other diagnoses treated in the early days were trigeminal neuralgia, Parkinson's Disease, small arteriovenous malformations, acoustic neurinomas and pituitary adenomas.

As stated above, the first Gamma Unit had been devised for producing disc shaped lesions appropriate for functional work. With the advent of dopamine, at the beginning of the 1970s, the number of Parkinson patient referrals decreased. At the same time, the widening of the indications for Gamma Knife surgery came to include tumours made the disc shape less than optimal. Moreover, the collimators were too small for most tumours and malformations, which might reasonably be treated by the method. Thus, it was deemed necessary to design a second Gamma Unit.

The Second Gamma Unit

In this unit 179 beams were obtained from 179 ^{60}Co sources, as in the first Gamma Unit, but in this new machine the collimators were circular in cross section and described as either 8 mm or 14 mm in diameter. These distances referred to the diameter of the 50% isodose. The larger and more spherical dose distributions, available with the newer collimators were more appropriate for the treatment of malformations and tumours. Indeed, the machine was constructed to accommodate a collimator size range from 8 to 14 mm. Subsequently, 4 mm collimators became available. Larger sizes were not used because the dose fall becomes more gradual with larger collimator sizes. This matter is dealt with in more detail in a later chapter. The new computer programme available with the new unit permitted the calculation of multishot dose-plans, for any of the collimator sizes in the above-mentioned range. This greatly increased the precision with which a dose distribution could be tailored to fit the shape of the lesion that was being treated. Usually, the aim was to fit the 50% isodose to the edge of the lesions. Figure 6.4 shows a diagram of the longitudinal section through this version of the Gamma Unit. This looks exactly like the section through the first Unit. The only difference is that the collimator shape is different and that is not shown in this diagram.

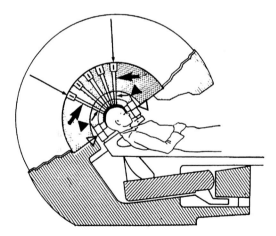

Fig. 6.4 This shows a longitudinal section through the machine with the patient in place. The patient is fixed to an inner helmet (*filled arrow heads*) and adjusted to bring the target to the focal point of the machine. The inner fixed to the couch of the machine which is driven by a hydraulic system in this model. The couch is driven into the machine and up so that the inner helmet docks with the outer helmet located within the machine. The channels in the inner and outer helmets are concordant and radiation can flow down them. In this way the dose delivered will develop on the diameter of the openings in the inner helmet and duration of the patient in the docked position

The Third Gamma Unit (Gamma Knives U and B)

This existed in two models. One was very like the second gamma unit illustrated in Fig. 6.4, but with new 18 mm collimators. It had the same helmets and hydraulic system.

The other version was called the B model after Bergen which had the first installation (Fig. 6.5). It had a different helmet shape and a simpler movement of the patient to the treatment position with the opening in the helmet at a simple right angle to the long axis of the bed of the machine. In this model the patient is only moved horizontally into the machine and not in and up as in previous models. More-over, the helmet is slightly larger than in the earlier models. The difference in distribution of sources in the U and B models did not affect the quality of the treatment or the results but had practical consequences for the users just the same, see Fig. 6.6. *However, please note that no matter which model is under discussion, all Gamma Units/Gamma Knives retain the basic pattern of a focal point where all the fine beams cross each other. Radiosurgery is performed by moving the target inside the head of the patient around this point and keeping it in position for suitable durations.*

Fixation of the Patient to the Gamma Knife

As described in Chap. 8 a frame is attached to the head. This frame functions as in other stereotactic procedures as both an axis system and a platform. The axes work as previously described. It is a platform for imaging indicators to secure accuracy of measurement of the axes. Moreover, the frame is a platform to which adapters to fix

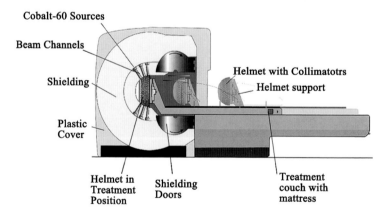

Fig. 6.5 The Gamma Knife "B" model. Horizontal couch movement and no hydraulics. Also the distribution of sources is different as reflected by the different pattern of collimators in the helmet. This is illustrated on the next page for clarity

Collimator Distribution

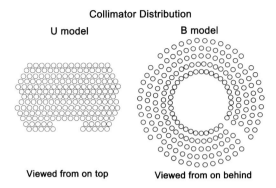

Fig. 6.6 In the U model the patient slides into the machine and then upwards. The sources and hence collimators are asymmetrically arranged in respect of the head in an upper quadrant of the machine as shown in the figure. The B model had the sources arranged symmetrically in circles around the top of the patients head. In view of the treatment positions in the two machines the views in the figure are from the top on the left and from behind in the patient. However, this is the same direction as in both instances the collimators are viewed looking at the top of the patient's head. Another consequence of this arrangement was that in the U model the asymmetry meant it was sometimes preferable to treat a patient prone, whereas in the B model the symmetry made this unnecessary

it to the helmet of the Gamma Knife maybe attached. These adapters, fixed to the same frame, in a position that has remained unchanged since the dose-planning X-rays were taken ensures that the axis system recorded on the X-rays and the axis system in the Gamma Knife are exactly **concordant**. In the U model and the first edition of the B model this fixation was done by means of bars called trunnions. The helmet and trunnions are shown in Fig. 6.7. Nonetheless, there is a practical problem relating to the application of the frame for use with the Gamma Knife, which does not apply for open stereotactic surgery. In this latter situation, instruments can gain access to any point within the cranium. This is not the case with the Gamma Knife. The size of the helmet restricts the degree of movement of the head with its attached frame so that targets with an eccentric intracranial location require special frame placement. The aim is to place the target as near the centre of the frame as possible, since in all cases the target MUST be brought to the focal point of the machines gamma rays without any part of the frame or skull coming into contact with the inner wall of the helmet.

A limitation of GKNS using the U or B models became apparent with the increase in the number of peripherally placed targets after metastases became a common indication for this form of treatment. The frame has to be assembled in an advantageous way and rotation as described in Chap. 8 may be required. It must be admitted that in the early days it was thought that a peripheral lesion location could represent a contraindication for the Gamma Knife. It was considered that they would be difficult to fit into the machine. This is almost invariably not true if the principles described in Chap. 8 are followed.

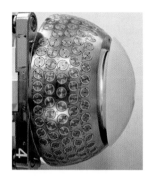

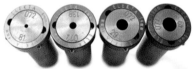

4mm   8mm   14mm   18mm

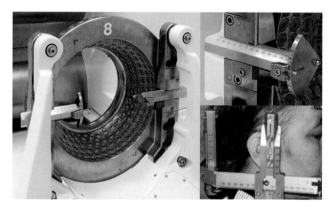

Fig. 6.7 Shows the B model helmet filled with 8 mm collimators and also shows the 4 collimator sizes. Shows the trunnions (*lower left*) and attachments (*lower right*) used to fasten the frame to the helmet. As can be seen there is limited space within the helmet, so correct frame placement is a priority with this Gamma Knife model

Automatic Positioning

With the continuing development of the Gamma Knife technology the "U" model gradually disappeared. However, experience suggested that the repeated manual repositioning of the patient with the trunnions and attachments shown in Fig. 6.7 was a potential source of error and very time consuming. It also in practice limited the number of shots given to a patient. This, in principle could lead to less accurate dose planning. A result of these concerns was the introduction of the "Automatic Positioning System" or APS. A robot which replaced the trunnions attachments. The APS is shown in Fig. 6.8. The improved speed of operation allows the use of far

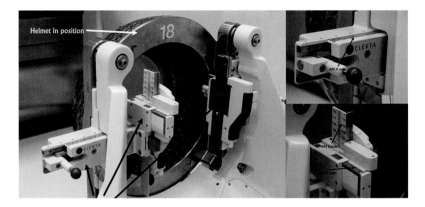

Fig. 6.8 The APS is fixed to the helmet. The *black arrows* indicate the scales. The patients head may be moved in the X, Y or Z directions by the motors in the APS from shot to shot (treatment position to treatment position). Thus, the only time the operator needed to enter the Gamma Knife room was if there was a need to change the helmet or the angle at which the treatment was delivered. It is very accurate and if there is enough strain in the frame that the sensors Régister a difference between the 2 sides of more than 0.3 mm the system will not function

more shots. In addition there is a tendency to use more small shots rather than a smaller number of bigger shots.

The use of the APS has co-incided with an increased interest in quality assurance measures during treatment planning. The APS contributes to better dosi-metry because it permits the use of a greater number of smaller shots. It also speeds up the treatment of small metastases a great deal as it allows the head to be taken from one location to another without having to detach the patient from the machine and adjust manually.

However, there is a disadvantage with the APS system. It takes up space and this is particularly a disadvantage with the treatment of cerebral metastases. This has become increasingly important of recent years because of the frequency with which metastases are treated. It means that in some cases the APS system must be removed and replaced with trunnions if certain targets are to be reached. There is also one other lesser problem. The patient lies on the couch while the APS moves the head. This puts a strain on the neck. These various disadvantages have eventually led to the development of a completely redesigned Gamma Knife called Perfexion.

Gamma Knife Perfexion

Introduction

This is not a modification of any existing gamma knife. It is a new design whereby the irradiation reaching the patient may have characteristics similar to earlier models. However, the new design permits more space, better patient comfort and faster treatments, since there are no helmets to change. It also in principle would allow the treatment of cervical lesions, though this possibility is not practically available at the time of writing.

Design Differences

1. There is no helmet.
2. Treatment occurs inside a tungsten mass through which have been drilled 192 collimator channels. The difference in the available space is shown in Fig. 6.9.
3. The sources are not mounted in a fixed position in an outer helmet. Instead they are mounted on 8 moveable sectors. Each of these sectors contains 24 sources given a total of 192. The arrangement is illustrated in the diagrams in Fig. 6.10. The 8 sectors surround the head. The holes in the tungsten cone section which sit over the collimators can be seen in Fig. 6.9.

In view of the very different geometry of this system compared with previous Gamma Knife models the system was extensively tested before being taken into commercial use. It unquestionably makes the use of the Gamma Knife speedier and more efficient for the user while permitting access to any location within the cranium and making the process more comfortable for the patient (Fig. 6.11).

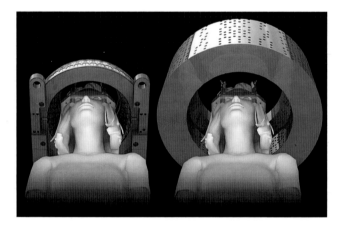

Fig. 6.9 Shows the different dimensions inside previous models of the Gamma Knife on the left and within the tungsten cone section on the right. Our experience is that patients who are impossible to treat for a variety of reasons (extreme eccentric location +/− craniotomy) in the earlier models of the Gamma Knife can easily be treated in Perfexion. The holes in the tungsten conic section lie over the deeper collimators which penetrate all the way through the metal but which cannot be seen in this image

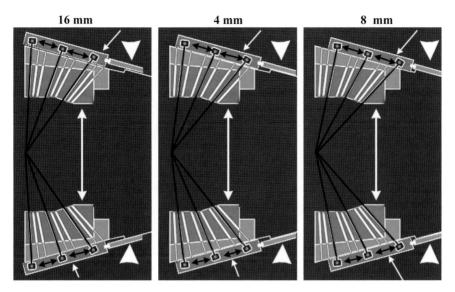

Fig. 6.10 Shows a diagrammatic longitudinal section through the Gamma Knife Perfexion (1). The *black straight lines* are the gamma rays meeting at a focal point (2). They pass through white tubes which are the collimators drilled through the tungsten conic section (3). The double headed long *white arrow* indicates the this tungsten conic section (4). The double headed *black arrows* indicate the sources embedded in the sectors (5). The single ended *white arrows* indicate the sectors (6). The *white arrowheads* indicate the motorised rods which may slide the sectors along the surface of the tungsten conic section so that sources are either over a collimator or not. (7). There are eight such sectors surrounding the conic section and each sector can be selected to irradiate through any one of the three available collimators or to take an intermediate position and thus be blocked (8). The position on the left with the front collimators is 16 mm, the intermediate is 4 mm and the posterior is 8 mm. (9). The blocked position between collimator locations is not shown (10). The sectors may be withdrawn away from the collimators altogether to a resting position which is also not shown

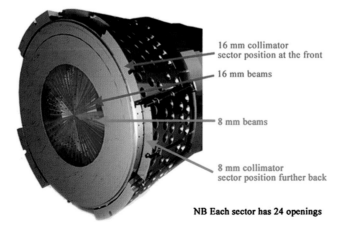

Fig. 6.11 Note the 3 D appearance of 2 of the 8 sectors. It can be seen each sector contains 24 openings. The 16 mm collimator sector is at the front and appropriately the 8 mm collimator sector is further back. The beams from both can be seen to cross at the centre of the system as described

The rest of this book is mainly aimed at users with Gamma Knife Perfexion. However, for some time to come the Gamma Knife "C" model will be extensively in use so a section is added concerning frame application for this model. The application of the frame with Perfexion is considerably simpler.

Chapter 7
Radiophysics, Radiobiology and the Gamma Knife

Introduction

The purpose of this chapter is to relate the general knowledge, outlined in Chaps. 3–5, to the particular conditions pertaining to Gamma Knife radiosurgery. One particularly important aspect that will be mentioned is the effects of a single session radiation treatment on living tissue. The term radiosurgery has been redefined over the years and with the official definition mentioned in chapter one the meaning has changed from the original intention of the inventors of the technique. Nonetheless, it is suggested that for Gamma Knife Neurosurgery, extremely precise localization and a single treatment session radiation should remain the two hallmarks of the technique.

Radiophysics and the Gamma Knife

Energy

Gamma radiation is of course electromagnetic radiation without mass, to be considered either as waves or photons. The gamma radiation produced by ^{60}Co has two energies, reflecting two distinct radioactive breakdown pathways. The gamma radiation from these two reaction series has an energy of either 1.17 or 1.33 MeV depending on which radioactive breakdown pathway is being considered. With radiation energy within this range, according to the description in Chap. 3, most of the interaction between radiation and irradiated tissue can be expected to be mediated by Compton scattering. The energy level of this radiation is sufficient to give it a high power of penetration. It has a low LET (see Chap. 3). The narrow beams, essential to the technique, are produced as described in Chap. 6.

J.C. Ganz, *Gamma Knife Neurosurgery*,
DOI 10.1007/978-3-7091-0343-2_7, © Springer-Verlag/Wien 2011

Radiobiology and the Gamma Knife

Factors Affecting Cell Survival

It must be clear that those elements of radiobiology related to fractionation are not relevant with a single session treatment. Thus, the 4 "Rs" of conventional fractionated radiotherapy lose much of their importance. The place of any cell in the cell cycle will be entirely random. By the same token reassortment will play no part in this sort of treatment. Repair and repopulation will not occur during a treatment, which takes in under an hour. Neither will reoxygenation be of importance. On the other hand, oxygenation at the time of radiation can play a part, although this is not usually considered during treatment. Moreover, a single treatment session should be more effective in reducing the chance of repair and repopulation after cessation of treatment compared with fractionated treatment using the same dose. This is because fractionation reduces the biological effect (cell kill) of a given dose. The cell kill must be achieved by a combination of single lesions and the summation of potentially lethal hits, in keeping with the linear quadratic concept. However, as explained below the situation is a little more complicated.

Dose

The most important biological parameter related to cell kill is the dose. As the individual beams are characterised by a low LET, little energy (or dose) is absorbed along their individual paths. However, where the 192/201 narrow beams meet, at the focal point of the Gamma Knife, there is a summation of dose, which gives a high target dose. The design of the machine, with the large number of narrow beams, enables the construction of very precise dose distributions, with a very sharp fall in dose at the 50% isodose. It is for this reason that the 50% isodose is most often made to conform with the edge of any lesion to be treated. It is the prescription isodose. Figure 7.1 shows the relative dose fall as a function of the distance from the central maximum dose. The very sharp dose fall, between the 80% and 30% isodoses, a result of the machine's geometry as stated above, enables the delivery of a high target dose to the lesion, within the 50% isodose and a low integral dose to the surrounding brain. It is necessary to determine a minimum acceptable target dose and place this at the edge of the lesion, at the 50% isodose. The appropriate dose for different types of lesion varies for each lesion and will be discussed subsequently. Thus, it is the geometry of the radiation dose distribution rather than the technique of fractionation, which spares normal tissue with the Gamma Knife.

Dose Rate

The half-life of ^{60}Co is 5.27 years. This means that with the passage of time, the dose rate for the Gamma Knife is steadily decreasing. Or put another way, the same

Fig. 7.1 Shows the relative dose fall as a function of the distance from the central maximum dose for the 3 Perfexion collimators. This is a diagram to show the principle. It is NOT a graph of real measurements

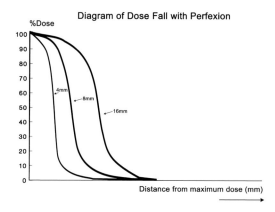

treatment with the same dose takes longer and longer the older the machine becomes. There is some evidence that reducing the dose rate reduces the biological effectiveness of radiation especially if the dose is less than 1 Gy/min. Doses as low as this are to be found at the lesion edge, with even a fairly new Gamma Knife, though their significance is not clear at this time. However, as the results of Gamma Knife surgery are so good it seems unlikely that low dose rate within the target is of any great importance.

One advantage of the geometry of the Gamma Knife is that since a lower isodose is associated with a lower dose rate a measure of protection is provided for the normal tissue outside the target volume. This is because the maximum dose rate is set by the activity level of the gamma source. Thus, for a single shot, the dose rate at the 50% isodose will be half that of the dose centre and the dose rate further out from the centre will decrease in proportion. This means that with a dose of 100 Gy at the centre, with a 3 Gy/min dose rate, the dose rate at the 50% isodose will be 1.5 Gy/min and at the 10% isodose 0.3 Gy/min, which is a dose rate low enough to reduce the effectiveness of the dose, thereby producing a measure of extra protection in the surrounding tissue.

Dose Volume

This is a factor under close scrutiny at the present time. This has been mostly concerned with the treatment of arteriovenous malformations and will be mentioned again during the chapter related to that topic. In general, the effect of lesion volume on therapeutic success in controlling the lesion should be considered to be the same as for radiotherapy. A larger lesion has a larger number of clonogenic cells to control, which for a given dose will make control less likely. It is logical to consider the effect of treatment volume on the surrounding tissue at this point. Van der Kogel found that correlating the length of rat spinal cord irradiated with the development of radiation induced paralysis showed that there was a relationship between these variables. Briefly, if the length of irradiated cord were 2 mm or less, no white matter necrosis developed, even with a single dose of more than 80 Gy. On the other hand for a length of 2 cm or more, 20 Gy consistently produced white matter necrosis. Between these two limits, there was a gradual increase in the occurrence of paralysis with increasing length of cord irradiated. One very relevant finding, consistent with these observations is that there is as yet no patient reported to have a facial palsy following treatment of an acoustic neurinoma, with a volume of less than 1,000 mm^3.

These findings are important and in keeping with clinical experience. It is also important to be clear about the fact that an increase in target volume automatically increases the volume of normal tissue receiving a significant dose of radiation; or in other words increases the integral dose to the normal brain. This is the factor, which limits the size of lesion, which can be treated by the Gamma Knife. The technique is fully capable of producing much larger radiation fields than are currently in use. So, it is not the machine design, which limits the target volume, which is appropriate for radiosurgery. It is the decreasing tolerance of normal brain with large integral doses.

Dose Homogeneity

The Gamma Knife radiation field is inherently inhomogeneous. This must be so, if the radiation dose is high and is distributed between a maximum and 50% of that maximum, across any given target. Clearly this does not matter all that much, since the technique works. However, during the early days of radiosurgery it was untraditional for teletherapy, where in conventional radiotherapy it was usual to strive for as homogeneous field as possible. Subsequently, conformal dose-planning has become much more usual in all forms of radiotherapy. Since it is impossible for a radiation dose to be both conformal homogeneous, homogeneity has become less of an issue than it used to be.

Delayed Radiation Damage of Nervous Tissue and the Gamma Knife

Inevitably any discussion of radiobiology must consider the particular characteristics of the tumour being irradiated and the characteristics of the tissue surrounding the tumour, or from which it grows. Some of the more specific biological tumour related topics will be mentioned in chapters related to individual tumours. However, there are some general considerations relating to tumours and it is clearly appropriate to discuss the radiobiological qualities of the normal tissue surrounding intracranial tumours, the tissues of the central nervous system.

Radiation Tolerance of the CNS

The effect of single shot radiation on the nervous system has received considerable attention, in particular from the late Professor Börje Larsson and from Professor

Albert Van der Kogel of Nijmegen Holland. What is presented in the following paragraphs relies heavily on the writings of these two experts.

Using a variety of mainly small experimental animals, it would seem that the following tentative conclusions may be drawn. Irradiation of central nervous tissue, either brain or spinal cord, produces damage which appears to be dose related and affects either or both the white matter myelin and the vascular endothelium. These changes are thought to be due to damage to the endothelial or glial cells, in particular oligodendroglia, which have a relatively high rate of cell division, in a tissue with an otherwise low rate of cell division. These processes appear to be interrelated in some ways, though the details of this interrelationship are not clear. There appears to be a threshold dose involved in the production of CNS necrosis. For conventional external beam fractionated radiotherapy the acceptable total brain dose in relation to an acceptable therapeutic index is 55 Gy [1]. For radiosurgery the situation is more complex. There is a lot of information about the reactions of very small volumes of brain tissue to single session radiation doses from the early work done prior to the development radiosurgery prior to the design of the first Gamma Unit. This is mentioned below. In terms of treating pathological lesions, the acceptable dose will be affected by neighbouring structures, target volume and the nature of the illness. The current appropriate doses will be mentioned in the specific chapters on individual diseases.

Dose Latency Relationships

What sorts of tissue reactions to radiation are seen in the CNS? Are they early or late? This is not entirely a straightforward matter. An early normal tissue reaction (within a week or two after treatment), consisting of reversible oedema has been described, but this is exceptional and will not be referred to again. According to the characteristics of early and late radiation complications, outlined in Chap. 5, the tissue reactions described in the preceding paragraph are late reactions. Nonetheless, it is just these reactions that are the basis of the lesion in thalamotomy, described in Chap. 6 and these lesions occur before 90 days. According to one of the accepted usages of the terms early and late, in this context, that would make the complications early. The other definition of early and late complications, related to duration of treatment is obviously not relevant, in respect of the Gamma Knife, with its total dose in a single session technique. All complications occur after cessation of treatment. On the other hand, in traditional, fractionated, radiotherapy a striking feature of the development of clinical CNS damage, following a total dose of the order of 55 Gy is the long latent interval from radiation to necrosis. The explanation of these apparent discrepancies of definition is that the latent interval is dose dependant and the terms early and late were defined in relation to the doses used in conventional radiotherapy, not those used in functional radiosurgery. What one is seeing after GKNS could be termed an accelerated late reaction. This is in keeping with the contents of Chap. 5 where it is described how since the latency of late reactions is dose dependent for "F" tissues, of which the CNS, at least to some extent is one. And indeed, it is consistent that a complication latency of many months is also seen with GKNS in the context of the lower doses used in the treatment of space occupying lesions.

The first work done on brain tolerance of single session focussed irradiation was the doctoral thesis of Börje Larsson working in the Werner Institute in Uppsala using a synchrocyclotron [2]. It was found that to produce a CNS lesion, appropriate for thalamotomy (2–5 mm diameter), within 1–2 weeks, a dose of 200–300 Gy was required. Lower doses produced the effect with a longer latency, down to a threshold of about 130–150 Gy. Below this level no lesions were noted. Using the same size of lesion, with dose levels above 400 Gy, there was a risk of hemisphere swelling, indicating a quite different set of biological processes at this dose level.

This brings us to the protection of the brain in a different but far more common pathophysiological situation. When using GKNS in the treatment of a visible target one of the aims is to protect the brain around the visible lesion. This is achieved by focussing the radiation, so that the brain outside the lesion receives an acceptably low dose. It has been mentioned earlier that the 50% isodose was placed at the edge of lesions produced with cross-firing techniques, whether proton beam or gamma ray. The reason for this was to limit the late spread of the lesion on the basis of two concepts. Firstly, the latency of the white matter necrotic effect was dose dependent. With a rapid dose fall there should also be a rapid rise in necrosis latency, concomitant upon the falling dose. Secondly, there was a lower threshold for white matter necrosis, below which no necrosis would occur. Thus, the smaller the volume enclosed within this threshold dose, the larger the volume outside this dose, which could not be damaged.

In the previous paragraphs the reactions to be expected in an F tissue are discussed. However, the brain is considered a mixed tissue with H elements and F elements. It is known that some of the glial cells of the normal brain are refurbished from a layer of subependymal stem cells. However, the contribution of the H component of the brain to its reactions to radiation is not clear at the time of writing.

CNS Radiation Tolerance and Fractionation

As the CNS behaves largely as an F-tissue, showing late complications, it is to be expected that it is sensitive to fractionation. This is indeed the case. On the other hand the significance of the duration of treatment is not at all clear. While fractionation sensitivity is an advantage, which the Gamma Knife surgeon has hitherto not used, this does not matter, since the advantage is related to preservation of normal tissue. This the Gamma Knife surgeon achieves through the accuracy and geometry of his instrument, as described above. Thus, single dose treatment strategies remain the standard for Gamma Knife surgery, as it is practised today. However, there is a debate within the milieu about the potential benefits of doses in two fractions for larger lesions. The importance of this remains to be seen. The author allows himself the reflection that there may well be situations where fractionated treatment has advantages but NOT fractionation to a whole target volume with the concomitant reduction in biological effect. In the case of AVMs it has been demonstrated that treating larger lesions segment by segment reduces the overall dose to the perilesional cerebral tissue. Each partial volume receives an adequate dose retaining the biological effect to that segment. This is explained in more detail in Chap. 19. The work is early and is not yet standard, but is seems a positive approach. This way of treating is the equivalent of staged surgical treatment of difficult lesions which was employed by Cushing for meningiomas, at the birth of modern neurosurgery. Moreover, it remains an acceptable option today, since it has been recently advocated by Spetzler, in the management of difficult arteriovenous malformations. Thus, for most relevant lesions, the Gamma Knife remains essentially a surgical tool, with its accurate application being dependent on surgical competence rather than the number of treatment sessions. Finally, while every physician should wish to improve his technique, the Gamma Knife's track record, when used as a single session radiosurgical tool is not lightly to be disregarded. The lack of advantage obtained by fractionating the dose will be considered further a little later.

Tumour Tissue and the Gamma Knife

All that has been mentioned so far in this chapter applies to the reactions of normal nervous tissue, nothing has been said about the reactions of the pathological tissue. In other words, single tissue radiation has been considered, rather than the more conventional arrangement of a pathological target, surrounded by a normal tissue at risk. Firstly, since the Gamma Knife has recently been applied to the treatment of malignant targets the tumour factors relating to such targets may be considered first. This is because the aim of treatment is identical with that of conventional radiotherapy. This aim is sterilization and disappearance of the tumour. This will require a very high dose and a higher rate of complications is acceptable, due to the poor prognosis of the condition being treated. Perhaps the most significant characteristic predicting success is tumour volume. The permitted volumes treated vary with the lesion being treated and the doses employed. However, one diagnosis requires particular attention in this regard. Cerebral metastases require a high dose for consistent control. Thus, it seems reasonable to suggest that a total volume of all metastases should not exceed 20 cm^3. The significance of volume is even more apparent in relation to glial tumours, whose visible volume is usually larger than this, and whose real volume is even bigger.

The technique allows a radiation dose, in one session, which may be the biological equivalent of the whole dose of conventional fractionated radiotherapy. It may be even more effective. Again, it is the rapid fall of dose at the edge of the lesion, which permits adequate single session treatment. Other factors related to the effect of treatment, such as oxygenation, tumour bed effect, and accelerated repopulation are of little interest with the Gamma Knife.

The aim of Gamma Knife treatment with benign tumours may be slightly different from that described in the previous paragraph. Firstly, it has been widely accepted that growth arrest without disappearance is an acceptable result. This has been applied for vestibular schwnnomas, meningiomas and pituitary adenomas. For such lesions, in particular where alternative therapies are available, it is imperative that there is a minimum of normal tissue complications. This restricts the doses that may be employed. Though let it be said, this has not hindered excellent results with the technique. Recently, Larsson has argued that the desired differential radio-sensitivity requirement for the treatment of cancers, with the implication of death to all malignant cells may not be a requirement for life-long tumour control of benign intracranial tumours. He points out that the doses current in radiosurgery (20–200 Gy) should reduce the probability of survival of irradiated cells to approximately 10^{-6}. He goes on to suggest this may produce adequate tumour control for all practical purposes. However, he adds a caveat that in vitro studies, from his and other laboratories have indicated a considerable variation in the radiosensitivity of both healthy and tumour cells, of the types likely to find themselves within a radiosurgical target volume [3].

Radiobiological Correlates with Single Session Radiosurgery

Relevance of the Linear Quadratic Equation

The linear quadratic equation was developed in relation to standard fractionated external beam radiotherapy or brachytherapy. The basic biological responses to ionising radiation are independent of the technique employed. However, there are some serious discrepancies which arise when trying to apply the linear quadratic equation and to single session treatments.

It is necessary to remember that mathematical formalisms, like the linear quadratic equation are not pieces of primary data but models which fit observed phenomena with consistency. Nonetheless, as they are only models it is not unexpected that they may have limitations. To begin with the linear quadratic equation has no component relating to time. Earlier equations did have a time factor however, the demonstrated usefulness of the equation has led to the belief that the time factor is, at least for most radiotherapy of secondary importance. Moreover, it is of very limited relevance in single session radiosurgery where the entire dose is given at once.

Another limitation of the linear quadratic equation is that it is considered to be relevant only for fraction doses up to around 5 Gy [4]. Above this value per fraction the equation is regarded as unreliable. Moreover, as the dose per fraction increases there is evidence that the survival fraction curve approaches a straight line [4]. This all means that for the survival fractions following single session radiosurgery using current doses, the linear quadratic equation is not reliable [5].

If the linear quadratic equation is not a reliable tool for the assessment of single session radiosurgery with current doses, it follows that the α/β ratio is also of limited use since its greatest relevance is in the design of fractionated dosimetry, where quickly reacting tissues (high α/β ratio) and slowly reacting tissues (low α/β ratio) permit fractionation patterns which optimise protection of the normal tissues.

Relevance of Fractionation

This brings us to the relevance of fractionation. The modern definition of radiosurgery includes fractionation up to 5 fractions. On the other hand the designers of the Gamma Knife considered fractionation unnecessary. The reasons are as follows and are simple. Fractionation is a technique whereby normal tissue is spared the damaging effects of the radiation to which they are exposed by means of dividing up the dose into fractions and using the various advantages as described above. However, with single session radiosurgery, the geometry of the focused radiation field means that the surrounding tissues are NOT receiving a harmful dose of radiation requiring the protection afforded by fractionation. In addition the dose to tissues at risk may be discovered by delineating volumes at risk and using the dose planning software to show the doses within these tissues. **Adjusting the shape of the dose plan is an effective method of minimising the dose to adjacent tissues at risk. Moreover, since the tolerated single session dose in most of the tissues at risk is now fairly well known, the measurement of that dose in those tissues seems to be a more secure method of procuring safety than guessing at a fractionation scheme**.

There is another issue. Many of the benign lesions treated with radiosurgery are late reacting tissues with a low α/β ratio and thus particularly fractionation sensitive if treated with conventional fractionated radiotherapy. This applies to meningiomas (α/β ratio 3) [6], vestibular schwannomas(α/β ratio 2.5) [7], pituitary adenomas (α/β ratio 2.5) [8], AVMs (α/β ratio 3.5) [9]. To fractionate the dose would in principle have a strong reduction in the biological effect of the dose, which in turn would seem to require an increase in the total dose. This is a process which rather defeats the object of the exercise. With regard to metastases, which might be expected to have a higher α/β ratio this is not predictably the case. Melanomas for example have been shown as mentioned earlier to have an α/β ratio of less than one. And yet again it is not possible to ignore the clinical success of single session treatment of metastases, considering the extensive literature confirming this effectiveness for them as well as for other indications.

Nonetheless, it must not be considered that the author is blindly suggesting that fractionation should be avoided at all costs. There are situations where it is not only desirable so much as mandatory. The whole notion of single session radiosurgery is built on a particular target property. That is the target must be well defined and distinguishable from surrounding adjacent tissues at risk. This is the case for meningiomas, pituitary adenomas, AVMs and vestibular schwannomas and indeed cerebral metastases. In the case of optic sheath meningiomas this is not the case and the tumour and normal tissue are intimately intermingled. Here fractionated radiotherapy is the treatment of choice. Moreover, with gliomas it is often preferable. This is particularly the case with brain stem gliomas. It is characteristic of these tumours that anatomical distortion and tumour volume increase alarmingly with relatively little clinical disturbance until the terminal phase. It follows that the tumour and functioning brain stem are intermingled. It would be impossible to damage tumour cells without risking concomitant damage to the blood supply, supporting astrocytes and insulating oligodendroglia of functioning neurones. In this situation fractionated radiotherapy is clearly preferable.

Conclusion

The point is to adjust the treatment to the specific disease, guided by the evidence to be found in the literature. Even so there are important questions which remain. One of these is, what is the reason that not all lesions respond to treatment? Is it because of innate biological variability such as variation in personal radiosensitivity? This is not an easy area in which to do research and very little if any information is available. On the other hand it is possible that treatment failure could be the result of less than optimal treatment strategies. The large amount of experience and the excellent results with the technique suggest that treatment strategies are fairly sophisticated, though clearly not perfect. The author suggests that there is a crying need for effort and investment into research aimed at providing tests for individual radiosensitivity.

References

1. Dörr W. Time factors in normal-tissue responses to irradiation. eds. Joiner M, van der Kogel A. Hodder Arnold and Hachette UK company, London: pp 149–157; 2009
2. Larsson B. On the Application of a 185 MeV Proton Beam to Experimental Cancer Therapy and Neurosurgery. Inaugural Dissertation Uppsalla University: pp 7–20; 1962
3. Larssson B. Radiobiological fundamentals in radiosurgery. ed. Steiner L. Raven Press, New York: pp 3–14; 2009
4. Joiner MC, Bentzen SM. Fractionation: the linear-quadratic approach. eds. Joiner M, van der Kogel A. Hodder Arnold and Hachette UK company, London: pp 102–134; 2009
5. Bentzen SM, Joiner MC. The linear-quadratic approach in clinical practice. eds. Joiner M, van der Kogel A. Hodder Arnold and Hachette UK company, London: pp 135–148; 2009
6. Colombo F, Casentini L, Cavedon C, Scalchi P, Cora S, Francescon P. Cyberknife radiosurgery for benign meningiomas: short-term results in 199 patients. Neurosurgery **64(2 Suppl)**: A7–A13; 2009

7. Niranjan A, Flickinger J. Radiobiology, Principle and Technique of Radiosurgery. In Modern Management of Acoustic Neuroma. eds. Régis J, Roche P-H. Prog Neurol Surg **21**: pp 32–42; 2008

8. Breen P, Flickinger JC, Kondziolka D, Martinez AJ. Radiotherapy for nonfunctional pituitary adenoma: analysis of long-term tumor control. J Neurosurg **89(6)**: 933–938; 1998

9. Kocher M, Wilms M, Makoski HB, Hassler W, Maarouf M, Treuer H, Voges J, Sturm V, Müller RP. Alpha/beta ratio for arteriovenous malformations estimated from obliteration rates after fractionated and single-dose irradiation. Radiother Oncol **71(1)**: 109–114; 2004

Chapter 8
Preparation for Treatment Planning

Introduction

While most of this book is concerned with the Gamma Knife Perfexion, this chapter contains some notes relative to models Gamma Knife B, C and 4 C. This is because the relatively limited space within these models can result in the stereotactic frame or the patient's head colliding with the helmet during treatment. This can make treatment impossible if necessary positions within the machine cannot be reached. A few simple principles will avoid this problem in nearly all cases. Occasionally, it is not possible to treat certain lesions and mention of this will be made during the chapter.

There are a number of methods taught about how the frame should be applied. In general if a user has found a method of application which is satisfactory, then there is no reason to change it. However, a particular method of application is outlined in Appendix A because it has proved useful to the author over the years. Its advantages are simplicity and independence. The method was devised at a time when no guarantee of a qualified assistant was possible. Thus, it was necessary to find a method of frame application which did not require assistance and yet which was reliable and quick.

Frame Application: General Method for Gamma Knife C Models

The design of the Gamma Knife is such that it is much simpler to treat lesions that are centrally placed in the frame. The Leksell frame's "Y" axes runs from values of 25–175 as illustrated in Fig. 8.1. The Z axis values are not marked on the frame but are calculated by the treatment planning software from fiducial markers (see below).

With the C model machines, with the automatic positioning system (APS) attached the axis of rotation in the "Y" direction is round a point below the centre of the "Z" axis. This means that the range in this direction can be extended.

J.C. Ganz, *Gamma Knife Neurosurgery*,
DOI 10.1007/978-3-7091-0343-2_8, © Springer-Verlag/Wien 2011

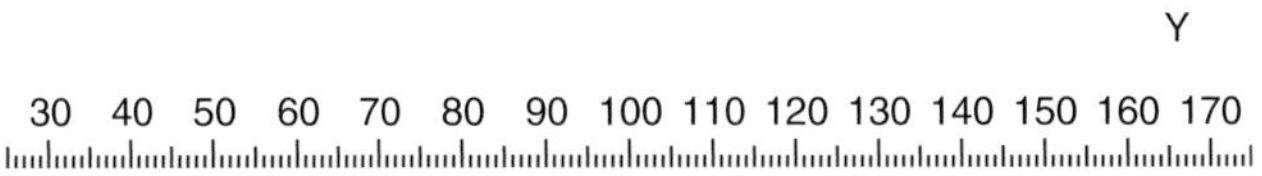

Y

30 40 50 60 70 80 90 100 110 120 130 140 150 160 170
|ıııl|ıııl|ıııl|ıııl|ıııl|ıııl|ıııl|ıııl|ıııl|ıııl|ıııl|ıııl|ıııl|ıııl|ıııl|ıııl|ıııl|ıııl|ıııl|ıııl|ıııl|ıııl|ıııl|ıııl|ıııl|ıııl|ıııl|ıııl|ıı|

Fig. 8.1 The lateral side of the frame showing the "Y" axis markings. As can be seen they run from 25 to 175. However, since the axis of rotation with the APS system is different from the axis of rotation of the frame it happens that lesions outside these boundaries can be reached. The detail of this process is outside the scope of this book

The "X" axis is similarly marked on the frame and runs from 40 to 160. However, in the X axis with some slight variation, the maximum available range within the Gamma Knife helmet is from 53 to 147 using the trunnions and from 60 to 140 using the APS. These are the physical limits available to the user. The application of the frame should take these limitations into account. If this is done following certain simple principles, single targets may be reached in almost any location within the cranium. In over 2,000 patients the author has had to stop a treatment because of an inaccessible lesion in 4 cases, using the C model or its predecessors. In one case the lesion was in the retina of the eye and the patient's head was extremely large. In the three remaining cases the lesions were laterally placed and a craniotomy defect prevented the application of the frame in a way which would make the lesions accessible. It is worth noting that all of these three patients were easily treated in Perfexion.

We must return to the C model. Since the patient is lying supine in the Gamma Knife the "X" axis remains from side to side but the "Y" axis runs from below to above. The "Z" axis is along the long axis of the couch or in other words reflects how far into the helmet the patient is placed. Figure 8.2 illustrates the relevant orientation of the patient in the machine.

Frame Placement in the Gamma Knife Helmet for Single Targets

While there are one or two exceptions, the information above indicates that the frame should be placed on the head in such a way as to place the target as close to the centre in the axial plane as possible. Moreover, the frame should be so placed that the value of the target centre in the "Z" axis should be as small as possible. In other words the target should be close to the mouth of the helmet. These relationships are illustrated in Fig. 8.2.

To achieve this consistently careful inspection of the images is needed. In principle the application of the frame can be standardised for most locations for the commoner indications using a knowledge of the relationship of surface anatomy to deep structures. In this context targets divide up into and extra and intra parenchymal. The intraparenchymal also subdivide into single and multiple. An occasional case of multiple meningiomas may also be a challenge but these are rare.

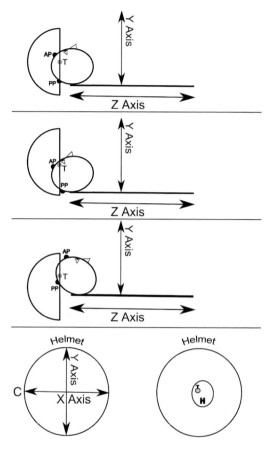

Fig. 8.2 (**a**) Diagram of Model C Gamma Knife from the side, showing "*Y*" and "*Z*" axis directions with the supine patient. "*T*" Target, The position is ideal from this point of view. *AP* Anterior Post and *PP* Posterior Post. with the target in the middle of the "*Y*" axis giving maximum manoeuvrability and also situated at the mouth of the helmet in the "*Z*" axis where the helmet diameter is a maximum of 33 cm. (**b**) Diagram of Model C Gamma Knife from the side, showing "*Y*" and "*Z*" axis directions with the supine patient. In this situation with the anterior target the head is extended to bring the posterior post outside the helmet thus avoiding collision. (**c**) Diagram of Model C Gamma Knife from the side, showing "*Y*" and "*Z*" axis directions with the supine patient. In this situation with the posterior target the head is flexed to bring the anterior post outside the helmet thus avoiding collision. (**d**) On the left a diagram of Model C Gamma Knife from the foot of the couch looking into the helmet, showing "*X*" and "*Y*" axis directions with the supine patient. On the right showing the frame placed with the target centred on both the "*X*" and "*Y*" axis or in other words in the axial plain. Again, this is optimal placement permitting maximum use of the space within the helmet

With lesions which are eccentric in the "*Y*" or "*X*" axes certain manoeuvres are necessary to avoid collision between the patient, posts and the helmet. The principle is illustrated in Fig. 8.2.

Intracranial Extracerebral Solitary Targets: Frame Displacement

Pituitary Adenoma

The anterior midline position of pituitary adenomas leads to a simple frame fixation: even more so now that most pituitary surgery is transsphenoidal. However, in some patients an older craniotomy may be present which will need to be taken into account. Otherwise the frame should be low and anterior and symmetrical about the midline. If a CT is required make sure that the pins of the frame are placed well above the chiasm so that there is no interference between CT artefact and the region of interest.

Vestibular Schwannoma

Vestibular Schwannomas can provide problems of frame placement if certain simple rules are not observed. In all the times the author has seen collisions between the frame and the helmet in the treatment of these tumours, the frame has ALWAYS been too far anterior and often not lateral enough. It is necessary to place the frame posteriorly and above all laterally. How it should be placed in practice is described below in the legend to Fig. 8.3. With correct frame application there should never be a problem with collisions and between the frame and the helmet with the Gamma Knife C model.

Parasellar Meningioma

While meningiomas appear in many regions something close to 70% are close to the cavernous sinus. The frame application for them is simple as they rarely extend laterally. How to place the frame for more laterally placed sphenoidal ridge meningiomas is described below. The majority of parasellar meningiomas, including the cavernous sinus tumour illustrated in this image lie in front of the midline of the head in the "Y" axis. Thus, the frame should be placed anteriorly. The lateral displacement of the tumour centre from the midline of the head is in good agreement with the location of the inner canthus of the eye. This can be used to guide the degree of lateral displacement. The frame is placed low on the head. This is a simple routine application.

   The above examples indicate the simple frame placement principles for reasonably centrally placed solitary lesions. In each case the frame is applied displaced in an appropriate direction, backwards or forwards or from side to side.

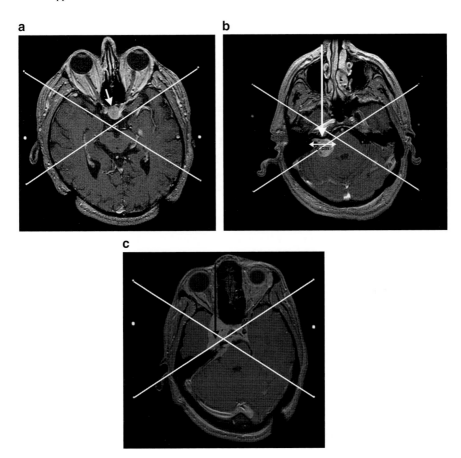

Fig. 8.3 (**a**) The *white arrow* shows the centrally anteriorly situated pituitary tumour. The fossa is midline at roughly the level of the lens of the eye. The application of the anteriorly placed frame is simple. The anterior fiducial markers can be seen placed anteriorly at the level of the outer canthus of the eye. The intersection of the white diagonals shows how close the centre of the axial plane is to the target with this frame position. (**b**) The *white single parasagittal arrow* confirms that the external wall of the nostril is close to the sagittal plane of the anterior wall of the internal opening of the internal acoustic canal. The double headed white arrow indicates that the lateral extent of the intrameatal portion of the tumour can easily be <2 cm from the middle of the frame with proper placement. Moreover the external auditory canal, while slightly caudad to the middle of the tumour is an indicator of the location in the anterior posterior direction (Y Axis). The displacement of the frame to the left is clearly visible. NB the anterior fiducial are displaced back behind the orbit. The intersecting white diagonals show that the axial plane centre is close to the tumour. (**c**) This image illustrates that the majority of a parasellar meningioma lies in front of the middle of the head as indicated by the intersection of the two *white lines*. The lateral location may be reasonably judged using the inner canthus of the eye as a guide. The intersection of the diagonals shows that the centre of the frame lies close to the target. The anterior fiducial markers are placed anteriorly. The frame is displaced to the right as shown by the distance between the fiducial markers and the side of the head on the two sides

Intracranial Extracerebral Solitary Targets: Frame Rotation

There are situations where displacement of the frame will still not permit access to the certain targets because they are too far lateral. Being far forward or backward is seldom a problem. Being low down is a relatively limited problem because the shape of the posterior fossa is such, the lower down a target lies the closest it must be to the axial midline, because of the shape of the walls of the posterior fossa.

For far lateral lesions mainly situated lateral to the temporal lobe, a further technique is required. The limitation is that in the "X" axis the maximum available distance from the midline is 47 mm using the trunnions, or 40 mm using the APS. There is no way this can be altered once the frame is applied. Thus to compensate for this limitation a different frame application method must be used and this is frame rotation. This must be applied according to a set of strict principles if it is to be useful rather than confusing. Figure 8.4 illustrates the principles of frame rotation.

The strengths and weaknesses of rotation to optimise frame position are shown in Figs. 8.5 and 8.6.

Lateral Sphenoidal Ridge Meningioma

This tumour fulfils the criteria for which rotation is useful. It may be rotated from in front of the centre of the "Y" axis and thus further forwards and closer to the centre of the critical "X" axis. This is illustrated in Fig. 8.5. When rotating the frame, it would seem the limitation of rotation of the frame is almost always contact between one of the anterior posts of the frame and the nose.

Glomus Jugulare Tumour

In this context it is worth mentioning that the glomus tumour is surprisingly close to the centre. The only problem with this entity is how high the head is. The "X" and "Y" axes should not be a problem. Before accepting a patient it is worth applying the Leksell frame with the MR adapter attached. Given that the tip of the mastoid process is close to the level of the foramen magnum, it is simple to see if the frame will reach that far down. In most cases it will. In a few it will not. The lateral extension of the glomus tumour to the middle ear may tempt one to rotate the frame to improve the position of the tumour. However, such rotation proves of little help as it is basically the kind illustrated in Fig. 8.4b. The effect is shown in Fig. 8.6.

Examples of the kind of rotation shown in Fig. 8.4c are not available since this rotation is never helpful so no images are available to demonstrate it.

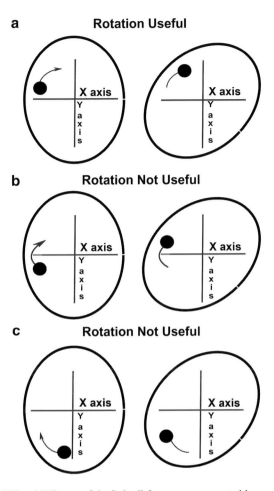

a **Rotation Useful**

b **Rotation Not Useful**

c **Rotation Not Useful**

Fig. 8.4 (**a**) The "X" and "Y" axes of the Leksell frame are represented by a cross. The lesion is shown by a *black circle*. The oval represents the skull. In example "**a**" with a lateral lesion the rotation to the opposite side brings the lesion closer to the middle of the "X" axis which is the object of the exercise. It works because target is rotated away from the centre of the "Y" axis and is thus able to become closer to the centre of the X axis while moving away from centre of the less critical "Y" axis. An example is shown in Fig. 8.5. (**b**) The "X" and "Y" axes of the Leksell frame are represented by a cross. The lesion is shown by a *black circle*. The oval represents the skull. In example "**b**" with a lateral lesion the rotation to the opposite side brings the lesion around the centre of the X axis so that it's distance from the centre of the "X" axis is not changed materially. An example is shown in Fig. 8.6. (**c**) The "X" and "Y" axes of the Leksell frame are represented by a cross. The lesion is shown by a *black circle*. The oval represents the skull. In example "**c**" with a posterior lesion the rotation to the opposite side brings the lesion closer to the centre of the less critical Y axis and at the same time it's distance from the centre of the "X" axis is increased, which is not a useful change

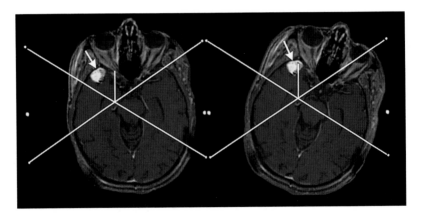

Fig. 8.5 Shows the lateral sphenoidal ridge meningioma indicated by the *white arrow*. On the left the head has been displaced maximally to the left and the lesion is still some way from the centre of the frame, as shown by the intersecting diagonal white lines. In the right sided image with rotation the lesion has moved to the centre of the crucial "*X*" axis as indicated by the *white line*

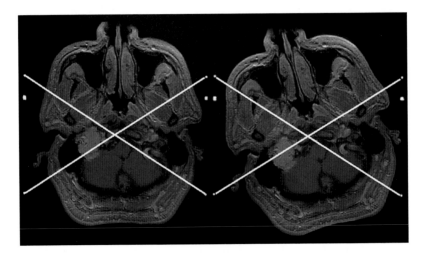

Fig. 8.6 The frame centre in the axial plane is shown by the intersection of the *white lines*. The image is non rotated on the left and rotated on the right. There is very little advantage gained by rotating the tumour towards the centre of the "*X*" axis as the rotation is around the centre of "*Y*" axis, thus keeping the target at the same distance from the centre. However, with the extreme low lateral position of the lateral border of the tumour, even this small

Intracranial Intracerebral Multiple Targets

With intracerebral targets, frame rotation is seldom appropriate because the fixed landmarks guiding such rotation are not as well defined as in the case of the skull

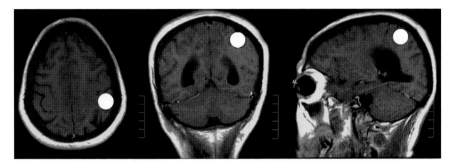

Fig. 8.7 A *white sphere* is shown in the three planes. Its position may be measured on the images with a ruler or micrometer screw gauge. The result can be converted to the true value using the scale shown on the images. The catch with this method when applied from image to patient is that it assumes the patient's position is orthogonal in respect of the plane of the image, which is not always the case

base lesions illustrated above. The commonest intracerebral solitary lesions are single metastases and arteriovenous malformations (AVMs). The identification of these lesions in relation to surface anatomy is fairly simple but involves the use of a slightly different technique. This will require the use of the images and a felt tip pen. Moreover, where possible, it is an advantage to fix the pins of the frame (see below) below the target in the "Z" axis. In this way all parts of the frame are outside the helmet so that collision with the helmet is not possible. However, such a pin placement is not always feasible and in these common instances, location of the frame is best guided by the use of axial and sagittal MR images, a felt tip pen and the scale on the side of the images. Images illustrating these principles are shown in Fig. 8.7. When a location has been determined it be may marked on the patient using a felt tip pen. Since the head is covered in hair, it will often be necessary to mark the side of the face or neck to indicate the correct location in the given plane. Clearly, this only applies to the "X" and "Y" axis. For the most part the "Z" axis location cannot be so marked.

Because the patient's position may be tilted in respect of the plane of the image there is another method which is harder to explain but easier to apply and is illustrated in Fig. 8.8. This is an outline of an axial skull MR image. It shows that the outline of the skull can be divided into portions which roughly consist of two lateral straight lines and two approximate semicircles at the front and the back.

It is a simple matter to determine where a lesion is in relation to these lines and curves. So for example a target could be located in relation to the posterior third of the right sided anterior curve and this can easily be identified on the head and the skin marked. In the actual diagram shown in Fig. 8.8, derived from the lesion shown in Fig. 8.7, the lesion is at the posterior end of the left sided straight portion just at the beginning of the posterior curve. To place a pen mark on the neck appropriate to this location both at the side and the back is simplicity itself. Moreover, experience in over 2,000 patients shows that this level of accuracy is more than enough to

Fig. 8.8 Looking at this image the division of the skull into anterior and posterior curves and straight angled sides is shown. For details see text

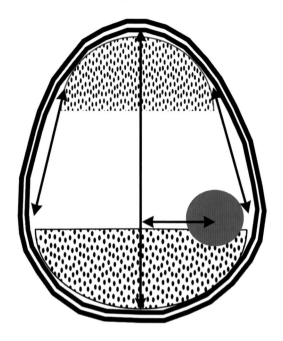

ensure appropriate frame placement for the Gamma Knife "C" model. The distance from the centre of the head to the centre of the lesion is also indicated as this is such a simple measurement and a useful additional check in keeping with the principles of redundancy, appropriate to accurate safe work with a therapeutic system.

Intracranial Intracerebral Multiple Targets: Frame Displacement and Rotation

There can be no fixed guidelines for multiple lesions. This mostly applies to cerebral metastases. In a few cases it will also apply to multiple meningiomas, however the size and distribution of these lesions make them less satisfactory Gamma Knife targets because they are often spread like a carpet rather than assembled like a lump. The images below show what is possible in a patient with multiple metastases, using the principles outlined below. Basically, the frame must be placed with relation to the most eccentric lesion and assessed as to the possibility of reaching the other tumours. Alternatively it can be centred round the largest local collection of tumours. In either case the patient is warned that maybe two frame applications will be necessary. If the frame is applied properly two should be all that is required (Fig. 8.9).

The patient shown above had ten metastases despite having received 5 × 4 Gy of conventional external beam fractionated radiotherapy. He was in otherwise in general good health with his primary tumour controlled. He was indeed informed that

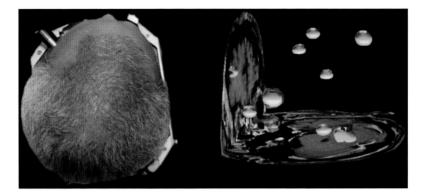

Fig. 8.9 The image on the left shows the rotated frame. It also shows a nice real life demonstration of how easy it is to see the curved and straight portions of the skull, permitting adequately accurate marking for guidance during frame application. The image on the left shows the distribution of the 10 metastases, which were treated in a single session

two treatment sessions would be necessary. In the event he was treated in one session. At 3 months after treatment all the tumours had either shrunk or disappeared.

Frame Application: General Method for Gamma Knife Perfexion

Frame Application

In Perfexion the increased space inside the machine makes the frame placement far less critical. However, there are a few details to which attention must be paid. The aim as before is frame application which will not produce a collision between the walls of the machine and some part of the head or frame. In Perfexion this is much easier.

The Frame Cap

It is important to know that the patient's head or the frame will not collide with the interior of the Gamma Knife during treatment. With the Perfexion model a new instrument has been introduced called the frame cap. A picture of the frame cap fixed to the patient's head is shown below. If the frame box is attached to the frame with no conflict between the head, posts or pins and the plastic box then in most situations the patient will fit in the Gamma Knife Perfexion. However, special care is needed if a lesion is very posterior or very anterior. In these situations it is wise to measure the lengths of the posts above and below the frame together with the length

Fig. 8.10 Shows the frame cap attached to the frame with no conflict between the head, posts or pins and the plastic box. This means the patient should will fit in the Gamma Knife Perfexion in most situations

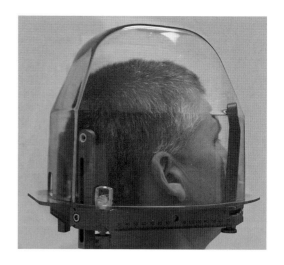

of the projecting pins. In general these measurements should be performed in all metastasis cases. This avoids difficulties if new eccentric metastases are discovered on the day of treatment (Fig. 8.10).

Imaging: MRI

After the frame is fixed the patient is taken to the imaging department for what today will usually be a stereotactic MR examination. This means an MR examination with a volume uptake or fine slices with no space between slices, through the region to be examined. The examination is rendered stereotactic by the stereotactic indicator box which is fixed to the frame. This contains the fiducial markers which indicate the stereotactic space. With an MR **indicator box** these are narrow tubes containing a weak solution of $CuSO_4$ which shows up on MR imaging as a bright signal (Fig. 8.11).

Details of radiology technique, practice, debate and quality control are beyond the scope of this book. The interested reader will find more information from the References attached at the end of this chapter.

Sources of Distortion on MR Images

Minor degrees of distortion could pass unnoticed on diagnostic images. When the images shall be used for therapy the requirements are stricter. The mechanical accuracy of the Gamma Knife is <0.3 mm. Distorted images could not support

Fig. 8.11 This image shows
the attached frame with the
MR indicator box attached.
The fiducial tubes are
indicated by the letters. *A*
anterior, *P* posterior and *D*
diagonal. The tubes are filled
with CuSO4 which shows up
on MR series as an intense
signal

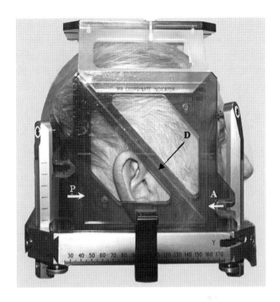

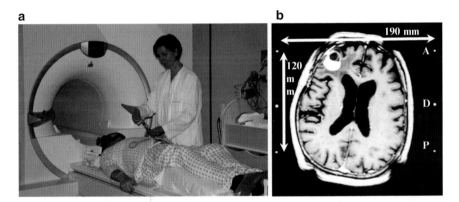

Fig. 8.12 (**a**) The patient is placed in the MR machine with a special **adapter** connected to the
indicator box, ensuring a stable position. Gadolinium is injected as shown in this picture and the
relevant images are taken. The major requirement is either a volume uptake or thin slices with no
inter-slice interval. The patient is in position in the MR receiving gadolinium. (**b**) On the right is a
typical image showing the 6 fiducial markers labelled as in Fig. 8.11. The distance from front to
back is 120 mm. The distance from side to side is 190 mm. This should be checked at every
examination to ensure that there is no distortion

that level of accuracy. By measuring the distances shown in Fig. 8.12 on the right
it will become apparent if distortion is present. If it is the MR machine must be
adjusted. The requirements are that measurement for the antero-posterior distance
should be between 119 and 121 mm and that the two sides should not differ from
one another by more than 1 mm. Furthermore, the requirements for the side to

side distance should be a measurement between 189 and 191 mm and that the two distances should not differ from one another by more than 1 mm. A common cause of sudden unexpected distortion can be a bra. Other sources of error include what the patients have in their pockets. Zips in clothing can also cause distortion.

Imaging: Angiogram

DSA Images

The treatment of AVMs requires DSA images in addition to MRI. Quite a lot of detail needs to be observed to obtain optimal images. The DSA is required to enable a more accurate distinction between feeding arteries, AVM nidus and draining veins. This is achieved because the serial DSA images permits resolution in time as well as space and as shown below improves the selection of tissue to be treated.

1. To begin with a different indicator box is used for angiograms. It contains marks on it in the form of crosses either X or +. Their location corresponds to known positions within the stereotactic system and can be read by the dose-planning software. The box is shown in Figs. 8.13 and 8.14.

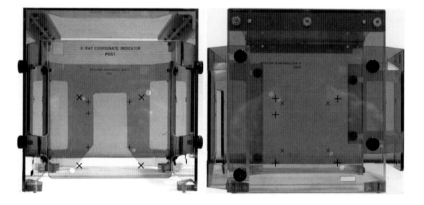

Fig. 8.13 *Front View.* The fiducial lines of the MRI box are replaced by crosses. The picture above is photographed from behind. This can be seen from the word "POST" at the top of the image but also from the size of the + and X symbols. As shown in Fig. 8.14, the larger cross is close to the camera or X-ray source and the smaller is closer to the film. There are 4 X at the back at the corners of a square and 4 + symbols at the corners of a square at the front. The 5th + is at the front on the left. *Side View.* This time the picture is taken from the left towards the right since the "+" symbols are larger and thus nearer to the camera or X-ray tube. Again the 5th "+" symbol is at the front on the left side look at Figs. 8.14 and 8.15

Fig. 8.14 Illustrates how the parts of the image close to the camera will appear larger on the film or screen than the parts at a distance from the camera. In this image, the camera is behind the indicator box so that the "X" marks appear larger and the "+" marks appear smaller. NB For the observant reader a little clarification is called for as there is a discrepancy between this image and that in Fig. 8.13. The left anterior fiducial on the left in this image appears on the right because the camera is behind the indicator box while the film is in front and the image is viewed as from in front. In Fig. 8.13 the same + appears on the left because both the camera and the film are behind the box and thus the box is viewed from behind

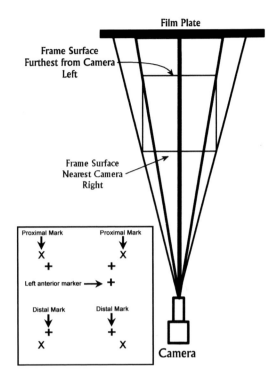

2. The films must be so positioned that the AVM with its feeding arteries and veins are visualised together with all the fiducial markers. This is shown in Fig. 8.15.

   (a) It is important that the image is coned in so that as little air as possible is included. If this is not done the exposure metre compensates for the bright air (See "M" in Fig. 8.15) and produces an unnecessarily dark image.

3. The Gamma Knife user agrees with the radiologist as to which arteries should be examined.

   (a) The author has seen internal and external carotid examinations and vertebral examinations required in the same patient; albeit very rarely.

   (b) When the images are complete the surgeon and the radiologist agree as to which images in each series best demonstrate the nidus. The concept is illustrated in Fig. 8.16.

   (c) The early filling vein is identified in a later image in the series and then the series is followed backwards until the image which shows the first shadow of this vein, as in image 4c below. This is the usual image in the series used to define the nidus.

The images to be used are exported to GammaPlan for use during dose planning. Details of radiology technique, practice, debate and quality control are beyond the scope of this book. The interested reader will find more information from the references.

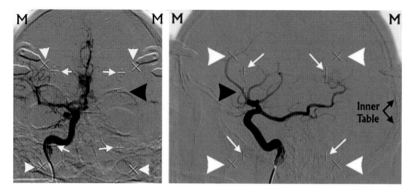

Fig. 8.15 *Front view. White arrows* indicate + indicators, *white arrowheads* indicate X indicators and the *black arrowhead* indicate the extra left anterior + mark. Since the X markers are larger the camera was behind the head and the film in front. Ideally, the smaller indicators should be reasonably symmetrically disposed within the larger indicators. The "M" marks indicate the area around the skull – see text. NB these images are straight antero-posterior (AP) and not Town's view and thus the quality is a little less good in the AP view. *Side view. White arrows* indicate + indicators, white arrowheads indicate X indicators and the black arrowhead indicate the extra left anterior + mark. Since the X indicators are larger than the "+" indicators, the camera was to the right of the head and the film in to the left. Ideally, the smaller indicators should be reasonably symmetrically disposed within the larger indicators. Thus, the radiologist must note the position of the indicators as well as the demonstration of the malformation. The "M" marks indicate the area around the skull. This region should be minimal – see text. The inner table is marked as it is important that this is shown where relevant to ensure that the detailed venous drainage of the AVM is visualised

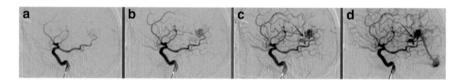

Fig. 8.16 (**a**) Early image no definite nidus seen. (**b**) Later image definite nidus seen. No early filling vein. (**c**) Later image definite nidus seen. Early filling vein just visible. (**d**) Later image definite nidus seen. Early filling vein clearly visible

A reference list follows for the interested reader who wishes to deepen his/her knowledge of the use of imaging techniques in radiosurgery.

References

1. Abe T, Matsumoto K, Horichi Y, Hayashi T, Ikeda H, Iwata T. Magnetic resonance angiography of cerebral arteriovenous malformations. Neurol Med Chir (Tokyo) **35(8)**: 580–583; 1995
2. Bednarz G, Downes B, Werner-Wasik M, Rosenwasser RH. Combining stereotactic angiography and 3D time-of-flight magnetic resonance angiography in treatment planning for arteriovenous malformation radiosurgery. Int J Radiat Oncol Biol Phys **46(5)**: 1149–1154; 2000

3. Bednarz G, Downes MB, Corn BW, Curran WJ, Goldman HW. Evaluation of the spatial accuracy of magnetic resonance imaging-based stereotactic target localization for gamma knife radiosurgery of functional disorders. Neurosurgery **45(5)**: 1156–1161; 1999

4. Berndt A, Beck J. Effect of skull shape approximations in Gamma Knife dose calculations. J Appl Clin Med Phys **8**: 2377; 2007

5. Borden JA, Tsai JS, Mahajan A. Effect of subpixel magnetic resonance imaging shifts on radiosurgical dosimetry for vestibular schwannoma. J Neurosurg **97(5 Suppl)**: 445–449; 2002

6. Cernica G, Wang Z, Malhotra H, de Boer S, Podgorsak MB. Investigation of gamma knife image registration errors resulting from misalignment between the patient and the imaging axis. Med Phys **33(4)**: 941–943; 2006

7. Chan AA, Lau A, Pirzkall A, Chang SM, Verhey LJ, Larson D, McDermott MW, Dillon WP, Nelson SJ. Proton magnetic resonance spectroscopy imaging in the evaluation of patients undergoing gamma knife surgery for Grade IV glioma. J Neurosurg **101(3)**: 467–475; 2004

8. Chavez GD, De Salles AA, Solberg TD, Pedroso A, Espinoza D, Villablanca P. Three-dimensional fast imaging employing steady-state acquisition magnetic resonance imaging for stereotactic radiosurgery of trigeminal neuralgia. Neurosurgery **56(3)**: E628; 2005

9. Chuang CF, Chan AA, Larson D, Verhey LJ, McDermott M, Nelson SJ, Pirzkall A. Potential value of MR spectroscopic imaging for the radiosurgical management of patients with recurrent high-grade gliomas. Technol Cancer Res Treat **6**: 375–382; 2007

10. Chung HT, Kim DG. Distortion correction for digital subtraction angiography imaging: PC based system for radiosurgery planning. Comput Methods Programs Biomed **71(2)**: 165–173; 2003

11. Crescenti RA, Scheib SG, Schneider U, Gianolini S. Introducing gel dosimetry in a clinical environment: customization of polymer gel composition and magnetic resonance imaging parameters used for 3D dose verifications in radiosurgery and intensity modulated radiotherapy. Med Phys **34**: 1286–1297; 2007

12. Donahue BR, Goldberg JD, Golfinos JG, Knopp EA, Comiskey J, Rush SC, Han K, Mukhi V, Cooper JS. Importance of MR technique for stereotactic radiosurgery. Neuro Oncol **5(4)**: 268–274; 2003

13. Engh JA, Flickinger JC, Niranjan A, Amin DV, Kondziolka DS, Lunsford LD. Optimizing intracranial metastasis detection for stereotactic radiosurgery. Stereotact Funct Neurosurg **85 (4)**: 162–168; 2007

14. Ertl A, Saringer W, Heimberger K, Kindl P. Quality assurance for the Leksell gamma unit: considering magnetic resonance image-distortion and delineation failure in the targeting of the internal auditory canal. Med Phys **26(2)**: 166–170; 1999

15. Griffiths PD, Hoggard N, Warren DJ, Wilkinson ID, Anderson B, Romanowski CA. Brain arteriovenous malformations: assessment with dynamic MR digital subtraction angiography. AJNR Am J Neuroradiol **21(10)**: 1892–1899; 2000

16. Guo WY, Chu WC, Wu MC, Chung WY, Gwan WP, Lee YL, Pan HC, Chang CY. An evaluation of the accuracy of magnetic-resonance-guided Gamma Knife surgery. Stereotact Funct Neurosurg **66(Suppl)**: 185–192; 1996

17. Guo WY, Nordell B, Karlsson B, Soderman M, Lindqvist M, Ericson K, Franck A, Lax I, Lindquist C. Target delineation in radiosurgery for cerebral arteriovenous malformations. Assessment of the value of stereotaxic MR imaging and MR angiography. Acta Radiol **34(5)**: 457–463; 1993

18. Guo WY, Pan HC, Chung WY, Wang LW, Teng MM. Do we need conventional angiography? The role of magnetic resonance imaging in verifying obliteration of arteriovenous malformations after Gamma Knife surgery. Stereotact Funct Neurosurg **66(Suppl 1)**: 71–84; 1996

19. Guo WY. Application of MR in stereotactic radiosurgery. J Magn Reson Imaging **8(2)**: 415–420; 1998

20. Heck B, Jess-Hempen A, Kreiner HJ, Schopgens H, Mack A. Accuracy and stability of positioning in radiosurgery: long-term results of the Gamma Knife system. Med Phys **34**: 1487–1495; 2007

21. Jursinic P, Prost R, Schultz C. A new magnetic resonance head coil and head immobilization device for gamma knife radiosurgery: an analysis of geometric distortion and signal/noise characteristics. J Neurosurg **97(5 Suppl)**: 563–568; 2002

22. Jursinic PA, Rickert K, Gennarelli TA, Schultz CJ. Effect of image uncertainty on the dosimetry of trigeminal neuralgia irradiation. Int J Radiat Oncol Biol Phys **62(5)**: 1559–1567; 2005

23. Kondziolka D, Dempsey PK, Lunsford LD, Kestle JR, Dolan EJ, Kanal E, Tasker RR. A comparison between magnetic resonance imaging and computed tomography for stereotactic coordinate determination. Neurosurgery **30(3)**: 402–406; 1992

24. Kondziolka D, Lunsford LD, Kanal E, Talagala L. Stereotactic magnetic resonance angiography for targeting in arteriovenous malformation radiosurgery. Neurosurgery **35(4)**: 585–590; 1994

25. Landi A, Marina R, DeGrandi C, Crespi A, Montanari G, Sganzerla EP, Gaini SM. Accuracy of stereotactic localisation with magnetic resonance compared to CT scan: experimental findings. Acta Neurochir **143(6)**: 593–601; 2001

26. Levivier M, Massager N, Wikler D, Goldman S. Modern multimodal neuroimaging for radiosurgery: the example of PET scan integration. Acta Neurochir Suppl **91**: 1–7; 2004

27. Levivier M, Massager N, Wikler D, Lorenzoni J, Ruiz S, Devriendt D, David P, Desmedt F, Simon S, Van Houtte P, Brotchi J, Goldman S. Use of stereotactic PET images in dosimetry planning of radiosurgery for brain tumors: clinical experience and proposed classification. J Nucl Med **45(7)**: 1146–1154; 2004

28. Levivier M, Wikier D, Goldman S, David P, Metens T, Massager N, Gerosa M, Devriendt D, Desmedt F, Simon S, Van Houtte P, Brotchi J. Integration of the metabolic data of positron emission tomography in the dosimetry planning of radiosurgery with the gamma knife: early experience with brain tumors. Technical note. J Neurosurg **93(Suppl 3)**: 233–238; 2000

29. Linskey ME, Lunsford LD, Flickinger JC. Neuroimaging of acoustic nerve sheath tumors after stereotaxic radiosurgery. AJNR Am J Neuroradiol **12(6)**: 1165–1175; 1991

30. Mack A, Czempiel H, Kreiner HJ, Durr G, Wowra B. Quality assurance in stereotactic space. A system test for verifying the accuracy of aim in radiosurgery. Med Phys **29(4)**: 561–568; 2002

31. Mack A, Wolff R, Scheib S, Rieker M, Weltz D, Mack G, Kreiner HJ, Pilatus U, Zanella FE, Bottchet HD, Seifert V. Analyzing 3-tesla magnetic resonance imaging units for implementation in radiosurgery. J Neurosurg **102(Suppl)**: 158–164; 2005

32. Massager N, Abeloos L, Devriendt D, Op de Beeck M, Levivier M. Clinical evaluation of targeting accuracy of gamma knife radiosurgery in trigeminal neuralgia. Int J Radiat Oncol Biol Phys **69**: 1514–1520; 2007

33. McGee KP, Ivanovic V, Felmlee JP, Meyer FB, Pollock BE, Huston JI. MR angiography fusion technique for treatment planning of intracranial arteriovenous malformations. J Magn Reson Imaging **23(3)**: 361–369; 2006

34. Mori Y, Hayashi N, Iwase M, Yamada M, Takikawa Y, Uchiyama Y, Oda K, Kaii O. Stereotactic imaging for radiosurgery: localization accuracy of magnetic resonance imaging and positron emission tomography compared with computed tomography. Stereotact Funct Neurosurg **84(4)**: 142–146; 2006

35. Morikawa M, Numaguchi Y, Rigamonti D, Kuroiwa T, Rothman MI, Zoarski GH, Simard JM, Eisenberg H, Amin PP. Radiosurgery for cerebral arteriovenous malformations: assessment of early phase magnetic resonance imaging and significance of gadolinium-DTPA enhancement. Int J Radiat Oncol Biol Phys **34(3)**: 663–675; 1996

36. Novotny J, Dvorak P, Spevacek V, Tintera J, Novotny J, Cechak T, Liscak R. Quality control of the stereotactic radiosurgery procedure with the polymer-gel dosimetry. Radiother Oncol **63(2)**: 223–230; 2002

37. Novotny J Jr, Vymazal J, Novotny J, Tlachacova D, Schmitt M, Chuda P, Urgosik D, Liscak R. Does new magnetic resonance imaging technology provide better geometrical accuracy during stereotactic imaging? J Neurosurg **102(Suppl)**: 8–13; 2005

38. Perks J, St George EJ, Doughty D, Plowman PN. Is distortion correction necessary for digital subtraction angiography in the Gamma Knife treatment of intra-cranial arteriovenous malformations? Stereotact Funct Neurosurg **76(2)**: 94–105; 2001

39. Perks JR, Liu T, Hall WH, Chen AY. Clinical impact of magnetic resonance imaging on Gamma Knife surgery for brain metastases. J Neurosurg 105(Suppl): 69–74; 2006
40. Piovan E, Dal Sasso M, Urbani GP, Sartori R, Foroni R, Benati A. Digital subtraction angiography for arteriovenous malformations in stereotactic radiosurgery. Stereotact Funct Neurosurg 66(Suppl 1): 57–62; 1996
41. Piovan E, Zampieri PG, Alessandrini F, Gerosa MA, Nicolato A, Pasoli A, Foroni R, Giri MG, Bricolo A, Benati A. Quality assessment of magnetic resonance stereotactic localization for Gamma Knife radiosurgery. Stereotact Funct Neurosurg 64(Suppl 1): 228–232; 1995
42. Pollock BE, Kondziolka D, Flickinger JC, Patel AK, Bissonette DJ, Lunsford LD. Magnetic resonance imaging: an accurate method to evaluate arteriovenous malformations after stereotactic radiosurgery. J Neurosurg 85(6): 1044–1049; 1996
43. Scheib SG, Gianolini S. Three-dimensional dose verification using BANG gel: a clinical example. J Neurosurg 97(5 Suppl): 582–587; 2002
44. Snell JW, Sheehan J, Stroila M, Steiner L. Assessment of imaging studies used with radiosurgery: a volumetric algorithm and an estimation of its error. Technical note. J Neurosurg 104 (1): 157–162; 2006
45. Soderman M, Picard C, Ericson K. An algorithm for correction of distortion in stereotaxic digital subtraction angiography. Neuroradiology 40(5): 277–282; 1998
46. St George EJ, Butler P, Plowman PN. Can magnetic resonance imaging alone accurately define the arteriovenous nidus for gamma knife radiosurgery? J Neurosurg 97(5 Suppl): 464–470; 2002
47. Taschner CA, Le Thuc V Reyns N, Gieseke J, Gauvrit JY, Pruvo JP, Leclerc X. Gamma Knife surgery for arteriovenous malformations in the brain: integration of time-resolved contrast-enhanced magnetic resonance angiography into dosimetry planning. Technical note. J Neurosurg 107: 854–859; 2007
48. Walton L, Hampshire A, Forster DM, Kemeny AA. Accuracy of stereotactic localisation using magnetic resonance imaging: a comparison between two- and three-dimensional studies. Stereotact Funct Neurosurg 66(Suppl 1): 49–56; 1996
49. Walton L, Hampshire A, Vaughan P, Forster DM, Kemeny AA, Radatz MW. Distortion in magnetic resonance images obtained for stereotactic localization. Case report. J Neurosurg 93 (Suppl 3): 191–192; 2000
50. Warren DJ, Hoggard N, Walton L, et al. Cerebral arteriovenous malformations: comparison of novel magnetic resonance angiographic techniques and conventional catheter angiography. Neurosurgery 61: 187–196; 2007
51. Watanabe Y, Han E. Image registration accuracy of GammaPlan: a phantom study. J Neurosurg 109(Suppl): 21–24; 2008
52. Watanabe Y, Lee CK, Gerbi BJ. Geometrical accuracy of a 3-tesla magnetic resonance imaging unit in Gamma Knife surgery. J Neurosurg 105(Suppl): 190–193; 2006
53. Watanabe Y, Perera GM, Mooij RB. Image distortion in MRI-based polymer gel dosimetry of gamma knife stereotactic radiosurgery systems. Med Phys 29(5): 797–802; 2002
54. Worthington C, Hutson K, Boulware R, Neglia W, Gibbons JP, Clark R, Rand J. Computerized tomography cisternography of the trigeminal nerve for stereotactic radiosurgery. Case report. J Neurosurg 93(Suppl 3): 169–171; 2000
55. Yan Y, Shu H, Bao X, Luo L, Bai Y. Clinical treatment planning optimization by Powell's method for gamma unit treatment system. Int J Radiat Oncol Biol Phys 39(1): 247–254; 1997
56. Yu C, Apuzzo ML, Zee CS, Petrovich Z. A phantom study of the geometric accuracy of computed tomographic and magnetic resonance imaging stereotactic localization with the Leksell stereotactic system. Neurosurgery 48(5): 1092–1098; 2001
57. Yu C, Petrovich Z, Apuzzo ML, Luxton G. An image fusion study of the geometric accuracy of magnetic resonance imaging with the Leksell stereotactic localization system. J Appl Clin Med Phys 2(1): 42–50; 2001

58. Yu C, Petrovich Z, Apuzzo ML, Zelman V, Giannotta SL. Study of magnetic resonance imaging-based arteriovenous malformation delineation without conventional angiography. Neurosurgery **54(5)**: 1104 discussion; 2004
59. Zeck OF, Fang B, Mullani N, Lamki LL, Gould KL, Kramer LA, Hac S, Walsh JW. PET and SPECT imaging for stereotactic localization. Stereotact Funct Neurosurg **64(Suppl 1)**: 147–154; 1995
60. Zerris VA, Noren GC, Shucart WA, Rogg J, Friehs GM. Targeting the cranial nerve: micro-radiosurgery for trigeminal neuralgia with CISS and 3D-flash MR imaging sequences. J Neurosurg **102(Suppl)**: 107–110; 2005

Chapter 9
Dose Plan Indices

Dose-Plan Finalisation

When a dose plan is completed it is useful to assess its quality using indices to quantify the dose in one of the following ways:

1. The degree to which the target is covered by the prescription dose
2. The degree to which the prescription dose is specific to the target and is not spread into to the surrounding tissue

The indices are as follows.

Conformity Index: RTOG PITV Index [1]

$$PITV = PIV/TV^*$$

Target Volume Ratio (TVR) [2]

$$TVR = TV/PIV$$

Clearly the TVR is the reciprocal of the PITV. Both indices reflect the proportion of the target covered by the prescription isodose. They say nothing about the dose outside the tumour.

Moreover, they contain an inherent flaw. The proportion relates the volume of the prescription isodose to the volume of the target. However, the equations reflect nothing of the location of the isodose and the volume.

---

*PIV $=$ Volume of the prescription isodose. TV $=$ Target Volume.

J.C. Ganz, *Gamma Knife Neurosurgery*,
DOI 10.1007/978-3-7091-0343-2_9, © Springer-Verlag/Wien 2011

Fig. 9.1 This shows how
different Each of Conformity
Index calculations gives a
value of one and yet can
reflect an unsuitable
prescription

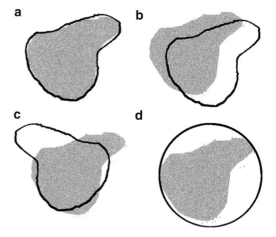

The perfect value for PITV or TVR would be one. However, the formulae permit
one in the situations illustrated in Fig. 9.1.

This discrepancy led Ian Paddick to propose a different formula which is now
called the Paddick Conformity Index (PCI) [2]

Paddick Conformity Index (PCI) [1]

The crucial new parameter is TV_{PIV} which is the volume of the target covered by
the prescription isodose. This compels the formula to be related to the location of
the target. For details on how the formula has its specific shape the reader is referred
to Paddick's original article [1].

$$\frac{TV_{PIV}^{2*}}{TV \times PIV}$$

Selectivity [3]

This is a simple index comparing the volume of the prescription isodose inside the
target with the total volume of this isodose. The formula is as follows.

$$\frac{TV_{PIV}}{PIV}$$

---

*TV_{PIV} = Volume of prescription isodose within the target.

Gradient Index

This index is devised to show the sharpness of the fall of dose outside a target. It was described by Paddick and Lippitz [4]. The formula is as follows.

In this formula, "x" is the isodose which carries the prescription isodose and x/2 is the isodose carrying half that dose. Thus in a typical situation x would be 50% and x/2 25%. One interesting result of the work underlying this index was the discovery that the dose fall outside a target was distributed a little differently than was previously thought. Based on the studies using single shots, it had been thought that the steepest dose gradient outside the target was with a prescription isodose of 50%. It has been stated that with multi shot dose plans the steepest gradient outside the target is associated with a slightly lower isodose somewhere between 40 and 50%. The author has not been able to confirm this.

$$\frac{PIV_{x\%}}{PIV_{(x/2)\%}}$$

Comment on the Use of Indices

The above mentioned indices are tools. They must be applied with sense. As Leksell himself famously stated "A fool with a tool is still a fool". Thus, it must be remembered these indices are aimed at helping the user to avoid complications of treatment. This is necessary. However, the main task is to control the pathological process. There may be situations where a dose plan with a poorer index will provide a better application of dose to the target even a safer dose to the target. A typical example would be in a patient with a cystic lesion. There excess radiation may be allowed to dissipate in fluid. A less well shaped dose plan may even so permit the delivery of a quicker and higher dose. In a world where more and more patients are treated with metastases, the duration of treatment becomes an important point for patient comfort. Maybe a slightly less than optimal set of indices may provide an adequate treatment with a shorter treatment time for a patient in considerable discomfort.

However, it should not be taken that the above means the author encourages less than optimal treatment. Quite the reverse is the case. It is however, necessary to remember we are treating people and not objects and that essential factor has to be included in the design of dose plans.

Nonetheless, the indices do serve one very vital and one useful purpose. The vital purpose is to encourage consistency of dose-planning up to standards that are perceived to be adequate. The useful purpose is in conveying information to colleagues when writing scientific papers.

Finally there is the question as to what are the acceptable values for the various indices. To be honest nobody knows for sure but any department using GKNS should work out a set of useable values and make sure they are up to date with current practice.

The author finds the following practice useful, expressing a preference for whole numbers, thereby inverting some of the indices. This is to some extent a matter of taste.

Target cover by PIV	$\geq$95%
1/Conformity Index	This value should not exceed 1.05 and will not do so if Target cover is >95%
1/Selectivity	This should not exceed 1.25
Gradient Index	This should be less than 3

None of these values are definitive, but are seen to provide adequate safe cover and consistent practice.

References

1. Paddick I. A simple scoring ratio to index the conformity of radiosurgical treatment plans. Technical note. J Neurosurg **93(Suppl 3)**: 219–222; 2000
2. Shaw E, Kline R, Gillin M, Souhami L, Hirschfeld A, Dinapoli R, Martin L. Radiation Therapy Oncology Group: radiosurgery quality assurance guidelines. Int J Radiat Oncol Biol Phys **27 (5)**: 1231–1239; 1993
3. Régis J, Hayashi M, Porcheron D, Delsanti C, Muracciole X, Peragut JC. Impact of the model C and automatic positioning system on gamma knife radiosurgery: an evaluation in vestibular schwannomas. J Neurosurg **97(5 Suppl)**: 588–591; 2002
4. Paddick I, Lippitz B. A simple dose gradient measurement tool to complement the conformity index. J Neurosurg **105(Suppl 1)**: 194–201; 2006

Part II
The Patient's Experience

Chapter 10
Gamma Knife Surgery and Computer Networks

Introduction

The internet and hospital intranets have had a very large effect on all hospital practice. Most of this has been useful. This brief chapter is merely to outline how it has changed the way patients are managed. These networks affect patient management in two major ways as outlined below.

The Effect of Computer Networks on the Physician

1. Administration of the patient's information
   (a) It is no longer necessary for the hospital's internal mailing system to deliver a patient's notes to a given place. Nor is there any longer competition between who shall have access to a given patient's file at a given time. Any authorised member of the hospital staff may view the information in the patient's file at any time. It enables rapid updating of notes, ordering investigations and requesting specialist advice
   (b) Data management programs facilitate the allocation of available resources of materials and expertise to the planning and execution of the tasks involved in managing patients
   (c) The data stored in these systems enables the tabulating and statistical analysis of health care offered by a hospital. It also enables analysis of the use to which the budget is made
2. Email has a number of effects
   (a) Between institutions it facilitates the exchange of experience and enables speedy advice in respect of the management of difficult cases
   (b) Between institutions it can facilitate the referral process by ensuring missing data is acquired or found and then sent
   (c) Within an institution it helps to optimise the use of facilities and the processes of referral.

J.C. Ganz, *Gamma Knife Neurosurgery*,
DOI 10.1007/978-3-7091-0343-2_10, © Springer-Verlag/Wien 2011

3. Library access is hugely improved
   (a) Easy access to journals with downloading of important texts facilitates the acquisition and maintenance of the physician's knowledge.
4. Imaging
   (a) The days of the physical image are long past. This has advantages in a number of respects

   - Before computer networks, images were supposed to be stored in an archive. In reality they often were not, having been borrowed by a professor or similar person and not returned. Data storage without hard copy avoids this trap. (In 1974 the Bristol Royal Infirmary had an extension number in its internal catalogue named Missing X-rays, indicating the problems with hard copy image storage).
   - The image may be viewed by the referring physician and the limitations imposed by the choice of window and level for a printed hard copy, no longer apply. The user may adjust the image at his own viewing station and perform measurements upon it.
   - The days of the images which are too small for sensible viewing are a thing of the past.

5. Scientific Journals
   (a) Journals are now available electronically
   (b) While journals are not in principle free with a journal subscription it is much easier to access and download papers both recent and ancient. They are mostly downloaded as pdf files and this permits the speedy searching for significant terms.
   (c) Purchase of a journal usually gives access to all the earlier editions of that journal, although there is one European publisher for whom this is regrettably not the case.
   (d) Increasingly there are free review articles published. The Journal of Neurosurgery is a pioneer of this with its monthly free review publication called Neurosurgical Focus.
6. Medline
   (a) This is now available free at NIH
   (b) The search engine has been sophisticated with searching getting easier and easier
7. Emedicine.com
   (a) This website has review articles which are constantly kept up to date. While not an everyday resource it is remarkably useful for reviewing really rare conditions.

There are many other facilities up on the net but the above outline gives an idea of how comprehensive the change in access to information has become. Google is surprisingly useful for physicians as well as patients if the specialist searches fail to deliver.

The Effect of the Computer Networks on the Patient

1. Information about the illness
   (a) This is widely available using Google. It can be helpful in enabling patients to understand their condition in a more relaxed location than a consulting room and with no time limits placed on how long the explanation can continue
   (b) Most responsible sites have somewhere a note informing the patient of the importance of consulting their own physician and not to use the information on the site as source of practical guidance but merely for information. Some of these sites can be more confusing than helpful
2. Information about the treatment
   (a) Searching for Gamma Knife on Google will lead the patient to many competent sites and there will often be elegant explanations of how the Gamma Knife works and what it can do
   (b) The patient may also end up on Elekta, the manufacturer's website which also has information for patients
   (c) Searching Google with the term radiosurgery will lead the patient to a variety of Gamma Knife or LINAC sites. On the whole this does not matter and anyway it cannot be avoided. However, the information available may be technique specific which could be confusing
   (d) The International RadioSurgery Association was founded in 1995. It is an independent organization dedicated to providing educational information and guidelines on stereotactic radiosurgery for brain tumours and brain disorders. Its panel of experts cover expertise for all the existing technologies which may be used for this purpose. It is a very helpful website for those seeking more information about intracranial radiosurgery. Its "url" is http://www.irsa.org/

Computer Networks and Medical Ethics

The last few years have seen the development of the internet in a variety of fascinating directions. One of these has been the development of social networks and another the capacity to upload video material which is thereby made available to the general public. This is in principle a wonderful way in which responsible simplified information can be communicated to colleagues and potential patients alike.

However, there is another less positive side to the possibilities which this new technology delivers to our doorsteps. In the USA a Federal Trade Commission ruling, upheld in the Supreme Court in 1981 compelled the AMA Council on Judicial and Ethical Affairs to unwillingly accept that the AMA must renounce its ban on advertising [1]. Even so this change has given rise to concern within the profession. It is refreshing to see that colleagues still feel uncomfortable with this ruling as indicated in a recent article [1]. Moreover, it was encouraging to read the statement from the Mayo Clinic's Webpage on the matter of advertising which is quoted here. "If advertising is a source of funding it will be clearly stated. A brief description of the advertising policy adopted by the Web site owners will be displayed on the site. Advertising and other promotional material will be presented to viewers in a manner and context that facilitates differentiation between it and the original material created by the institution operating the site".

The extent to which these changes regarding license to advertise have changed our practice is well illustrated in an excellent recent biography of Harvey Cushing. It is there recounted how the young Cushing was impecunious to the extent that his wife commented on it in relation to his gangliectomy for trigeminal neuralgia. She is quoted as saying "Why are all ganglions impecunious I wonder? Anyhow all ours are" [3]. Her husband had performed 16 gangliectomies for trigeminal neuralgia before he found a paying patient. All the previous cases had been charity patients. However, the following embarrassment occurred as the book recounts "...one of William Randolph Hearst's newspapers, immediately sensationalised Cushing's JAMA report in the Sunday feature story entitled 'How Toothache and Neuralgia are cured'". The book goes on to say "Notoriety like this deeply embarrassed doctors, who are forbidden by all their codes of ethics from advertising their skills" [4].

It seems the author of this book is not alone amongst neurosurgeons in wishing that some of the modern changes could be reversed, even while acknowledging how unlikely this is to happen. The distinguished Dr. Patrick Kelly wrote a passionate review of times past and lost values last year in Surgical Neurology [2].

It thus seems fair to claim that there are many concerned colleagues who are worried about the way commerce and commercial practice has infiltrated our profession. One example which is relevant in a chapter on computer networks is the discovery of the results of a search of "YouTube" with the terms "radiosurgery" or "Gamma Knife". It is distastefully easy to happen upon self-serving self-congratulatory videos, whose sole purpose would appear to be to attract referrals.

Dr. Kelly asked "How did we lose it – and can we ever get it back? [2]" The answer would appear to be when the AMC was compelled against its will to bow to a court ruling in favour of the Federal Trade Commission. "Sic transit gloria mundi".

Conclusion

Despite the concerns expressed in the previous paragraph, the existence of the computer networks has completely changed the doctor patient relationship within the field of Gamma Knife neurosurgery and mostly for the better. In practice, while some patients have been confused by what they read on the internet, the majority are much better informed than they were in the past. This is helpful. The easy access to information and advice make the doctor's work both less arduous but also stimulates a higher quality. Moreover, the common paternalism which senior physicians employed and enjoyed 20 years ago is now thankfully a thing of the past. Also the improved administration of patient information has made a huge difference. The author remembers only 20 years ago that referring physicians from abroad were advised not to send X-ray images rolled up in tubes as customs officials tended to suspect concealed weapons and delay the package. He can also remember from Cairo the local practice where it is patients who store their images in plastic bags from supermarkets. This system is in many ways more efficient in terms of image access than the old fashioned hospital archive. However, it suffers from the disadvantages that the images may not remain in the right order, they may stick together from coffee and they may disappear when exposed to the sun. Nonetheless, it is a less than optimal system which computer networks can circum-navigate.

References

1. Jones JW, McCullough L. Surgical infomercials: the ethical price of stardom. J Vasc Surg **50(1)**: 215–216; 2009
2. Kelly PJ. How did we lose it – and can we ever get it back? Surg Neurol **72(3)**: 306–310; 2009
3. Bliss M. Harvey Cushing. A Life in Surgery. Oxford University Press, Oxford: pp 184; 2007
4. Bliss M. Harvey Cushing. A Life in Surgery. Oxford University Press, Oxford: pp 130; 2007

Chapter 11
Aims of Gamma Knife Surgery

Introduction

The purpose of this chapter is to introduce a small number of important concepts. These should be kept in mind when treating the patients. They are concepts concerned with what we want to do, what we can do and what is in the patient's best interest.

What We Want to Do and What We Can Do

The aim of any treatment is the eradication of a disease and the resolution of all the symptoms caused by the disease. In the case of the Gamma Knife sometimes these aims can be met and sometimes not.

1. Disease eradication
   (a) AVMs can often be eradicated
   (b) Most tumours are not eradicated but made to shrink or stop growing. They are controlled not eradicated
2. Relief of symptoms
   (a) In the treatment of functional indications the Gamma Knife can relieve symptoms. In practice the most common functional indication by far is trigeminal neuralgia. The other functional indication which has gained a following is temporal lobe epilepsy.
   (b) It is also true that the epilepsy associated with visible targets such as AVMs or tumours may improve. In the case of skull base tumours where the brainstem and cranial nerves are affected there are good chances of resolution of symptoms. However, this improvement remains unpredictable.
   (c) Symptoms with vestibular schwannomas will not improve – in common with all other interventional treatments.
   (d) Loss of vision which has been present more than 4 weeks prior to treatment is very unlikely to improve.

J.C. Ganz, *Gamma Knife Neurosurgery*,
DOI 10.1007/978-3-7091-0343-2_11, © Springer-Verlag/Wien 2011

(e) Pituitary endocrinopathies do improve in some instances but the rate of normalisation is not as high as one could wish.

What Is in the Patient's Best Interest?

The question mark is introduced into the subheading because it is proposed to suggest a somewhat controversial though not altogether original notion. It is controversial because it goes against the grain of current surgical teaching and indeed against the grain of the competent surgeon's psychology. However, let us consider that maybe our attitudes are still coloured by the teachings of our ancestors who had different worries from us, because they did not have access to the technology which we can use. Two diagnoses may be used to illustrate this point.

1. Vestibular Schwannoma
   (a) Maybe the treatment aim of eradicating the disease is not necessarily in the patient's best interest. Lownie and Drake reporting on 11 patients with vestibular schwannomas more than 3 cm in diameter could record 82% preserved facial function following intracapsular surgery. Tumour recurrence occurred in two patients. In nine patients there was no recurrence and there were no late recurrences [1]. The point is that since even in the best hands, facial palsy occurs in over 30% of patients with radical surgery of tumours more than 3 cm in diameter, there would appear to be a case for a less radical operation [2].
   (b) Vestibular schwannomas are excellent for illustrating the current concept. The early neurosurgical pioneers, practicing prior to the introduction of computerised imaging techniques had no way of assessing either the radicality of their surgery or the course of the operated tumour. This led to the teaching that radical removal was the optimal treatment to prevent recurrence and death. However, the patients had to pay a heavy price in the form of new neurological deficits following discharge from hospital. Facial palsy was the commonest such complication with a high degree of concomitant social maladjustment.
   (c) Today MRI permits the follow up of these tumours so there is no urgency to be radical. The Drake paper suggests a more modest surgical approach which failed to fulfil the aim of radical removal of disease permitted the persistence of a desired function. It is more than probable that many patients would prefer such an approach even if a retreatment were required some years later. Moreover, after intracapsular removal of a vestibular schwannoma, the tumour shrinks facilitating Gamma Knife treatment of the residual lesion.
2. Prolactinoma
   (a) The aim of treatment is to normalise the serum prolactin level. This is often achieved adequately with dopamine agonists. However, sometimes the tumour is resistant and sometimes the medication's side effects are intolerable to the patient.

(b) The next stage is surgery but a high recurrence rate is by no means unknown. Jules Hardy's group recorded a late recurrence rate of 36% [3]. In this author's experience it is very difficult to normalise a hyperprolactinaemia with Gamma Knife radiosurgery following failed microsurgery. However, in our unpublished material in Cairo it was not so hard to achieve a good functional result in a slightly indirect way. It would seem that the decreased prolactin secretion following Gamma Knife treatment enabled dopamine agonists to normalise the prolactin at doses the patients could tolerate. Function was restored not by the Gamma Knife but by a multimodality treatment.

Conclusion

The concepts that arise out of this short presentation are as follows.

1. It is necessary to be clear about what is desirable and what is possible and inform the patient accordingly.
2. A hallmark of a modern University Centre is that complex diseases are managed by teams of physicians covering multiple areas of expertise. Gamma Knife competence should be represented on these teams where relevant. Then the rational safe treatment of difficult tumours could be planned from the start, instead of the currently familiar practice of calling in the Gamma Knife surgery team when radical surgery has proved too hazardous.
3. To put the final concept in the vernacular, for some diseases it may be better to nibble than to bite. A surgeon's instinct is to remove all the pathological tissue he can get his hands on without threatening life. However, with the safety available with modern computerised imaging methods, the surgeon could consider becoming more interested in staged procedures. This is a noble tradition following in the footsteps of none other than Harvey Cushing. If this is correct it raises the possibility that not only could mortality be kept low but appropriate staged procedures could lead to a reduction in avoidable surgical morbidity.
4. The above notions are in no way meant to indicate a lack of respect or admiration for the talents of many gifted colleagues. It is however a call to reassess how we use our modern technology to adapt our methods for the best interest of our patients.

References

1. Lownie SP, Drake CG. Radical intracapsular removal of acoustic neurinomas. Long-term follow-up review of 11 patients. J Neurosurg **74**: 422–425; 1991
2. Samii M, Gerganov V, Samii A. Improved preservation of hearing and facial nerve function in vestibular schwannoma surgery via the retrosigmoid approach in a series of 200 patients. J Neurosurg **105**: 527–535; 2006
3. Serri O, Rasio E, Beauregard H, Hardy J, Somma M. Recurrence of hyperprolactinemia after selective transsphenoidal adenomectomy in women with prolactinoma. N Engl J Med **309(5)**: 280–283; 1983

Chapter 12
Principles of Information and Follow Up

Introduction: The Processes of Referral

The patients requiring Gamma Knife neurosurgery will usually be suffering from a dangerous, potentially life threatening and thus intensely worrying condition. To become someone who is assessed for referral to the Gamma Knife involves a process which varies greatly with the condition to be treated. The details of presentation are considered under the chapters about the specific diseases. Nonetheless, the nature of the conditions treated, their rarity and the variety of opinions about optimal treatment induce frustration and anxiety in these patients. Most referring physicians know relatively little about the details of a radiosurgery treatment. However, there is also a wealth of information available on the internet which can be helpful but may also be confusing. Thus, a Gamma Knife centre's staff must always be aware that the pathway to referral has in most cases been a troubled route for patients suffering from a dangerous illness.

While most patients are referred by an experienced medical practitioner, a significant minority arrange a referral because they want to avoid surgery at all costs. Some patients will be refused as unsuitable. The most usual reason for refusal is that the Gamma Knife is not the patient's best treatment option. In some cases surgery is clearly more appropriate. Surgery produces a result overnight and is advised when technically simple. Moreover, some lesions are too large to be treated safely with radiosurgery. In others cases, for example a large number of metastases or a brain stem glioma, radiotherapy is more appropriate.

Finally, we come to the point where the patient has been accepted for treatment. This current chapter is concerned with how these patients shall be informed.

J.C. Ganz, *Gamma Knife Neurosurgery*,
DOI 10.1007/978-3-7091-0343-2_12, © Springer-Verlag/Wien 2011

Information After Acceptance

The Nature of the Technique

Firstly, how does the Gamma Knife work, irrespective of the illness being treated? Well, to begin with it is not a laser and there is no requirement to open the head to apply it. Even today, after 25 years of use and over 500,000 patients treated worldwide, few new patients have a clear idea of how the machine works. There are still people who believe a Gamma Knife is some sort of laser machine. Clearly, the mechanism of action has already been explained in some detail in previous chapters. However, not all patients are interested in this degree of detail. One analogy, which is useful, is to compare the Gamma Knife's focussing of gamma rays to the effect of a magnifying glass on the rays of the sun. An important feature to emphasise is that the amount of damage done with a magnifying glass, focussing the sun's rays depends on how long it is held in position and the same applies, in essence, to the Gamma Knife.

The Safety of the Technique

Patients are naturally concerned as to the nature of the rays involved. They should be informed that gamma rays are more or less just like X-rays. Like X-rays they penetrate the body, without it being necessary to open the body, so that surgery is avoided. However, such rays are clearly very powerful and thus potentially dangerous. The safety of the treatment is based on the ability of the machine to focus radiation where it is needed and keep it away from normal functioning brain and nerves. However, it is important to mention that a technique capable of treating serious intracranial illness is a powerful treatment and has unavoidably some complications. However, it is true to say that the risks with the Gamma Knife are really small compared to the untreated disease; otherwise the patient would not be advised to receive the treatment. Moreover, a most advantageous feature of the Gamma Knife is that while the treatment may have a low morbidity, properly used the mortality of a Gamma Knife treatment is zero.

The Degree of Disruption to the Patient's Life

The pattern of daily life disruption varies from centre to centre. It will to some extent depend on the distance the patient has to travel to reach the centre and the means of transport available. The patterns of management seem to follow one of two patterns. In the first, the patient is admitted on one day, treated the next and discharged on the third. Sickness benefit, related to the treatment procedure itself need not be extended beyond the weekend following discharge from hospital. Some would say even that was generous. In other centres the treatment is simply an outpatient procedure without admission. Both systems seem to work admirably and the choice of treatment arrangement is dependent on a cultural rather than a medical basis.

The Waiting

Both the patient and the referring physician will need to expect some degree of waiting, between the referral and the acceptance of the patient. This delay may be of the order of a few days to weeks depending on the waiting list and the urgency of treatment. It is advised that all metastasis patients must be treated not later than 4 weeks after their most recent MR examination. If the delay is much more than this a new MR will be advantageous.

It is important to let the physicians and departments who refer to a Gamma Knife Center to know what investigations are required and what sort of imaging will be necessary for a decision to be made. For most diagnoses MR images with T1 +/− contrast and a T2 series are necessary. For AVMs an angiogram is helpful. MRA is often less satisfactory than an MRI study. Sometimes a DSA will be needed, especially with smaller lesions. Where relevant, if the images are sent on a CD and the accompanying reports describe changes through the different examinations all the image series should be included on the CD.

In addition to images there is other vital information that should be included with a referral. For all patients details of previous intracranial radiation treatments should be included. For patients with metastases this is mandatory and absence of this information could lead to delays.

For patients with vestibular schwannomas a current audiogram including tone and speech registration should be included. For any patient with a tumour somewhere near the visual pathway a written visual field examination and its report should be available. The visual field examination in this situation can be nearly as useful for optimal dose-planning as the images. The most common tumours where this is a requirement are meningiomas and pituitary adenomas.

Information on Admission to Hospital

The Brochure

It is a good idea to design a brochure covering the major steps of the procedure. In addition as a centre matures the brochure can contain information of the number of patients treated and maybe some of the therapeutic successes. It can be sent out to patients at the same time as they receive a letter confirming their appointment. Where relevant the brochure should be written in all the languages of the peoples referring to the centre.

The Day Before

The patient is admitted to the department in the usual way and a clinical examination is undertaken and documented. Then a detailed explanation is given which has two main elements. Firstly, the aims of treatment, the risks and the expected final results are discussed. Thereafter, the sequence of events that the patient will undergo the following day is explained. It goes without saying that children are spared much of this information. For adults it is usual to explain that most of the treatment is painless. However, the stereotactic frame application is uncomfortable or even painful and there is a sensation of marked compression at the end of frame application which resolves in roughly 5 min.

The Day of Treatment

The patient may receive premedication, though this should be done with some judgement and not as a routine. If necessary, 10 mg diazepam is useful as a sedative. On the other hand 4 mg dexamethasone, half an hour prior to applying the frame is useful in relieving the nausea and vomiting that some patients experience after radiation treatment. In some cases, with critically placed large tumours, the surgeon may wish to place the patient on full dosage dexamethasone, for a couple of days, followed by gradual withdrawal of the drug over a week or so. The purpose of this is to reduce the risk of acute swelling following Gamma Knife surgery. It should be stated that at the present time this is merely a precaution. To the best of the author's knowledge it is extremely rare for such a swelling to occur with this technique.

The frame is applied with the patient sitting in a chair or bed. The hair is washed in an alcohol based disinfectant solution. No shaving of hair is required; a popular detail this. After the frame is applied the rest of the day is essentially tedious. The next stage is an MR examination; the sequences selected to suit the individual disease. If an arteriovenous malformation is to be treated an angiogram follows the MRI and this may be slightly uncomfortable, though not markedly so with modern contrast media. The images are then sent to the dose planning computer. When the dose planning is completed the patient comes to the Gamma Knife suite and treatment is performed. This may involve several turns in and out of the machine, depending on the site and shape of the lesion and the type of Gamma Knife. With Perfexion most treatments are performed with a single entry into the machine. The actual treatment while again rather tedious is entirely painless. After it is over the frame is removed. At this stage some patients require a mild analgesic for the temporary headache which follows removal of the frame. If the patient has undergone angiography, this will determine the period of immobilization. Other patients may mobilize at their convenience. A plaster is placed over the pin holes in the forehead and the patient is advised not to wash the hair for 2 days. Very occasionally a pin will have pierced and artery leading to bleeding when the pin is removed. Usually this will stop with pressure over 5–6 min. If not a single suture will solve the problem. The suture can be removed after a couple of days.

After the treatment is completed is a good time to give information on the further outlook and especially the plans for a follow-up, which is necessarily detailed and long term. This is also the time to discuss unwelcome restrictions in activity, though clearly such decisions are more appropriately the responsibility of the referring physician. Finally, a very few patients may experience pain related to the fixation of the frame, especially where one of the posterior pins has been in contact with an occipital cutaneous nerve. Explanation of the reason for this discomfort and that it is due to the frame and not to some unwelcome intracranial complication seems to go a long way to reconciling the patient to the discomfort, which would appear to be almost invariably short term.

Follow-Up

The follow up routines vary a bit with each disease and divergences from the routines outlined below are detailed with the chapters about specific diseases. There is no general agreement but the following suggestions ensure that important changes are not missed, which can occur if the examinations are less frequent. What follows is merely a useful outline it is by no means considered definitive.

Benign Tumours

1. 3D MR T1 sequence every 6 months for the first 2 years with and without contrast together with a T2 series through the region of interest
2. Same sequences annually for the next 3 years
3. Same sequences every 5 years for the rest of the patient's life

Malignant Gliomas

1. Same sequence every 3 months

Metastases

1. Same sequences at 4 weeks and subsequently every 3 months starting 3 months after treatment.

AVMs

1. Same sequences every 6 months until the AVM disappears then a final DSA. Very small AVMs are not seen on MRI. Then a decision has to be taken about when to take the first DSA.

Other Follow Up Measurements

1. With pituitary micro-adenomas associated with an endocrinopathy it is essential to perform an endocrinological follow up every 6 months until normalisation occurs. Thereafter annual follow up is adequate to make sure pituitary insufficiency does not develop undetected. MR examinations are largely unnecessary in this situation.
2. Any patient with a benign tumour where vision is at risk should have a visual field examination done at the same time as the follow up imaging or earlier if visual symptoms develop.
3. Any patient with useful hearing after the treatment of a vestibular schwannoma or cerebro-pontine angle meningioma should have audiograms performed at the same time as MR imaging for the duration of follow up.

Conclusion

The most important principle to remember is this. Treatment with the Gamma Knife is not definitive and time limited like surgery. It is the first step in a process. The patient must be made aware of this. The advice outlined above is just the detailed specifics of the application of this concept in varying situations.

Part III
The Gamma Knife and Specific Diseases: Tumours

Chapter 13
Vestibular Schwannomas

Unilateral Vestibular Schwannomas: History and Microsurgery

Introduction

Vestibular Schwannomas (VSs) have always been considered difficult lesions to treat. The routine diagnosis and investigation will not be mentioned as this information is easily available in standard neurosurgical texts. The evolution of treatment may be considered briefly in 2 periods. The first stage was the development of life saving surgery for large dangerous tumours. The first operation of modern times with a successful outcome for a cerebello-pontine angle tumour is attributed to Sir Charles Balance [1]. He made what seems to us the rather alarming statement "a finger had to be insinuated between the pons and the tumour to get it away." This remarkable event occurred on November 19th 1894. Cushing was later of the opinion that the tumour was a meningioma [2]. The first true VS was removed by Annandale from a pregnant woman, who subsequently gave birth to a healthy baby [3]. This operation was performed on May 3rd 1895. These two operations can be regarded as successful if isolated first attempts. The first person to produce a series with decent results was Cushing who in 1917 had operated 30 cases with a mortality of 15.4% [2]. Cushing opened with a broad bilateral posterior fossa approach with a T shaped incision. He also performed an intracapsular removal. Dandy opted for a unilateral approach, reducing the time of the surgery and aimed at total tumour removal [4]. This became the accepted method and other famous surgeons including Olivecrona in Stockholm built on it. He operated on 349 patients with an operative mortality of 19.2% [5]. The great majority of the deaths were caused by damage to the pons. Atkinson pointed out that most pontine injury resulted from damage to the anterior inferior cerebellar artery. For our purposes, this era while

---

This chapter is also contributed by Erling Myrseth.

J.C. Ganz, *Gamma Knife Neurosurgery*,
DOI 10.1007/978-3-7091-0343-2_13, © Springer-Verlag/Wien 2011

producing impressive achievements has little relevance for current practice, which has a superior technology available for diagnosis, therapy and follow-up.

The second period of the development developed gradually through the 1970s to the 1990s. It involved the introduction of the operating microscope, bi-polar diathermy and the application of computerised imaging, first CT and later MRI. Monitoring of nerve function during surgery was introduced. In addition, other sophistications were employed including standardised audiometry and the introduction of semi-quantitative scales to register facial and hearing function before and after surgery. A comprehensive review of the existing literature published in 1991 documented a tumour removal in 95–99% of cases [6]. There were minor variations in removal percentage related to the technique of surgery. The authors advised choice of operation was not critical and was up to the surgeon.

Debates About Function After Treatment

This second period has been characterised by debates about post operative function especially facial palsy and retained hearing. Loss of function is no longer acceptable.

Facial Nerve Function

This has come to be reported in a standard way using the House Brackman Scale [7] as shown in Table 13.1.

Table 13.1 House Brackman grading system

Grade	Features
1	Normal symmetrical function in all areas
2	Slight weakness noticeable only on close inspection Complete eye closure with minimal effort Slight asymmetry of smile with maximal effort Synkinesis barely noticeable, contracture, or spasm absent
3	Obvious weakness, but not disfiguring. May not be able to lift eyebrow. Complete eye closure and strong but asymmetrical mouth movement with maximal effort. Obvious, but not disfiguring synkinesis, mass movement or spasm
4	Obvious disfiguring weakness. Inability to lift brow. Incomplete eye closure and asymmetry of mouth with maximal effort. Severe synkinesis, mass movement, spasm
5	Motion barely perceptible. Incomplete eye closure, slight movement corner mouth. Synkinesis, contracture, and spasm usually absent

Table 13.2 Koos grading of vestibular schwannomas

Grade	Definition
1	Intracanalicular
2	Tumour in the cerebello-pontine angle but not reaching the pons
3	Tumour reaching the pons, perhaps deforming it but not shifting it
4	Tumour deforming the pons and shifting the fourth ventricle

Sometimes facial nerve preservation is documented in terms of anatomical continuity, not function [6]. However, with time it has become usual to report facial nerve function as demonstrated in a distinguished paper published in October 2006 [8]. The House Brackman Grades 1 and 2 are classified as excellent and Grade 3 as good. Calling grade 3 a good result might be questionable to some. The paper reports 59% Grades 1 and 2, 2 weeks after surgery and Grade 3 in 16%. At 1 year the facial function was Grades 1–3 in 81%. However, there is no mention of the distribution between these grades. Moreover, the well known relationship between tumour volume and permanent facial palsy is confirmed. However, the facial palsy rate is not reported in respect of tumour volume group by group. A more recent paper from Japan reports that only Grades 1 and 2 are good results, which is more reasonable [9]. This paper is published in 2003 and is a meta-analysis of the treatment of various groups of patients including 5,005 who received microsurgery through different approaches. In the vast majority of series there was 93% total removal or more. Poor facial function was recorded in an average of 13% of cases with a range of 5–34%. The average risk of poor facial function for small to medium tumours was 10% with a range of 1–20%. Their small to medium roughly correspond to Koos grades 1–3 (see Table 13.2), The findings of these three major papers are described in slightly more detail than usual to underline how difficult it can be to interpret the significance of reporting for this particular condition. The feature most consistently associated with permanent loss of facial function after microsurgery is tumour volume [10–14]. Another feature associated with a poor result is a cystic tumour [12].

Intracanalicular tumours are a special sub-group that have become familiar with the increasing awareness, and early diagnosis of these lesions together with a proportion of incidentally found tumours during an MR examination for something else. Modern rates of facial preservation (House Brackman Grades 1–2) vary between 90 and 100% for the retrosigmoid approach and 72–98.9% for the middle fossa approach [12]. These differences are not statistically significant.

Preservation of Hearing After Surgery

In 1992 it could be stated that a major problem with hearing preservation was the small number of patients with useful pre-operative hearing [10, 15–18]. A changing

Table 13.3 Gardner Robertson grading of hearing

Grade	Description	Pure tone audiogram (dB)	Speech discrimination
1	Good, excellent	0–30	70–100
2	Serviceable	31–50	50–69
3	Non-serviceable	51–90	5–49
4	Poor	90–100	1–4
5	None	0	

world and improving technology has produced papers covering microsurgery aimed at retaining hearing in a substantially larger proportion of the total population of vestibular schwannomas presenting for treatment [13, 19]. One paper describes the intimate relationship between the tumour and the cochlear nerve even with smaller tumours [20]. The difficulty in retaining hearing has been attributed to this.

In addition to the technical surgical difficulties, the reporting of hearing preservation has been dogged by inconsistency. Today the preservation of hearing has been codified and the most popular grading system in current use is that of Gardner and Robertson [21]. It is shown in Table 13.3. The Gardner Robertson classification is essential. It is shown for this parameter also that there is a consistent relationship between tumour volume and post-operative hearing deterioration [18, 19, 22–24]. Moreover, the percentage of hearing retention in modern series is consistently moving in the direction of 50% for small tumours [19, 24–28].

Intracanalicular tumours can be considered here too as a separate subgroup as in the case of preservation of facial nerve function. Serviceable hearing preservation has been recorded between 12 and 57% for the retrosigmoid approach. On the other hand serviceable hearing is preserved between 38 and 66% for the middle fossa approach. These differences are not statistically significant.

Unilateral Vestibular Schwannomas: Gamma Knife Neurosurgery

Gamma Knife and Vestibular Schwannomas

As with microsurgery, Gamma Knife radiosurgery has had to develop and become more sophisticated over the 30 years since it was introduced for the treatment of this condition [29]. At the start it was usual to say that Gamma Knife neurosurgery was appropriate for the treatment of patients who would be at high risk for surgery, of advanced age or who refuse open surgery for whatever reason [6]. More recent publications that there is support for the use of the Gamma Knife as the primary treatment of VSs up to a certain size [30, 31]. There would be broad agreement that Koos Grades 1, 2 and even 3 can be safely treated with the Gamma Knife. This leaves Grade 4 as the continuing province of the surgeon [31]. This in fact may raise a dilemma for surgeons trying to perform radical surgery with total tumour removal of Grade 4 tumours. The increasing use of radiosurgery for smaller tumours makes it difficult for the tyro surgeon to learn his/her trade on the easier lesions. There is a risk that this competence may diminish in the future. This is a worry perceived by others [32]. However, as will be discussed later, there is a way round this problem.

The Early Days

VS was one of the original Gamma Knife indications basing target definition on metrizamide cisternography and then CT. The dose planning was necessarily primitive compared with the current dose-planning software. Yet the results were surprisingly good. Fourteen patients were treated with tumours varying from 7 to 30 mm in diameter. They received by modern standards the very high prescription dose of 25–35 Gy. Five of the fourteen patients suffered transient facial palsies. Four tumours retained some hearing. In 1979, one patient required a second irradiation. All tumours were controlled. The results were outstanding seen against the backdrop of what could be achieved with surgery in 1979.

The next step forward was the publication of a series of VSs from Pittsburgh. The material was very important because of its simple logical presentation and its transparent honesty with regard to complications. The Pittsburgh group were using a new machine with bigger collimators and they initially used relatively few large collimators [33] and a prescription dose of 20Gy which is high by modern standards [34]. In consequence they were seeing a high frequency of facial and trigeminal neuropathies [35]. In this they were deviating little from the then known published patterns of treatment. What was important was that they firstly published their complications and then set about adjusting their methodology until the complications stopped. The publication of this experience was immensely useful to other Gamma Knife users. At that time it must also be remembered that the dose planning software was a great deal less sophisticated than that available to us today. These initial difficulties are mentioned to illustrate that radiosurgery like microsurgery was travelling along a learning curve in the 1980s and 1990s.

Current Gamma Knife Treatment

The selection of patients for treatment is a somewhat complex process. The optimal situation is once again that these patients are managed by a team, this time consisting of an otolaryngologist, a neurosurgeon, a Gamma Knife surgeon and a neuroradiologist. The primary referral will usually be to the otolaryngologist. The decisions for any given case may be wait and see, microsurgery, radiosurgery. The rationale behind these discussions may be deferred until later in the chapter.

The current section takes up when the patient has been accepted for Gamma Knife treatment. The procedure then enters a series of well known stages.

Information

The patient is informed that the Gamma Knife will not improve any symptoms and that its purpose is to prevent clinical deterioration and to prevent the tumour from becoming a source of risk. He/She is further informed that there is with modern treatment a very small perhaps 1–2% risk for a temporary slight (House Brackman Grade 2) facial palsy some months after treatment. Patients with useful hearing are informed that the treatment can damage the hearing but every effort will be made to avoid this. Tinnitus, vertigo, periaural pain, facial symptoms of numbness or tingling will not be reliably improved. The patient is informed that the advantages of radiosurgery are the short time in hospital, the short disruption to life and the low complication rate.

Preparation for Treatment

The frame is applied as usual. With the Gamma Knife Perfexion there is no particular need to be careful about frame placement. With the "C" model it is as well that the frame is as far over to the side of the tumour as possible and as far back as possible without the anterior post on the opposite side compressing the face.

Imaging

The patient will be sent to MRI. There are a few departments who prefer to add a CT to the examination series [36, 37]. This has not been the authors' practice since we find the MR adequate as others have done before us [38, 39]. However, it must be respected that some users feel they trust the anatomical accuracy of the CT better than the MR. The preferred series with the MR is a gradient echo 3D series with Gadolinium. Then a 3D CISS series is taken after the contrast has been given for patients with smaller tumours and useful retained hearing. With this series the contrast makes the tumour slightly more translucent and highlights the position of the slightly darker nerves in the CSF in Koos 2 and 3 tumours. The CT with bony window accurately delineates the confines of the internal auditory meatus.

Dose Planning

Today, it is not enough to just produce a conformal dose that gives adequate cover of the tumour and adequate selectivity and a good gradient index (see Chap. 9). It is also necessary to attempt to protect several normal anatomical structures at risk, especially if it is intended to preserve hearing. Linskey in particular has drawn attention to the various structures that must be considered [39]. Apart from the cochlear nerve these include the cochlea itself. He points out that the inferior basal turn and the modiolus are particularly at risk. He also points out that the ventral and dorsal cochlear nuclei, lying at the surface of the pons and close to the tumour are also at risk as had been described by Paek [40]. Thus, it seems necessary to be aware that hearing may be threatened at a variety of different locations which include, the cochlear nerve, the cochlea (particularly its basal turn and modiolus) and the cochlear nuclei in the brainstem. It has become clear that a most important controllable variable in this situation is the prescription dose. The practice in our centre since 1988 has been to use a prescription dose of 12 Gy. Many others have used higher doses. By 1995 the tendency to lower dose was expressed at the 7th International Gamma Knife Meeting held in Hawaii, where there was a discussion session on low and high dose and the doses were 12 and 14 Gy respectively. Today most people are using 12–13 Gy with a noticeable improvement in the rate of complications, particularly hearing loss [37, 41–48].

Follow Up

It is recommended that patients are followed every 6 months with a 3D T1 weighted MRI with contrast. At the same time, in patients where hearing preservation is a concern an audiogram with pure tone and speech discrimination is registered and classified according to the Gardner Robertson grading system. These two examinations are repeated at 6 monthly intervals for 2 years. They are then repeated annually for 3 years and thereafter every 5 years. To the best of current knowledge there is no clear cut off point when there is no longer a risk for hearing so the audiograms should continue with the MR imaging for the life of the patient. Only then will we accumulate more precise knowledge on which to base the advice given to patients.

Tumour Control

Tumour control is achieved in over 90% of patients in series published during the last 5 years [38, 40, 41, 45, 49–62]. In many cases the cure rate is over 95% [38, 40, 41, 45, 49, 51, 52, 54, 55, 58, 59, 61, 63]. It is a common finding at 6 months after treatment that there is loss of central contrast enhancement which will subsequently resolve within the following 6 months or so. This is usually in indication that the tumour is under control, see Fig. 13.1.

Where the control rate was less than 95% there was usually a reason. These reasons included secondary treatment following surgery [57, 62], large tumours [50, 56, 60], repeat GKNS [53] and unconventional dosimetry [64]. It is important to bear in mind that VSs quite often swell up after GKNS, without this having

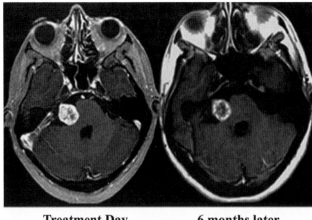

Treatment Day   6 months later

Fig. 13.1 This shows the same tumour with possible shrinkage at 6 months. A more striking finding is the loss of central contrast enhancement suggesting a good result

clinical significance or requiring treatment. The most comprehensive documentation of this phenomenon was made by Nagano et al [65] who recorded a transient increase in tumour volume in 74% of patients. This high figure reflects the method of measuring tumour volume. In stead of using the measurements available within in a standard MR unit the images were imported into the dose-planning software permitting precise volume measurements. Volume measurements are more sensitive and accurate than tumour size assessments based on diameters. These volume increases were associated with facial symptoms in the form of facial spasms or dysesthesias. The trigeminal symptoms were invariably associated with contact between the tumour and the nerve. They resolved when the tumour volume reduced again. In no case was this volume increase a cause for extra treatment of anything except the symptoms. The awareness of this volume increase is important for GK users who are informing patients and referring physicians.

Possible Complications and Problems

Facial Palsy

In recent series, preservation of facial nerve function after Gamma Knife surgery is found in between 95 and 100% of cases [38, 40, 41, 46, 49–51, 54, 55, 57, 66–71]. In practically all instances where there was a facial nerve deficit it was transient. Where the deficit was more than 1% of patients the most probable explanation was either a large volume [69] or the material while published recently included patients treated with an earlier form of dose-planning software [70]. Moreover, in the few cases where facial palsy did occur, it was nearly always transient [38, 66, 71]. These results compare more than favourably with the results of microsurgery described above.

There is a necessary tendency within the radiosurgery community to strive for ever more sophisticated imaging and dose planning to perfect the distribution of the radiation dose and minimise the dose outside the target in unwanted places. Nonetheless, in one series of 132 patients with VS, followed for a minimum of 2 years, eight suffered adverse radiation effects (AREs) [72]. Of these seven suffered facial numbness which persisted in 3 cases. Two patients had transient House Brackman grade 2 pareses. All these patients together with one asymptomatic patient had an increased T2 signal in the adjacent brainstem. All the patients received the same prescription dose of 12 Gy. The occurrence of the AREs were NOT related to the total volume of the tumours. This has relevance for the dosimetry mentioned in the next section. It may also reflect variations in individual radiosensitivity which is a parameter for which at present there is no useful test.

Trigeminal Dysfunction

Trigeminal symptoms, mainly numbness but occasionally dysesthesia or neuralgia were noted in 0–12% of patients [38, 41, 42, 51, 52, 57, 60, 61, 63, 67, 69, 73]. In a number of series a relationship is shown between tumour volume and the persistence of trigeminal symptoms [42, 61, 63]. There is no current explanation for the variation in trigeminal symptoms reported in different series.

Hearing Loss

There has been a growing tendency for hearing to be preserved in 50% of cases or more in recently reported series [30, 38, 40–42, 50–52, 54, 55, 60, 61, 63, 66–68, 71, 74–77]. The range in these series is 50–92.3%. However, in a number of papers the authors merely report the maintenance of a given Gardner Robertson grade, irrespective of whether the hearing is useful or not. The results clearly indicate how well damage to hearing can now be avoided. However, for the present purpose we shall concentrate on the preservation of useful hearing (Gardner Robertson grades 1 and 2). The first thing that must be acknowledged is that preservation of hearing has been more difficult to achieve than preservation of the function of the Vth and VIIth nerves.

The possible reasons for the preferential vulnerability of hearing function are many. Some of what follows will necessarily be speculative as there are lacunae in our understanding. Firstly, the vestibular cochlear nerve has an unusual anatomical arrangement in that oligodendroglia extend along it much further than for other nerve, reaching as far as the opening to the internal auditory meatus. While this part of the nerve is not the portion most at risk in the early stages of a vestibular schwannoma, this difference may nonetheless be of significance. It is a biological parameter, the significance of which is currently not known. Another difference related to hearing anatomy concerns the arterial supply to the cochlea which comes exclusively from the labyrinthine artery. This is a branch usually of the anterior inferior cerebellar artery but occasionally the basilar artery. The point is that the cochlea receives its blood supply only from the basilar or its branches. The rest of the labyrinth receives its blood supply not only from the labyrinthine artery but form the stylomastoid branch of the posterior auricular branch of the external carotid artery. In other words the semicircular canals have a double blood supply while the cochlea has a single supply. The facial and trigeminal nerves also have blood supply from the internal and external circulations. The subject of ischaemia in relation to radiation damage is a closed subject. The most comprehensive monograph on the subject of radiation pathology currently available does not have the word ischaemia (or ischemia) in the index [78]. It is emphasised that while hypoxia has a protective effect against radiation damage, ischaemia is a very different pathophysiological situation form hypoxia and at present little is know about it. Thus, while speculative, the single blood supply could be relevant in this situation in terms of the relative ease with which hearing may be lost following treatment of vestibular schwannomas.

This is enough speculation. We must return to the topic of how to adjust the dose plan to obtain an optimal result. The Marseille group have reported 77% retained useful hearing in patients with a pre-operative Grade 1 function. They emphasise moreover that the presence of tinnitus improves the chances of retained useful hearing [30, 75]. Table 13.4 shows the preservation of useful hearing in series published during the last 5 years. In the Delsanti paper [74] the tumours were cystic, which is a condition known to be associated with worse results. It is necessary to consider the structures other than the cochlear nerve which could produce hearing loss.

Cochlear Nuclei

In the Paek paper the authors consider the cochlear nuclei. They point out the mean dose to the cochlear nuclei was 11.1 Gy where hearing was lost and 6.9 Gy where

Table 13.4 Hearing preservation results

Hearing preservation last 5 years	
Reference	Preserved useful hearing
Chopra et al. [41]	74.0
Chung et al. [38]	60.0
Delsanti et al. [74]	53.0
Flickinger et al. [42]	78.6
Fukuoka et al. [50]	71.0
Gabert et al. [75]	60.0
Hasegawa et al. [66]	67.6
Lunsford et al. [54]	78.6
Massager et al. [76]	65.0
Niranjan et al. [55]	64.5
Paek et al. [40]	52.0
Régis et al. [30]	60.0
Roche et al. [60]	60.0

hearing was preserved [40]. However, the authors express some surprise at the degree of the poor result. They note the results in series with similar dosimetry and state "the hearing rate preservation after GK SRS using our current protocol is unexpectedly poor and difficult to explain". Nonetheless, they did observe a relationship between increasing volume in the internal auditory meatus with loss of hearing, although statistical significance was not demonstrated. The Marseille group could not confirm this finding [79] as with their dosimetry, the dose to the brain stem never reached the levels noted in the Paek paper.

Cochlea

The subject of the cochlea and its dosimetry has been reviewed three times by Linskey [39, 80, 81], and examined by the Brussels group [76, 82] and the Marseille Group [79]. There seems to be broad agreement between these writers and the reviewers of the most recent Marseille paper [79] that the desirable dose to the cochlea should not exceed 4 Gy. Linskey is of the opinion that special care should be taken with the modiolus and basal turn of the cochlea [39].

The Intrameatal Tumour Volume

The Brussels group found a relationship between the volume of tumour within the meatus and incidence of hearing deterioration [76]. In addition they found a relationship between the integral dose to that part of the tumour and the development of hearing loss. These findings were specifically not confirmed by the Marseille group [79]. They discuss the possibility that this may be due to variations in the populations in the two studies. However, they also point out that in their material the lateral extension of the tumour in the internal auditory meatus correlated with deterioration of hearing. The variation in lateral extension is illustrated in Fig. 13.2. This might well be relevant for the findings in the Brussels study but expressed in a different way.

Other Symptomatic Problems and Occasional Complications

Tinnitus is a common symptom with a VS. In the past it has been regarded with a kind of therapeutic nihilism. It is generally accepted that the effects of GKNS on tinnitus is totally unpredictable and in most cases the symptom will remain unchanged. The management of the symptom will fall to the otolaryngologist who is responsible for following up the patient. Since the origin of tinnitus is somewhere between the dorsal cochlear nucleus and the auditory cortex, (as indicated on PET scans) it is hardly surprising that a treatment aimed at an extra axial target will have no effect on this symptom. The Gamma Knife user should explain that the Gamma Knife will have no effect but should refrain from indulging

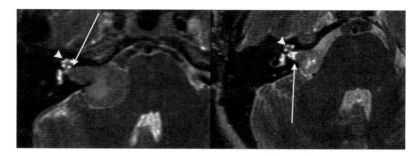

Fig. 13.2 Two MR images are shown of different 2 small VSs. In the image on the left the tumour has grown as far laterally as possible in the internal auditory meatus. On the right the tumour extends less far laterally leaving space between it and the cochlea. The cochlea is indicated by the *arrow head* and the lateral extension of the tumour by the *white arrow*

in negative comments about a symptom which will be the responsibility of another colleague. Various treatments exist, even if no sure fire simple method is yet available.

Hydrocephalus is associated with VSs. It is however uncommon being reported between 1 and 5% in some recent large series [50, 83, 84]. Awareness of the possibility is the most important aspect of avoiding this rare complication. It is not certain whether GKNS increases the natural tendency for patients with VSs to develop hydrocephalus.

Ataxia in the context of VSs is associated with larger tumours unsuitable for radiosurgery or indeed as a consequence of the surgery of such tumours.

Vertigo is often associated with VSs. To date there is no evidence that the Gamma Knife improves vertigo. There are even reported cases of vertigo starting up first after Gamma Knife treatment [51, 85, 86]. In one paper where there were 11 patients with vertigo, three had persistent intermittent vertigo after treatment. The point about vertigo is its effect on quality of life (QOL).

Quality of Life

During the last thirty years a revolution has taken place in respect to quality of life to be expected after treatment of a VS. In the 1960s surgeons were concerned with saving life. Ataxia and severe facial palsies were the prices the patient had to pay. Today facial palsy effectively is a thing of the past with GKNS used in association with modern computerised imaging techniques. Hearing retention has improved greatly. Recent work from Haukleand Hospital in Bergen has shown that today, one of the most important causes of reduced QOL is persistent vertigo [87]. In this context, the Gamma Knife has no certain effect. The treatment of vertigo today is with medicines and no universally effective medicament exists. The other common symptom which can affect QOL today is tinnitus and that has been mentioned above.

Gamma Knife or Microsurgery

The following remarks are limited to Koos 1–3 tumours. There are five retrospective case controlled series comparing surgical resection and GKNS [70, 88–91]. These studies found that GKNS had improved VIIth and VIIIth nerve results. Moreover, patients returned to work faster and the cost of GKNS was lower. In addition there are two level 2 prospective cohort studies of adult patients with unilateral VSs, less than 3 cm in diameter who were allocated to either a microsurgery or GKNS arm [58, 63]. GKNS was superior in terms of facial and hearing function. Patients who underwent microsurgery had a decline in physical functioning from 3 months to a year after treatment. It is contended that for VSs of the size under advisement, GKNS may now be considered the treatment of choice.

Intracanalicular Vestibular Schwannomas

These may be observed or treated. It is taken as a given that the only appropriate treatment on offer would be GKNS, using the dosimetry and imaging and tissue protecting practises outlined in this chapter. The decision to treat must be considered in relation to the patient's post-treatment quality of life. Various factors will affect the decision, and it is one to which no simple consensus currently applies.

It is clear that tinnitus and vertigo while of importance to QOL will not be affected by the treatment and thus should not be factors in the decision making process. Since the facial nerve can be expected to suffer no dysfunction with modern treatment methods, it is not a factor in the decision making process. Thus, in effect the decision boils down to the preservation of hearing with a wait and see policy and an active treatment policy.

The Marseille group have evidence to support the notion that avoiding treatment is associated with tumour growth and hearing loss. Moreover, they indicate that hearing loss can occur in the absence of tumour growth [31]. The Pittsburgh group are also convinced protagonists for the treatment of intracanalicular tumours early to avoid hearing deterioration [42, 55, 92]. The Brussels group also shares this view [76]. Yamakami et al. are less certain, but suggest observation must be followed with frequent clinical and MR examinations. Bakkouri et al. also favour a conservative wait and see policy [93]. Our own group has suggested a conservative approach to non-growing tumours less than 20 mm in diameter which of course included intracanalicular tumours [94].

It is suggested on the basis of the material described above that this approach could be the subject of a modification. In view of the currently generally agreed sensitivity of the cochlea to radiation damage, with intracanalicular tumours the dose to this structure must not exceed 4 Gy. For those patients with intracanalicular tumours which do not reach the lateral extent of the internal meatus it is a simple matter to import non stereotactic MR images into the Gamma Knife treatment planning system. It would then be easy to design a dose plan and assess if adequate tumour cover could be achieved while at the same time keeping the dose to the cochlea modiolus and basal turn at or below 4 Gy. Patients in whom this could be achieved, who had useful hearing (Gardner Robertson Grades 1 or 2) could then be offered GKNS on the grounds that the existing evidence indicates this would be the best chance for them to retain their pre-treatment level of hearing.

Large Vestibular Schwannomas

It has already been noted that larger VSs have a lower control rate following GKNS [50, 56, 60]. Thus, surgery will remain a component of the management of these tumours. Since the time of Dandy most surgeons have advocated radical removal of these tumours. This is certainly a view which is still current amongst distinguished colleagues [8, 95]. However, of recent years this view has been questioned. The first to consider a change of direction was Charles Drake of London Ontario. His aim was to reduce the inevitable frequency of facial nerve palsy which followed the surgery of tumours in excess of 3 cm in diameter [96]. Dr. Drake was no proponent of the increased use of radiosurgery, but his paper reports improved facial nerve function after microsurgery for larger tumours. The matter of facial nerve function was further questioned following the publication of the most recent results from one of the world's best centres for the treatment of VSs [8]. Even with the expertise available at this centre good or excellent results were obtained in only 81% of patients at 1 year. Moreover, a good result was viewed as a House Brackman Grade III, which is not a description of Grade III with which everyone would agree. Nor is this result clarified in terms of tumour size but applies to the whole series. There is no need to belabour this point but clearly this paper underlines the fact that even in the best hands the risk of a poor facial result after radical surgery for a large tumour remains high even in the most expert hands. It was suggested that maybe we should consider a policy of subtotal or intracapsular removal as Drake suggested and follow this up with GKNS some months after the surgery [97]. It was also indicated that VSs shrink over the early months after intracapsular operations thus facilitating safer GKNS [97]. The first to suggest a two stage treatment with microsurgery followed by GKNS was Iwai et al from Osaka [98]. Their tumours were treated with intracapsular or subtotal removal. The House Brackman Grade I to II for facial function with tumours with a mean maximum diameter of over 4 cm was 85.7%. This is a great improvement and the management paradigm received support from another centre. The most recent report is from the Marseille group where a two stage treatment was planned from the start. There were only eight patients but 7 (87.5%) retained Grades 1 to 2 and the remaining patient retained grade III [99].

It would seem from the material outlined in this subsection that large tumours may advantageously be treated by a planned two stage procedure with intracapsular microsurgery followed after a few months by GKNS. It is contended that this should be the treatment of the future. It has a further advantage. It was mentioned above that good results with the microsurgery of large tumours required that the trainee surgeon becomes familiar with smaller tumours which are easier to operate. However, with the ever growing popularity of GKNS for smaller VSs, this experience is less and less available. If the surgeon returns to the intracapsular operation, this lack of surgical experience is less of a problem, since the intracapsular procedure is quite a bit simpler. This would suit the available experience of the neurosurgeon of the future very well.

Patients with Bilateral Tumours

Neurofibromatosis 2

Bilateral tumours are usually a component of neurofibromatosis 2, shortened hereafter to NF2. These tumours are difficult in a variety of ways. Firstly, because they are bilateral the consequences for hearing are far more important than with unilateral tumours. Secondly, they often have a tougher consistency, making conventional surgery more difficult. Thirdly, the nerves whose function should be preserved are frequently not separated from the tumour by a clear anatomical plane [100]. This places the facial and acoustic nerves at risk both during open surgery and following Gamma Knife treatment.

It should further be noted that NF2 is not a single entity but consists of differing variations with dissimilar prognoses. The first type of NF2 was described by Wishart in 1822 [101]. This form is aggressive, occurs at a younger age and is associated with multiple brain and spinal cord tumours. Hearing is lost early. Then there is the form of Feiling and Gardner described in 1920 and 1930 respectively [101]. This characteristically starts in the third to fourth decade and runs a milder course often without associated brain and spinal cord tumours. Hearing may be retained until late in life. A third type was described by Lee and Abbott. This type can present at a variable age. It is characterised by early morbidity from associated tumours.

Samii suggests that radiosurgery is not an optimal primary treatment for NF2 VSs. This is based on his extensive experience with 165 patients [100]. This is sensible but then neither is microsurgery an optimal treatment. In this condition there is to date no optimal primary treatment. The Sheffield group reported their experience with 96 patients and 123 treatments GKNS [102]. Overall growth control was around 50% at 8 years. While not all of these required repeat treatment at 8 years this figure is a measure of the difficulty of treating these tumours. In addition the more severe phenotypes did less well. Five percent had persisting facial palsy and 2% had trigeminal neuropathies. The dosimetry used was similar to that reported elsewhere in this chapter, with a mean of 13.4 Gy. Thirty eight percent preserved hearing, 42% had some decrease in grade and 20% became totally deaf. This is not as good as with unilateral VSs but the results are good in terms of the results obtained with surgery.

These patients are so complex, that it is not possible to give a recommendation for treatment that covers all patients. They must be treated on a case by case basis.

Addendum Related to Dosimetry

This chapter has been at pains to point out that precise dosimetry with specific parameters are necessary to obtain the excellent results which have recently been recorded. There is for the Gamma Knife user a remaining dilemma. The prescription dose should ideally cover 100% of the target. If it does so it will automatically have a conformity index close to the perfect unity. There should be a high degree of selectivity. The gradient index should be as low as possible. However, to spare the surrounding tissues, in particular to keep the dose to the cochlea as low as possible, some degree of compromise is necessary between an optimal dose plan which covers the 100% of the tumour volume with excellent therapeutic indices and a suboptimal dose plan which, while providing good values of indices is less than optimal in order to spare the normal anatomy. The details of this compromise and which limits are acceptable are at present not defined. Merely as an example, we have endeavoured to keep the prescription dose covering 95% of the tumour with an inverse selectivity of 1.25 or less and a gradient index of less than 3. However, we are all too aware that this is a practice of convenience for which there is no scientific data to lend support or to confute.

References

1. Balance C. Some points in the surgery of the brain and its membranes. London. MacMillan & Co.: pp 276; 1907
2. Cushing H. Tumor of the nervus acousticus and the syndrome of the cerebellopontine angle. Philadelphia. WB Saunders Edit; 1917
3. Ramsden RT. Annandale's case, one hundred years on a brilliant surgical result, the first recorded: in Sterkers JMCR. Sterkers O (eds) Acoustic Neuroma and Skull Base Surgery. Amsterdam, New York. Kugler Publications: pp 7–10; 1996
4. Dandy W. An operation for the total removal of cerebello-pontine angle (acoustic tumors). Surg Gynecol Obstet 41: 129–148; 1928
5. Olivecrona G. Acoustic tumors. J Neurosurg 26: 6–13; 1967
6. Moskowitz N, Long DM. Acoustic neurinomas. Historical review of a century of operative series. Neurosurgery Quarterly 1: 2–18; 1991
7. House JW, Brackmann DE. Facial nerve grading system. Otolaryngol Head Neck Surg 93(2): 146–147; 1985
8. Samii M, Gerganov V, Samii A. Improved preservation of hearing and facial nerve function in vestibular schwannoma surgery via the retrosigmoid approach in a series of 200 patients. J Neurosurg 105: 527–535; 2006
9. Yamakami I, Uchino Y, Kobayashi E, Yamaura A. Conservative management, gamma-knife radiosurgery, and microsurgery for acoustic neurinomas: a systematic review of outcome and risk of three therapeutic options. Neurol Res 25(7): 682–690; 2003
10. Arriaga MA, Chen DA, Fukushima T. Individualizing hearing preservation in acoustic neuroma surgery. Laryngoscope 107(8): 1043–1047; 1997

11. Darwish BS, Bird PA, Goodisson DW, Bonkowski JA, MacFarlane MR. Facial nerve function and hearing preservation after retrosigmoid excision of vestibular schwannoma: Christchurch Hospital experience with 97 patients. ANZ J Surg **75(10)**: 893–896; 2005

12. Noudel R, Ribeiro T, Roche P-H. Facial microsurgical treatment of intracanalicular vestibular schwannomas. Régis J, Roche P-H (eds) Modern Management of Acoustic Neuromas. Basel, Karger. Prog Neurol Surg **21**: pp 103–107; 2008

13. Shelton C, Brackmann DE, House WF, Hitselberger WE. Middle fossa acoustic tumor surgery: results in 106 cases. Laryngoscope **99(4)**: 405–408; 1989

14. Wiet RJ, Mamikoglu B, Odom L, Hoistad DL. Long-term results of the first 500 cases of acoustic neuroma surgery. Otolaryngol Head Neck Surg **124(6)**: 645–651; 2001

15. Cohen NL, Ransohoff J. Hearing preservation – posterior fossa approach. Otolaryngol Head Neck Surg **92(2)**: 176–183; 1984

16. Hinton AE, Ramsden RT, Lye RH, Dutton JE. Criteria for hearing preservation in acoustic schwannoma surgery: the concept of useful hearing. J Laryngol Otol **106(6)**: 500–503; 1992

17. Moffat DA, da Cruz MJ, Baguley DM, Beynon GJ, Hardy DG. Hearing preservation in solitary vestibular schwannoma surgery using the retrosigmoid approach. Otolaryngol Head Neck Surg **121(6)**: 781–788; 1999

18. Rowed DW, Nedzelski JM. Hearing preservation in the removal of intracanalicular acoustic neuromas via the retrosigmoid approach. J Neurosurg **86(3)**: 456–461; 1997

19. Mohr G, Sade B, Dufour JJ, Rappaport JM. Preservation of hearing in patients undergoing microsurgery for vestibular schwannoma: degree of meatal filling. J Neurosurg **102(1)**: 1–5; 2005

20. Sekiya T, Iwabuchi T, Suzuki S, Hatayama T, Ishii M, Oda N. Failure to preserve hearing in acoustic neuroma surgery: experiences after introduction of MRI. No Shinkei Geka **17 (12)**: 1111–1117; 1989

21. Gardner G, Robertson JH. Hearing preservation in unilateral acoustic neuroma surgery. Ann Otol Rhinol Laryngol **97(1)**: 55–66; 1988

22. Baldwin DL, King TT, Morrison AW. Hearing conservation in acoustic neuroma surgery via the posterior fossa. J Laryngol Otol **104(6)**: 463–467; 1990

23. Dornhoffer JL, Helms J, Hoehmann DH. Hearing preservation in acoustic tumor surgery: results and prognostic factors. Laryngoscope **105(2)**: 184–187; 1995

24. Yang J, Grayeli AB, Barylyak R, Elgarem H. Functional outcome of retrosigmoid approach in vestibular schwannoma surgery. Acta Otolaryngol **128(8)**: 881–886; 2008

25. Levo H, Blomstedt G, Pyykko I. Is hearing preservation useful in vestibular schwannoma surgery? Ann Otol Rhinol Laryngol **111(5 Pt 1)**: 392–396; 2002

26. Maw AR, Coakham HB, Ayoub O, Butler SR. Hearing preservation and facial nerve function in vestibular schwannoma surgery. Clin Otolaryngol Allied Sci **28(3)**: 252–256; 2003

27. Shiobara R, Ohira T, Inoue Y, Kanzaki J, Kawase T. Extended middle cranial fossa approach for vestibular schwannoma: technical note and surgical results of 896 operations. Régis J, Roche P-H (eds) Modern Management of Acoustic Neuromas. Basel, Karger. Prog Neurol Surg **21**: 65–72; 2008

28. Yamakami I, Yoshinori H, Saeki N, Wada M, Oka N (2009) Hearing preservation and intraoperative auditory brainstem response and cochlear nerve compound action potential monitoring in the removal of small acoustic neurinoma via the retrosigmoid approach. J Neurol Neurosurg Psychiatry **80(2)**: 218–227

29. Hirsch A, Noren G, Anderson H. Audiologic findings after stereotactic radiosurgery in nine cases of acoustic neurinomas. Acta Otolaryngol **88(3–4)**: 155–160; 1979

30. Régis J, Tamura M, Delsanti C, Roche PH, Pellet W, Thomassin JM. Hearing preservation in patients with unilateral vestibular schwannoma after gamma knife surgery. Régis J, Roche P-H (eds) Modern Management of Acoustic Neuromas. Basel, Karger. Prog Neurol Surg **21**: 142–151; 2008

31. Roche PH, Soumare O, Thomassin JM, Régis J. The wait and see strategy for intracanalicular vestibular schwannomas. Régis J, Roche P-H (eds) Modern Management of Acoustic Neuromas. Basel, Karger. Prog Neurol Surg **21**: 83–88; 2008

32. Marouf R, Noudel R, Roche P-H. Facial nerve outcome after microsurgical resection of vestibular schwannoma. Régis J, Roche P-H (eds) Modern Management of Acoustic Neuromas. Basel, Karger. Prog Neurol Surg 21: pp 103–107; 2008

33. Ganz JC, Mathisen JR, Thorsen F, Backlund E-O. Acoustic neuromas: early results related to radiobiological variables. Lunsfor LD (ed) Stereotactic Radiosurgery Update. New York, Amsterdam. Elsevier: pp 359–364; 1992

34. Linskey ME, Lunsford LD, Flickinger JC. Radiosurgery for acoustic neurinomas: early experience. Neurosurgery **26(5)**: 736–744; 1990

35. Linskey ME, Lunsford LD, Flickinger JC, Kondziolka D. Stereotactic radiosurgery for acoustic tumors. Neurosurg Clin N Am **3(1)**: 191–205; 1992

36. Borden JA, Tsai JS, Mahajan A. Effect of subpixel magnetic resonance imaging shifts on radiosurgical dosimetry for vestibular schwannoma. J Neurosurg **97(5 Suppl)**: 445–449; 2002

37. Régis J, Tamura M, Wikler D, Porcheron D, Levrier O. Radiosurgery: operative technique, pitfalls and Tips. Régis J, Roche P-H (eds) Modern Management of Acoustic Neuromas. Basel, Karger. Prog Neurol Surg **21**: pp 54–64; 2008

38. Chung WY, Liu KD, Shiau CY, Wu HM, Wang LW, Guo WY, Ho DM, Pan DH. Gamma knife surgery for vestibular schwannoma: 10-year experience of 195 cases. J Neurosurg **102(Suppl)**: 87–96; 2005

39. Linskey ME. Hearing preservation in vestibular schwannoma stereotactic radiosurgery: what really matters? J Neurosurg **109**: 129–136; 2008

40. Paek SH, Chung HT, Jeong SS, Park CK, Kim CY, Kim JE, Kim DG, Jung HW. Hearing preservation after gamma knife stereotactic radiosurgery of vestibular schwannoma. Cancer **104(3)**: 580–590; 2005

41. Chopra R, Kondziolka D, Niranjan A, Lunsford LD, Flickinger JC. Long-term follow-up of acoustic schwannoma radiosurgery with marginal tumor doses of 12 to 13 Gy. Int J Radiat Oncol Biol Phys **68(3)**: 845–851; 2007

42. Flickinger JC, Kondziolka D, Niranjan A, Maitz A, Voynov G, Lunsford LD. Acoustic neuroma radiosurgery with marginal tumor doses of 12 to 13 Gy. Int J Radiat Oncol Biol Phys **60(1)**: 225–230; 2004

43. Flickinger JC, Kondziolka D, Pollock BE, Lunsford LD. Evolution in technique for vestibular schwannoma radiosurgery and effect on outcome. Int J Radiat Oncol Biol Phys **36(2)**: 275–280; 1996

44. Hirato M, Inoue H, Zama A, Ohye C, Shibazaki T, Andou Y. Gamma Knife radiosurgery for acoustic schwannoma: effects of low radiation dose and functional prognosis. Stereotact Funct Neurosurg **66(Suppl 1)**: 134–141; 1996

45. Hudgins WR, Antes KJ, Herbert MA, Weiner RL, DeSaloms JM, Stamos D, Barker JL, Echt GA, Nichols TD, Schwarz DE. Control of growth of vestibular schwannomas with low-dose Gamma Knife surgery. J Neurosurg **105(Suppl)**: 154–160; 2006

46. Inoue HK. Low-dose radiosurgery for large vestibular schwannomas: long-term results of functional preservation. J Neurosurg **102(Suppl)**: 111–113; 2005

47. Iwai Y, Yamanaka K, Shiotani M, Uyama T. Radiosurgery for acoustic neuromas: results of low-dose treatment. Neurosurgery **53(2)**: 282–287; 2003

48. Niranjan A, Lunsford LD, Flickinger JC, Maitz A, Kondziolka D. Dose reduction improves hearing preservation rates after intracanalicular acoustic tumor radiosurgery. Neurosurgery **45(4)**: 753–762; 1999

49. Dewan S, Noren G. Retreatment of vestibular schwannomas with Gamma Knife surgery. J Neurosurg **109(Suppl)**: 144–148; 2008

50. Fukuoka S, Takanashi M, Hojyo A, Konishi M, Tanaka C, Nakamura H Gamma knife radiosurgery for vestibular schwannomas Yamamoto M (ed) Japanese Experience with Gamma Knife Radiosurgery. Basel, Karger. Prog Neurol Surg **22**: 45–62; 2009
51. Hempel JM, Hempel E, Wowra B, Schichor CH, Muacevic A, Riederer A. Functional outcome after gamma knife treatment in vestibular schwannoma. Eur Arch Otorhinolaryngol **263(8)**: 714–718; 2006
52. Huang CF, Tu HT, Lo HK, Wang KL, Liu WS. Radiosurgery for vestibular schwannomas. J Chin Med Assoc **68(7)**: 315–320; 2005
53. Liscak R, Vladyka V, Urgosik D, Simonova G, Vymazal J. Repeated treatment of vestibular schwannomas after gamma knife radiosurgery. Acta Neurochir (Wien) **151(4)**: 317–324; 2009
54. Lunsford LD, Niranjan A, Flickinger JC, Maitz A, Kondziolka D. Radiosurgery of vestibular schwannomas: summary of experience in 829 cases. J Neurosurg **102(Suppl)**: 195–199; 2005
55. Niranjan A, Mathieu D, Flickinger JC, Kondziolka D, Lunsford LD. Hearing preservation after intracanalicular vestibular schwannoma radiosurgery. Neurosurgery **63(6)**: 1054–1062; 2008
56. Park CK, Jung HW, Kim JE, Son YJ, Paek SH, Kim DG. Therapeutic strategy for large vestibular schwannomas. J Neurooncol **77(2)**: 167–171; 2006
57. Pollock B.E., Link M.J. Vestibular schwannoma radiosurgery after previous surgical resection or stereotactic radiosurgery. Régis J, Roche P-H (eds) Modern Management of Acoustic Neuromas. Basel, Karger. Prog Neurol Surg **21**: 163–168; 2008
58. Pollock BE, Driscoll CL, Foote RL, Link MJ, Gorman DA, Bauch CD, Mandrekar JN, Krecke KN, Johnson CH. Patient outcomes after vestibular schwannoma management: a prospective comparison of microsurgical resection and stereotactic radiosurgery. Neurosurgery **59(1)**: 77–85; 2006
59. Régis J, Delsanti C, Roche PH, Thomassin JM, Pellet W. Functional outcomes of radiosurgical treatment of vestibular schwannomas: 1000 successive cases and review of the literature. Neurochirurgie **50(2–3 Pt 2)**: 301–311; 2004
60. Roche PH, Robitail S, Pellet W, Deveze A, Thomassin JM, Régis J. Results and indications of gamma knife radiosurgery for large vestibular schwannomas. Neurochirurgie **50(2–3 Pt 2)**: 377–382; 2004
61. Wowra B, Muacevic A, Jess-Hempen A, Hempel JM, Muller-Schunk S, Tonn JC. Outpatient gamma knife surgery for vestibular schwannoma: definition of the therapeutic profile based on a 10-year experience. J Neurosurg **102(Suppl)**: 114–118; 2005
62. Yang SY, Kim DG, Chung HT, Park SH, Paek SH, Jung HW. Evaluation of tumor response after gamma knife radiosurgery for residual vestibular schwannomas based on MRI morphological features. J Neurol Neurosurg Psychiatry **79(4)**: 431–436; 2008
63. Myrseth E, Møller P, Pedersen PH, Lund-Johansen M. Vestibular schwannoma: surgery or gamma knife radiosurgery? A prospective, nonrandomized study. Neurosurgery **64(4)**: 654–661; 2009
64. van Eck AT, Horstmann GA. Increased preservation of functional hearing after gamma knife surgery for vestibular schwannoma. J Neurosurg **102(Suppl)**: 204–206; 2005
65. Nagano O, Higuchi Y, Serizawa T, Ono J, Matsuda S, Yamakami I, Saeki N. Transient expansion of vestibular schwannoma following stereotactic radiosurgery. J Neurosurg **109**: 811–816; 2008
66. Hasegawa T, Fujitani S, Katsumata S, Kida Y, Yoshimoto M, Koike J. Stereotactic radiosurgery for vestibular schwannomas: analysis of 317 patients followed more than 5 years. Neurosurgery **57(2)**: 257–265; 2005
67. Hayashi M, Ochiai T, Nakaya K, Chernov M, Tamura N, Maruyama T, Yomo S, Izawa M, Hori T, Takakura K, Régis J. Current treatment strategy for vestibular schwannoma: image-guided robotic microradiosurgery. J Neurosurg **105(Suppl)**: 5–11; 2006
68. Iwai Y, Yamanaka K, Kubo T, Aiba T. Gamma knife radiosurgery for intracanalicular acoustic neuromas. J Clin Neurosci **15(9)**: 993–997; 2008

69. Liu D, Xu D, Zhang Z, Zhang Y, Zheng L. Long-term outcomes after Gamma Knife surgery for vestibular schwannomas: a 10-year experience. J Neurosurg **105(Suppl)**: 149–153; 2006
70. Myrseth E, Moller P, Pedersen PH, Vassbotn FS, Wentzel-Larsen T, Lund-Johansen M. Vestibular schwannomas: clinical results and quality of life after microsurgery or gamma knife radiosurgery. Neurosurgery **56(5)**: 927–935; 2005
71. Régis J, Roche PH, Delsanti C, Thomassin JM, Ouaknine M, Gabert K, Pellet W. Modern management of vestibular schwannomas. Szeifert GT, Kondziolka D, Levivier M, Lunsford LD (eds) Radiosurgery and Pathological Fundamentals. Basel, Karger. Prog Neurol Surg **20**: 129–141; 2007
72. Ganz JC, Reda WA, Abdelkarim K. Adverse radiation effects after Gamma Knife Surgery in relation to dose and volume. Acta Neurochir **151**: 9–19; 2009
73. Tamura M, Murata N, Hayashi M, Roche PH, Régis J. Facial nerve function insufficiency after radiosurgery versus microsurgery. Régis J, Roche P-H (eds) Modern Management of Acoustic Neuromas. Basel, Karger. Prog Neurol Surg **21**: 108–118; 2008
74. Delsanti C, Régis J. Cystic vestibular schwannomas. Neurochirurgie **50(2–3 Pt 2)**: 401–406; 2004
75. Gabert K, Régis J, Delsanti C, Roche PH, Facon F, Tamura M, Pellet W, Thomassin JM. Preserving hearing function after Gamma Knife radiosurgery for unilateral vestibular schwannoma. Neurochirurgie **50(2–3 Pt 2)**: 350–357; 2004
76. Massager N, Nissim O, Delbrouck C, Devriendt D, David P, Desmedt F, Wikler D, Hassid S, Brotchi J, Levivier M. Role of intracanalicular volumetric and dosimetric parameters on hearing preservation after vestibular schwannoma radiosurgery. Int J Radiat Oncol Biol Phys **64(5)**: 1331–1340; 2006
77. Yang I, Aranda D, Han SJ, Chennupati S, Sughrue ME, Cheung SW, Pitts LH, Parsa AT. Hearing preservation after stereotactic radiosurgery for vestibular schwannoma: a systematic review. J Clin Neurosci **16(6)**: 742–747; 2009
78. Fajardo LF, Berthrong M, Anderson ME. Radiation Pathology. Oxford. Oxford University Press; 2001
79. Tamura M, Carron R, Yomo S, Arkha Y, Muraciolle X, Porcheron D, Thomassin JM, Roche PH, Régis J. Hearing preservation after gamma knife radiosurgery for vestibular schwannomas presenting with high-level hearing. Neurosurgery **64(2)**: 289–296; 2009
80. Linskey ME, Johnstone PA, O'Leary M, Goetsch S. Radiation exposure of normal temporal bone structures during stereotactically guided gamma knife surgery for vestibular schwannomas. J Neurosurg **98(4)**: 800–806; 2003
81. Linskey ME, Johnstone PA. Radiation tolerance of normal temporal bone structures: implications for gamma knife stereotactic radiosurgery. Int J Radiat Oncol Biol Phys **57(1)**: 196–200; 2003
82. Massager N, Nissim O, Delbrouck C, Delpierre I, Devriendt D, Desmedt F, Wikler D, Brotchi J, Levivier M. Irradiation of cochlear structures during vestibular schwannoma radiosurgery and associated hearing outcome. J Neurosurg **107(4)**: 733–739; 2007
83. Roche PH, Ribeiro T, Soumare O, Robitail S, Pellet W, Régis J. Hydrocephalus and vestibular schwannomas treated by Gamma Knife radiosurgery. Neurochirurgie **50(2–3 Pt 2)**: 345–349; 2004
84. Unger F, Walch C, Schrottner O, Eustacchio S, Sutter B, Pendl G. Cranial nerve preservation after radiosurgery of vestibular schwannomas. Acta Neurochir Suppl **84**: 77–83; 2002
85. Bertalanffy A, Dietrich W, Aichholzer M, Brix R, Ertl A, Heimberger K, Kitz K. Gamma knife radiosurgery of acoustic neurinomas. Acta Neurochir **143(7)**: 689–695; 2001
86. Vermeulen S, Young R, Posewitz A, Grimm P, Blasko J, Kohler E, Raisis J. Stereotactic radiosurgery toxicity in the treatment of intracanalicular acoustic neuromas: the Seattle Northwest gamma knife experience. Stereotact Funct Neurosurg **70(Suppl 1)**: 80–87; 1998
87. Myrseth E, Møller P, Wentzel-Larsen T, Goplen F, Lund-Johansen M. Untreated vestibular schwannomas: vertigo is a powerful predictor for health-related quality of life. Neurosurgery **59(1)**: 67–76; 2006

88. Karpinos M, Teh BS, Zeck O, Carpenter LS, Phan C, Mai WY, Lu HH, Chiu JK, Butler EB, Gormley WB, Woo SY. Treatment of acoustic neuroma: stereotactic radiosurgery vs. microsurgery. Int J Radiat Oncol Biol Phys **54(5)**: 1410–1421; 2002

89. Pollock BE, Lunsford LD, Kondziolka D, Flickinger JC, Bissonette DJ, Kelsey SF, Jannetta PJ. Outcome analysis of acoustic neuroma management: a comparison of microsurgery and stereotactic radiosurgery. Neurosurgery **36(1)**: 215–224; 1995

90. Régis J, Pellet W, Delsanti C, Dufour H, Roche PH, Thomassin JM, Zanaret M, Peragut JC. Functional outcome after gamma knife surgery or microsurgery for vestibular schwannomas. J Neurosurg **97(5)**: 1091–1100; 2002

91. van Roijen L, Nijs HG, Avezaat CJ, Karlsson G, Linquist C, Pauw KH, Rutten FF. Costs and effects of microsurgery versus radiosurgery in treating acoustic neuroma. Acta Neurochir **139(10)**: 942–948; 1997

92. Niranjan A, Mathieu D, Kondziolka D, Flickinger JC, Lunsford LD. Radiosurgery for intracanalicular vestibular schwannomas. Régis J, Roche P-H (eds) Modern Management of Acoustic Neuromas. Basel, Karger. Prog Neurol Surg **21**: 192–199; 2008

93. Bakkouri WE, Kania RE, Guichard JP, Lot G, Herman P, Huy PT (2009) Conservative management of 386 cases of unilateral vestibular schwannoma: tumor growth and consequences for treatment. J Neurosurg **110(4)**: 662–669

94. Myrseth E, Pedersen PH, Moller P, Lund-Johansen M. Treatment of vestibular schwannomas. Why, when and how? Acta Neurochir **149(7)**: 647–660; 2007

95. Samii M, Matthies C. Gamma surgery for vestibular schwannoma. J Neurosurg **92(5)**: 892–894; 2000

96. Lownie SP, Drake CG. Radical intracapsular removal of acoustic neurinomas. Long-term follow-up review of 11 patients. J Neurosurg **74(3)**: 422–425; 1991

97. Ganz JC. Surgery or gamma knife. J Neurosurg **106(5)**: 937–938; 2007

98. Iwai Y, Yamanaka K, Ishiguro T. Gamma surgery combined with radiosurgery of large acoustic neuromas. Surg Neurol **59(4)**: 283–289; 2003

99. Fuentes S, Arkha Y, Pech-Gourg G, Grisoli F, Dufour H, Régis J. Management of large vestibular schwannomas by combined surgical resection and gamma knife radiosurgery. Régis J, Roche P-H (eds) Modern Management of Acoustic Neuromas. Basel, Karger. Prog Neurol Surg **21**: 79–82; 2008

100. Samii M, Gerganov V, Samii A. Microsurgery management of vestibular schwannomas in neurofibromatosis 2: indications and results. Régis J, Roche P-H (eds) Modern Management of Acoustic Neuromas. Basel, Karger. Prog Neurol Surg **21**: 169–175; 2008

101. Eldridge R, Parry DM. Neurofibromatosis 2: evidence for clinical heterogeneity based on 54 individuals studied by MRI with gadolinium, 1987–1991. Tos M and Thomsen J (eds) Acoustic Neuroma, Amsterdam, New York, Kugler Publications: pp 801–804; 1992

102. Rowe J, Radatz M, Kemeny A. Radiosurgery for Type II neurofibromatosis. Régis J, Roche P-H (eds) Modern Management of Acoustic Neuromas. Basel, Karger. Prog Neurol Surg **21**: 176–182; 2008

Chapter 14
Meningiomas

Introduction

It was stated in the preface that the purpose of this book was not to set up one treatment against another. Rather, the aim is examine the principles of treatment and maybe stimulate thought about the optimal way to combine the existing therapeutic methods into a harmonious multi modality management protocol in the best interests of the patient. There are general aspects of meningiomas which provide difficulties for surgeon and Gamma Knife user alike and this chapter is aimed at describing these difficulties with a view to providing a current baseline to which reference may be made. The major causes of complications following microsurgical procedures relate to the following:

1. Ischaemia
   (a) From vessel damage
   (b) From prolonged retraction
2. Post operative Oedema
   (a) A primary complication of the tumour
   (b) A result of retraction or interruption of venous drainage
3. Damage to a cranial nerves

Oedema may be the consequence of ischaemia or may result from the effects of the tumour. Cranial nerve function loss obviously relates to skull base surgery. The regions of potential risk are well known. They include the sagittal sinus, particularly behind the Rolandic Fissure with parasagittal tumours. They include also the brain stem and lower cranial nerves in the posterior fossa and the upper cranial nerves around the sella turcica. Surgery aimed at avoiding the regions of danger and leaving tumour in these locations to the Gamma Knife cannot but improve the

J.C. Ganz, *Gamma Knife Neurosurgery*,
DOI 10.1007/978-3-7091-0343-2_14, © Springer-Verlag/Wien 2011

quality of results. However, this approach will work best if planned prior to surgery rather than if left to chance as is commonly the situation today.

Natural History of Meningiomas

All rational treatment has to be based on the knowledge of the natural history of the disease to be treated. As always the risks of treatment must be weighed against the risks of leaving a disease untreated. In the current instance this relates to the size of a tumour at the time of its discovery and the speed at which a given meningioma may be expected to grow. In some instances this assessment will take place in the context of a tumour which causes symptoms. However, since the introduction of computerised imaging techniques in the early 1970s the question will also arise in respect of asymptomatic tumours which are discovered by chance.

Contribution of Computerised Imaging

In the age of CT and MRI it would be natural to think that there is plenty of information on this topic in the literature. However, a perusal of the said literature shows that there are many gaps in our knowledge, for understandable reasons [1]. There does seem to be broad agreement on the notion that hypointense T2 MR images and intratumoural calcification on CT suggest a tumour with a small potential for growth. With the exception of this agreement the topic is bedevilled with methodological problems. The follow up period of many of the series assessing the chance of growth in incidental asymptomatic tumours is short. In a series of 47 incidental meningiomas of whom six underwent surgery, 41 were followed conservatively for the unusually long period of 105 months. All the tumours grew to some extent though the growth rate was very variable being between 0.03 and 2.62 cm^3 per year. This translates into a tumour doubling time of 1.27–143.5 years. Nonetheless, in over 66% of cases tumour growth did not exceed 1 cm^3 per year, justifying continuing observation. In one series of 351 patients with asymptomatic meningiomas managed conservatively, there were 67 tumours followed for more than 5 years and there was tumour growth in 37.3% and symptoms developed in 16.4%. In this same series it was found that morbidity was doubled for patients operated who were over 70 years of age. Many other series have shorter observation periods [1–4]. These series consistently report a significant number of tumours which have not grown. It has to be considered that the risk of growth should not be considered in terms of a published frequency after a short follow up but in terms of the probability of growth over the expected lifetime of the individual patient.

Factors Concerning Who When and How to Treat Intracranial Meningiomas

Tumour Size

Meningiomas can of course vary in size from over 100 cm^3 to almost invisible on imaging. Obviously a bigger tumour will tend to be involved with more local structures and will in general require a longer and possibly more complex operation. Moreover, larger tumours can only be treated by open surgery although where the cut off goes between surgery and radiosurgery remains a matter of debate. Nonetheless the size as such is not the biggest problem in the surgery of these lesions.

The assessment of tumour growth is hardly precise. Most centres measure specific tumour diameters in different directions. This is known to be an insensitive method [5]. The measurement of volumes is required to obtain reasonably accurate results. This is time consuming and usually requires financing a dedicated staff to take on a task which lies outside the remit of a busy imaging department.

Patient Age and General Health

Over the last few years, there have been a number of papers on the possibility of operating on patients of 65 years of age or more with acceptable results. However, there are factors which mitigate against success including poor general health, low Karnowsky score, tumours with symptoms and tumour location. Skull base tumours have a worse prognosis. High age is more often associated with worse surgical results. There would seem to be broad agreement in the published reports that it is not the age as such which increases the risk. It is more the higher incidence of poor general health among the aged which has a negative effect on the results of surgery [6–17]. These quoted publications report not only the risks directly associated with the surgery but also the management risks in the elderly related to systemic complications including pulmonary embolus and other respiratory problems. There is one paper where age is not a determinant of the results of surgery [18].

Decision Making in the Treatment of Meningiomas: To Treat or Not to Treat

The decision to operate a meningioma will be made on the basis of what is known of the natural history as outlined above. Absent growth of asymptomatic meningiomas over a period of several years represents adequate grounds to be cautious with exposing a patient to surgery. The same principles may also apply to symptomatic tumours which produce tolerable symptoms and represent no immediate threat to life. The universal principle first formulated as an aphorism by Thomas Sydenham of London is applicable (primum non nocere). The slow growth of meningiomas [1] means that immediate treatment is not a matter of urgency in many cases [19]. Thus, asymptomatic tumours may well be observed say by MRI once a year. However, just in case the tumour is more aggressive than expected and especially if the T2 image shows a high signal, the patient can in addition be advised to contact the doctor any time unexpected possible tumour related symptoms should occur.

Radicality of Surgery

If surgery is deemed indicated then its aim is total removal. This aim is based on the notion that total removal will result in reducing or obviating the possibility of recurrence, with the concomitant threat to a patient's life and or function. The ability to perform radical surgery depends partly on size and consistency but even more on location and the relationship to surrounding structures. The definition of the radicality of surgery derives from a seminal paper on this subject was written by Donald Simpson at the Ratcliffe Infirmary in Oxford back in 1956 [20]. He developed a classification of five grades which have become familiar. Grade 1 was total removal of all tumour tissue including the dural attachment. Grade 2 was removal of all visible tissue and coagulating the dural attachment. Grade 3 was removing all intradural tumours but leaving extra dural remnants – a so called subtotal removal. Grade 4 was a partial removal and grade 5 was basically a decompression with or without biopsy. Simpson recorded clinical recurrence in that era before computerised imaging. The recurrence rate for grade 1 was 9% and for grade 2 was 19% and for the other grades appreciably higher. The main reason for recurrence after apparent radical removal is said to be "unnoticed invasion of a dural venous sinus or spread across a free dural septum". Other reasons could be fragments of the subdural fringe described in the paper, infiltration of the bone or multiple primary tumours. These recurrences relate to tumours which were apparently completely resected. It is emphasised that in Simpson's material 2 tumours were malignant, four others showed microscopic signs of rapid growth but 13 were unremarkable. This paper was an important contribution. It remains relevant today in terms of the definition of radicality of removal. However, the terms of definition of post operative recurrence have changed. The weakest part of Simpson's paper was that the definition of recurrence was based on clinical criteria. Not only that, but the clinical picture was often assessed at hospitals and by colleagues who were at some distance from the neurosurgeons responsible for the operations. The criteria of recurrence today are findings on computerised images. Thus, the rates of recurrence and residual tumour would be expected to differ from those described by Simpson. Another weakness of the Simpson paper is that the length of follow up and the relationship of morbidity to length of follow up are not described in detail. Thus, while it is a useful guide and thus is still reflected in current reporting, it is necessary to look at more recent papers where recurrence rates are based on computerised images, if up to date information is desired.

Tumour Location and Its Effect on Choice of Treatment

There can be little doubt that location, size and consistency are crucial character-istics affecting the possibilities of uncomplicated radical tumour removal. While there are a great many sites where meningiomas may occur for those interested in GKNS the major locations of interest are shown in the table below. In general the non basal tumours will do better with microsurgery. There are a fair number of papers indicating that a non basal location is associated with a relatively high frequency of complications when GKNS is used as a primary treatment [21–31]. Moreover, many of the convexity and falx meningiomas are considered relatively safe and simple to operate as assessed by the Co-morbidity, tumor Location, patient Age, tumor Size and neurological Signs and symptoms. The so called "CLASS" system devised at the Cleveland Clinic (Table 14.1). Thus, location when viewed alone indicates that GKNS is preferable for basal tumours and microsurgery for non-basal tumours. Location is not however the only parameter to consider. The other factors including symptoms and age have been mentioned above. However, the existence of co-morbidity is a bit of a wild card and there is no real system related to its effect on the choice of treatment except in so far as it is commoner amongst older patients. Otherwise each patient is assessed on a case by case basis.

Changing Technology and the Effect on Surgical Mortality

The influence of advancing technology is another factor which must be considered when reviewing results and comparing methods of treatment. The next table indicates that there has been a noticeable drop in surgical mortality in series reported after 2000 (Table 14.2).

Table 14.1 Surgical risk for various relevant meningioma locations

Location	Risk rate according to "Class" [32]	Basal/ non-basal
Convexity	0	Non-basal
Parasagittal	1	
Falx	1	
Olfactory groove	1	Basal
Medial sphenoidal ridge	2	
Tuberculum sellae	2	
Cavernous sinus	2	
Cerebello pontine angle	1	
Petrous bone	½	
Petroclival	2	
Foramen magnum	1/2	

Table 14.2 Changing pattern of surgical mortality over the last few years [11, 14, 18, 33–96]	Year of publication	Number of articles	Mean reported mortality
	<2000	21	5.7%
	≥2000	38	1.9%

The Morbidity and Mortality of Microsurgery and GKNS

The next tables shows summaries of the surgical and GKNS results for papers covering comparable lesions treated within the last 10 years (Tables 14.3 and 14.4).

In all cases major morbidity means permanent significant loss of function or epilepsy. Treatable or treated complications like diplopia, CSF leak, haematoma successfully treated and wound and bone flap complications are NOT included in the above figures. It should be noted that the mortality rate is generally low especially in larger series. The morbidity is significant but the avoidability of this will be discussed below. The recurrence rate in large measure reflects the difficulty of performing total resections of difficult tumours. This is another essential point to which we shall return.

Other Factors that Are Relevant to the Choice of Treatment

Tumour Consistency

The hardness of a tumour is a major consideration, because while the ultrasound knife facilitates the microdissection and removal of hard tissue it does not affect the interface between the tumour and normal tissue. A hard tumour is more difficult to separate from normal tissue and the possibilities for morbidity are thereby greater. Tumour consistency is of no consequence for GKNS.

Tumour Vascularity

This is clearly a major consideration during surgery. Blood loss is a danger in itself. Brisk haemorrhage obscures the operating field and delays the removal of a tumour. Vascularity has little if any certain effect on the success of GKNS

Peritumoral Oedema

This is today perceived to indicate a breakdown in the membranes surrounding the brain [133]. It is generally b believed the oedema is produced by the tumour and is associated with various tumour secreted peptides not least vascular endothelial growth factor (VEGF). There is an association between the presence of oedema

Table 14.3 Surgical mortality morbidity and recurrence over the last 10 years

Paper	Case no.	FU (months)	Mortality %	Major morbidity%	Recurrence %	Location
Sade et al. [97]	52	37.0	2.0	2.0	NA	Anterior clinoid
Jacob et al. [98]	30	24.0	0.0	30.0	NA	Cavernous
Sindou et al. [34]	100	100.0	5.0	48.0	13.3	sinus
Tomasello et al. [91]	13	48.3	0.0	7.7	0.0	
Nakamura et al. [14]	21	57.5	0.0	19.0	0.0	CPA
Bassiouni et al. [43]	25	73.2	4.0	8.0	8.0	Foramen
Boulton et al. [99]	10	33.0	0.0	10.0	10.0	magnum
Nakamura et al. [71]	8	58.3	0.0	0.0	0.0	IAM
Bassiouni et al. [40]	56	67.2	5.4	7.1	8.9	Olfactory
Hentschel and DeMonte [59]	13	24.0	0.0	0.0	16.0	groove
Turazzi et al. [92]	37	48.0	0.0	0.0	0.0	
DiMeco et al. [53]	108	79.5	1.9	10.1	13.9	Parasagittal
Zevgaridis et al. [148]	62	65.0	3.2	6.4	8.0	Parasellar
Bambakidis et al. [39]	46	43.2	0.0	30.0	15.2	Petroclival
Kawasawe et al. [100]	70	NA	0.0	18.6	NA	
Ramina et al. [79]	18	41.8	0.0	0.0	NA	
Bassiouni et al. [41]	51	60.0	0.0	14.0	3.9	Petrous
Sade and Lee [82]	56	NA	0.0	21.0	0.0	
Wu et al. [101]	82	54.0	0.0	19.0	6.0	
Abdel-Aziz et al. [33]	38	96.0	0.0	16.0	10.5	Sphenoidal
Nakamura et al. [69]	108	79.0	0.0	8.3	20.4	ridge
Ringel et al. [80]	63	54.0	3.0	9.5	NA	
Russell and Benjamin [81]	35	153.6	0.0	6.0	9.0	
Bassiouni et al. [42]	81	71.0	2.5	13.5	8.6	Tentorium
Hostalot et al. [60]	25	64.0	8.0	4.0	16.0	
Chi et al. [102]	21	3.0	0.0	11.0	0.0	Tuberculum
Cook et al. [48]	3	3.0	0.0	0.0	33.3	sellae
Fahlbusch and Schott [55]	47	51.0	0.0	20.0	4.2	
Jallo and Benjamin [61]	23	112.0	8.7	19.0	4.0	
Kim et al. [3]	27	22.2	0.0	22.2	7.0	
Nozaki et al. [73]	22	59.5	0.0	13.6	NA	
Pamir et al. [74]	42	37.5	2.3	21.4	2.4	
Park et al. [75]	30	75.9	0.0	16.7	13.3	

and the development of pial blood vessels and a destruction of the pia-arachnoid. The disappearance of these membranes results in a tumour which no longer has a clear cut plane between itself and the meningeal coverings of the surrounding brain. This makes dissection more difficult as the tumour becomes more adherent and there is an increased risk of leaving tumour cells behind.

While the presence of oedema will not make GKNS more difficult it does have relevance for the choice of treatment modality. Extensive oedema may represent

Table 14.4 GKNS morbidity and recurrence over the last 10 years

Author(s)	Case no.	FU (months)	Prescription dose (mean/median)	Target volume (mean/median)	Major morbidity% (mean/median)	Minor morbidity % (mean/median)	Recurrence% (mean/median)	Location
Hasegawa et al. [103]	115	62	13	14	0	4	**12**	Cavernous
Iwai et al. [104]	43	49.4	11	**14.7**	0	2.4	**9.5**	sinus
Lee et al. [105]	159	60	13	6.5	3.1	0	2.8	
Liscak et al. [106]	53	19	12	7.8	0	0	0	
Nicolato et al. [107]	122	48.9	14.6	8.3	0.8	0	3.5	
Nicolato et al. [108]	111	48.2	14.8	8.1	0.9	1	2.7	
Pollock et al. [109]	49	58	**15.9**	**10.2**	2	**10.2**	0	
Roche et al. [110]	80	30.5	28	5.8	3.8	1.3	5	
Kondziolka et al. [111]	34	31	14.2	8.5	0	2.9	2.9	Convexity WHO I
Muthukumar et al. [112]	5	36	10	**10.5**	0	0	0	Foramen Magnum
Kim et al. [113]	9	64	16	3.9	0	0	0	Intraventricular WHO 1
Bledsoe et al. [114]	116	70	15	**17.5**	7	**19**	**8**	Mixed
Chang et al. [21]	179	37.3	**15.1**	**10.1**	0	**35**	2.9	
DiBiase et al. [52]	162	54	14	4.5	0.7	**6.6**	**8.3**	
Flickinger et al. [115]	219	29	14	5	5	0.5	2.3	
Ganz et al. [116]	97	54	12	15.9	0	3.1	0	
Haselsberger et al. [117]	20	90	12	33.3	0	0	**10**	
Kondziolka et al. [118]	99	60 – 120	16	4.7	3	0	**7.0**	
Iwai et al. [119]	78	30	12	Diameter 2.2 cm	0	0	**7.2**	
Malik et al. [120]	277	44	**19.7**	7.3	0	1.4	**12**	
Pollock [121]	190	43	16	7.3	**3.2**	**10.5**	0	
Flannery et al. [122]	168	72	13	6.1	1.8	**6.5**	6	Petroclival
Roche et al. [123]	32	56	13	2.3	3.1	**6.3**	0	
Aichholzer et al. [124]	46	48	15.9	4.2	0	0	4.3	Skull base

Davidson et al. [125]	36	81	**16**	4.1	1	**9**	2.8
Eustacchio et al. [126]	121	60	13	6.8	1.7	3.3	0.8
Iwai et al. [127]	73	25	11.2	9.8	0	5.5	4
Iwai et al. [57]	108	86.1	12	8.1	0.9	5.6	**14.8**
Kreil et al. [128]	200	60	12	6.5	1	0	3.1
Nakaya et al. [129]	11	35.7	10	9.4	0	0	0
Pendl et al. [130]	164	55	12	8.3	0.6	0	3.7
Pollock et al. [131]	62	64	**17.7**	7.4	3.2	6.5	**12**
Zachenhofer et al. [132]	36	103	**16.8**	4	0	**8.3**	2.8

the major space occupying component associated with a given tumour. GKNS cannot produce a rapid reduction in raised intracranial pressure which will enable improved cerebral perfusion. In such a situation surgery may be preferred to GKNS even if GKNS would be technically simple to perform.

WHO Grade

WHO grade 2 and 3 tumour do a lot less well than grade 1 and this intrinsic biological characteristic affects all forms of treatment. In many instances today tumours are treated without prior biopsy because of the reliability of MR diagnosis, where the diagnosis is correct in up to 97% of cases [115]. Nonetheless, these patients will be treated currently without knowledge of tumour grade. This is considered acceptable since high grade tumours are relatively less common. Moreover, the comprehensive follow up system into which every patient treated with GKNS is entered should be adequate to permit early diagnosis of the relatively few patients whose tumours are more aggressive and thus permit appropriate extra measures.

Multiple Tumours

Multiple meningiomas are happily rare. There is obviously no simple surgical solution to these lesions, especially if they are widespread. They is moreover considerable disagreement about their pathogenesis. The term multiple meningiomas here refers to benign tumours in the absence of NF2. There is broad agreement that these tumour arise mostly around the convexities of the cerebrum or cerebellum.

In terms of surgical management one group suggests that multiple asymptomatic small lesions may be observed and followed with annual MRI. The mere presence of multiple tumours does not justify their removal. Thus, these tumours are still treated on a case by case basis with thorough consultation with the patients. Obviously radiosurgery is a simple answer up to a point. However, it may often need to be used in association with microsurgery since some of the tumours may by reason of size or location be unsuitable for GKNS.

With GKNS there is no mortality and almost no major morbidity. All forms of morbidity registered in Table 14.4 refer to permanent untreatable consequences of treatment. Recurrence rates in general have some relationship to number of patients and duration of follow up. Of course WHO grading is important as well.

Results of Microsurgery Compared with GKNS

These results should NOT be compared. That is like comparing chalk and cheese. Figure 14.1 shows why. This patient was treated many years ago before the Gamma Knife was available. He had a large sphenoidal ridge meningioma. This would never be a case for radiosurgery until after his operation.

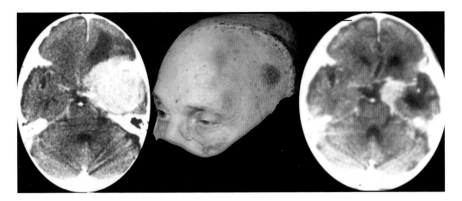

Fig. 14.1 On the *left* is a preoperative CT. In the *middle* is the patient 10 days after surgery. A well healed scar is seen. There is a mild left ptosis which subsequently recovered. There is some minor ecchymosis in the left lower eyelid. The patient had other wise lost no function. He was 71 years old. The CT on the *right* shows the post-operative result. Today we would have offered him GKNS but at that time the treatment was not available. These two images illustrate what would also today be considered as suitable candidates for microsurgery and GKNS

The tables show different things for different situations. The surgical mortality is remarkably low even if not zero. But the surgery is directed against large and dangerous lesions. The radiosurgery retains a noteworthy minor morbidity, treating as it does smaller lesions but often in very difficult places. In both instances the morbidity described concerns permanent loss of function.

How to Improve the Results

Making the Surgery Easier

The complications and mortality following surgery relate to attempts to separate tumour tissue from normal anatomy and in so doing damage the normal anatomical structures. Reducing the radicality of the surgery would reduce the risk. The situation is analogous to the preservation of facial nerve function with vestibular schwannomas by means of performing intracapsular surgery for larger tumours. With meningiomas, removing the centre of the tumour and leaving the margin will not work as with schwannomas because the rigid tumour wall will not collapse and the end result will still be a large mass with a central cavity. With meningiomas however other techniques already exist to solve this problem Black describes his conservative approach to the sagittal sinus when operating parasagittal meningiomas [134]. Other authors advise limiting the dissection of the cavernous sinus when operating on tumours which invade its walls and interior [33, 34, 98, 135]. Stealth technology is useful in this situation because as the tumours are fixed to the base of the skull they do not move during surgery. Thus, structures at risk like facial and

Table 14.5 Thirteen papers where larger tumours have been treated with GKNS with good results

Reference	Maximum target volume
Aichholzer et al. [124]	33.5
Bledsoe et al. [114]	48.6
Chang et al. [21]	45.0
DiBiase et al. [52]	80.0
Eustacchio et al. [126]	89.9
Flickinger et al. [115]	56.5
Haselsberger et al. [117]	79.8
Iwai et al. [119]	58.0
Kreil et al. [128]	89.8
Lee et al. [105]	52.4
Pendl et al. [130]	89.9
Pollock [121]	50.5
Zachenhofer et al. [132]	33.0

cochlear nerves or the basilar artery may be avoided leaving a remnant for GKNS at a later date without compromising the important structures which could be damaged by more radical surgery. Table 14.5 shows a list of papers which record the treatment of quite large tumours in some cases. It seems fair to say that surgeons without experience of GKNS underestimate the size of tumours which may be treated by this technique.

The author published a series of meningiomas treated with the GKNS where the smallest volume was 10 cm^3 and the largest 43.2 cm^3. In this series only 3 patients suffered adverse radiation effects all of which were reversible [116]. More of this will be mentioned. It might be considered this paper was an isolated example but that would be far from the truth. There have been a number of publications in which larger tumours have been treated with GKNS as shown in Table 14.5. On occasion staged procedures have been used [104, 117, 119, 127, 136]. The point is that surgeons can in reality probably be even more conservative about what they remove than is currently the case. This is at least a notion worth pursuing. It also brings the argument back to the starting point. The treatment of these lesions could be improved by planning a two stage procedure starting with surgery and ending with GKNS.

Improving the Results of GKNS

Dose and Complications

There are a number of areas where improvement could be achieved. The reader should peruse Table 14.4 taking particular note of the bold type figures. It is not appropriate to apply statistical analysis to data derived from so many diverse sources. However, there would seem to be at least one tendency suggested by this table. The highest rates of complications were associated with doses in the higher range. The author's experience is that 12 Gy is adequate for tumour control but that less than 12 Gy was associated with a reduction in tumour control [137]. Inevitably some tumours will be less radiosensitive than others and at present there is no means of measuring the radiosensitivity in individual tumours. However, 12 Gy at the margin seems to work adequately and moreover permit the treatment of larger tumours with safety [116].

WHO Grade and Recurrence Rate

It is not easy to tabulate the influence of this on recurrence from the available literature. There is an almost universal agreement that atypical and malignant meningiomas are associated with a worse prognosis and a more frequent recurrence after a shorter interval. Most of the documentation of this expected finding comes from LINAC centres but there is an LGK paper which confirms it for GKNS [111]. There remains a possibility that in papers where WHO grade is not specified, a higher recurrence rate may reflect innate but unrecorded tumour aggression.

Maximising the Safe Tumour Control Rate

Keeping the margin dose to around 12 Gy seems to be effective and in general over the years there has been a tendency to reduce the dose to this level. Retreatment following the minority of cases where there is recurrent growth after treatment may be considered and is of minimal inconvenience to the patient [138, 139]. Perusal of Table 14.4 shows with one exception that 12 Gy would seem to be an adequate dose. The exception is the paper from Osaka [140] Iwai et al. reporting on 108 patients treated with a low dose regime. This paper reports loss of tumour control in two patients "in field" and seven patients "out of field". Thus 6% of tumours were not adequately covered. Moreover, the maximum and median doses were 12 Gy but the minimum dose was 8 Gy. The paper does not report the relationship between dose and recurrence. The current author's earlier work, as cited above would expect recurrence where the dose was less than 12 Gy [137].

However, much of the current assessment of control rates is based on Kaplan Meier statistics rather than raw data. In the future there will be more raw data to give a more reliable assessment. At present, on the basis of available information it is suggested that a prescription dose of 12 Gy is adequate.

Minimising the Complication Rate

Non-basal Tumours

As indicated above, except in special cases meningiomas at the skull base do better than non-basal tumours. There is particular reason to believe that this is true for parasagittal tumours. It has been recorded that tumours can swell up temporarily

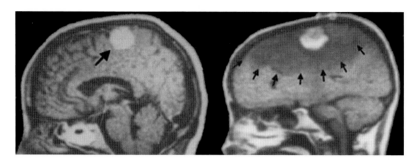

Fig. 14.2 This shows the sort of oedema that can arise together with contrast leakage with a non basal tumour. This patient had 12 Gy to the margin. The tumour diameter 25 mm. Hemiparesis for months

after GKNS [141]. This can compress or occlude adjacent veins with neurological deficit as a consequence. In general it would seem that this effect is of lesser significance if the patient has had a craniotomy and the treatment is directed at residual tumour [23]. A typical non-operated case is shown in Fig. 14.2. Patients must be warned of the risk of oedema after GKNS for residual parasagittal meningiomas. A venogram can be useful to demonstrate the proximity of the tumour to cerebral veins. It is considered possible that the temporary occlusion of veins connected to an occluded sinus may not produce symptoms as easily as in cases where the sinus is patent. However, there is no current evidence on this point.

Vascular Injury

Three cases of injury to perforating vessels inducing clinical damage have been reported from Marseille, following GKNS to three petroclival meningiomas with mean diameters between 2 and 2.5 cm. They were treated with prescription doses of 14 or 15 Gy. In one case there was no MR change and the clinical problem resolved. In the other two there were marked increased T2 signals from the adjacent brainstem. Both these patients were left with residual permanent clinical neurological deficit. Unfortunately, the article concerned does not comment on the two patients' general health and medication. A patient from Osaka was reported to suffer occlusion of a middle cerebral artery perforating branch 32 months after radiosurgery for a meningioma, the location of which is not mentioned. The specific prescription dose is not mentioned, but the mean prescription dose for the series was 12 Gy. Again the patient's age and pre-treatment medical condition are not mentioned [140]. A further patient with a petroclival meningioma and a post-treatment pontine infarct has been reported from the Mayo Clinic [114]. The specific dose is not mentioned but the mean dose for the series was 15 Gy (range 12–18 Gy).

A further case from Marseille recorded a transient central facial palsy associated with carotid occlusion in the cavernous sinus, following treatment of a cavernous sinus meningioma where the prescription dose had been 18 Gy to the 50% isodose [142]. There are a further three cases of carotid stenosis/occlusion reported from the Mayo Clinic [114]. In one the symptoms were temporary in the others permanent. The specific dose is not mentioned but the mean dose for the series was 15 Gy (range 12–18 Gy) [114].

In none of the cases of vascular damage mentioned above is there any adequate account of the patients' age, general clinical condition, tumour volume, specific dosimetry or medication. Nor is there comment on the anatomical status of the intracranial vascular tree prior to radiosurgery. Thus, it is not unreasonable to suggest that interpretation is not easy. Were the vascular changes recorded and published "post hoc" or "propter hoc". There is one other case of carotid occlusion associated with radiosurgery which is much better documented. It concerns the radiosurgery of a pituitary adenoma with an intracavernous tumour extension following craniotomy [143]. This occurred in a normotensive man of 35 years of age with no aggravating medical condition. The concerned artery was encased in tumour prior to treatment. The paper shows an illustration of a marked tumour shrinkage following GKNS with a prescription dose of 12 Gy. It does not show nor comment upon the detailed anatomy of the affected internal carotid artery prior to treatment. There is no angiogram, merely loss of flow void on the MRI.

The comments above indicate there may be a small risk for ischaemic injury following radiosurgery to intracranial vessels. It is certain that such occurrences are rare. It would also be desirable in the future that reports will improve our understanding if where possible they contain information about the pre-treatment vascular anatomy. This may of course be information that is not always available. On the other hand, information on the specifics of dosimetry, age, general health and medication should be a sine qua non for the acceptance for publication of such a report.

Cranial Nerve Injury

The optic and facial nerves and to an extent the trigeminal nerve have a special place in this context. Injury to the lower cranial nerves following treatment of petroclival meningiomas occurred in 3 of 168 patients treated in a recent series [122]. Injuries to the nerves controlling eye movement may improve of themselves or be helped by muscle balance surgery. The loss of hearing in one ear is a nuisance but not a tragedy and is unusual with GKNS for meningiomas. The loss of facial movement, specifically if visible at rest is a major problem to the patient. This has also been rare following the treatment of meningiomas. Vertigo may arise and is a very disturbing symptom to the patient as recorded in the chapter on vestibular schwannomas. Its frequency in the context of skull base meningiomas is not documented. Damage to the trigeminal nerve may give rise to numbness or pain. Both can in principle be treated. The pain can be a major problem in a minority of patients but is usually possible to manage with medication. The numbness is generally well tolerated.

The cranial nerve that causes most concern is the optic nerve and its connections, otherwise known as the optic or visual pathway. There have been various attempts to define the acceptable dose to this structure using vague definitions. The Mayo Clinic has been a pioneer in the adequate definition of what is an acceptable dose and how to measure it. Further work from Sheffield has indicated that unorthodox dosimetry may be helpful [144]. The Sheffield notions have been reinforced by a newer publication which demonstrates that acceptable dosimetry statistics (see Chap. 9) may be ignored in this situation. The details of this method lie outside the range of this book but are described in detail in the papers concerned [145].

Comments on Fractionation

There is a notion abroad that fractionation will enable safer treatment to preserve visual function for meningiomas **adjacent** to the optic pathways. This not only doesn't make great radiobiological sense, but there is not at the time of writing any published evidence to support the notion. The point about radiosurgery is that it delivers an adequate dose to the pathological tissue and a safe dose to surrounding tissue. It is not easy to understand how replacing GKNS with fractionated radiotherapy will improve the results. The α/β ratio for meningiomas and brain are similar so that there is no reason to believe that fractionating involves an inherent advantage. Fractionation is most useful when the surrounding tissue receives a similar dose to the that received by the tumour. This is not the case with GKNS. Moreover, if fractionation were used a higher total dose would be needed to offset the fact that fractionated treatments require a greater total dose to achieve the same biological effect as a single dose. Thus, for tumours **adjacent** to but not within the normal tissue at risk, there is no theoretical basis for fractionating the dose, on the basis of knowledge available today. For further details on this topic the reader is referred back to Chaps. 4 and 5

The reason that the word adjacent in the previous paragraph was printed in bold type is that it is the key term for meningiomas in relation to the optic pathways. There is one type of meningioma which involves the optic pathways and which is not adjacent to them but intermingled with them. For this tumour GKNS is NOT a suitable treatment as there is no way to distinguish the optic nerve fibres from the tumour. The treatment of choice here is fractionated radiotherapy which will increasingly be stereotactically guided. The reason is GKNS is not suitable when pathological tissue and normal anatomy cannot be distinguished from each other.

Optic Nerve Sheath Meningiomas

For these unusual tumours surgery is used for intracranial extension and disfiguring or distressing proptosis [146, 147]. For patients with retained vision fractionated radiotherapy is chosen. GKNS has no place in the treatment of these tumours since

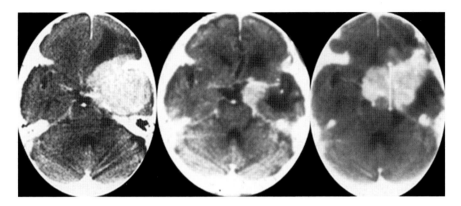

Fig. 14.3 On the *left* is a preoperative CT. In the *middle* is CT 6 months after treatment. The CT was taken 6 months after the one in the *middle*. It demonstrates aggressive growth which extends the tumour outside its original boundaries towards the opposite side. The lesion proved resistant to further treatment. As stated above no GKNS was given as it was not available outside Stockholm at the time this patient was treated

it is effectively impossible to separate the nerve and the tumour on imaging and fractionation in this instance offers a distinct benefit.

Malignant Change

Iwai et al. in their recent report document a malignant transformation of 6%. They attribute this finding to a spontaneous change in the tumour as documented by other workers [148–150]. A dramatic illustration of this phenomenon applies to the patient illustrated above in Fig. 14.3. Six months after the post operative image shown above, without any further intervention the tumour had become malignant without any other outside interference and he swiftly succumbed.

Conclusion

The chapter closes as it began with the suggestion that optimal treatment involves groups consisting of colleagues from various disciplines with varied expertise planning the treatment of these difficult lesions before treatment is begun. This should minimise damage, increase the flow of technical information between the responsible physicians and hopefully improve the results of the treatment of meningiomas above even the high levels of excellence that are documented in the papers and books to be found in the following references.

References

1. Cho KG. Natural history, growth rates, and recurrence. In: Lee JH (ed) Meningiomas: Diagnosis, Treatment and Outcome. Springer Verlag London Limited, Godalming: pp 45–51; 2008
2. HersoviciZ, Rappaport Z, Sulkes J et al. Natural history of conservatively treated meningiomas. Neurology **63**: 1133–1134; 2004
3. Kim TW, Jung S, Jung TY, Kim IY, Kang SS, Kim SH. Prognostic factors of postoperative visual outcomes in tuberculum sellae meningioma. Br J Neurosurg **22(2)**: 231–234; 2008
4. Olivero WC, Lister JR, Elwood PW. The natural history and growth rate of asymptomatic meningiomas. J Neurosurg **83**: 222–224; 1995
5. Nievas MN. Volume assessment of intracranial large meningiomas and considerations about their microsurgical and clinical management. Neurol Res **29**: 787–797; 2007
6. Arienta C, Caroli M, Crotti F, Villani R. Treatment of intracranial meningiomas in patients over 70 years old. Acta Neurochir **107**: 47–55; 1990
7. Awad IA, Kalfas I, Hahd JF et al. Intracranial meningiomas in the aged: surgical outcome in the era of computed tomography. Neurosurgery **24**: 557–560; 1989
8. Buhl R, Hasan A, Behnke A, Mehdorn HM. Results in the operative treatment of elderly patients with intracranial meningioma. Neurosurg Rev **23**: 25–29; 2000
9. Cornu P, Chatellier G, Dagreou F, Clemenceau S, Foncin JF, Rivierez M, Philippon J. Intracranial meningiomas in elderly patients. Postoperative morbidity and mortalityFactors predictive of outcome. Acta Neurochir **102**: 98–102; 1990
10. D'Andrea G, Roperto R, Caroli E, Crispo F, Ferrante L. Thirty-seven cases of intracranial meningiomas in the ninth decade of life: our experience and review of the literature. Neurosurgery **56**: 956–961; 2005
11. Kallio M, Sankila R, Hakulinen T, Jaaskelainen J. Factors affecting operative and excess long-term mortality in 935 patients with intracranial meningiomas. Neurosurgery **31(1)**: 2–12; 1992
12. Lieu AS, Howng SL. Surgical treatment of intracranial meningiomas in geriatric patients. Kaohsiung J Med Sci **14**: 498–503; 1998
13. McGrail K, Ojemann RG. The surgical management of benign intracranial meningiomas in patients 70 years of age and older. Surg Neurol **42(1)**: 2–7; 1994
14. Nakamura M, Roser F, Dormiani M, Vorkapic P, Samii M. Surgical treatment of cerebellopontine angle meningiomas in elderly patients. Acta Neurochir **147**: 603–609; 2005
15. Pompili A, Cacciani L, Cattani F, Caroli F, Crecco M, Mastrostefano R, Mazzitelli MR, Raus L. Intracranial meningiomas in the elderly. Minerva Med **88**: 229–236; 1997
16. Proust F, Verdure L, Toussaint P, Bellow F, Callonec F, Menard JF, Freger P. Intracranial meningioma in the elderly. Postoperative mortality, morbidity and quality of life in a series of 39 patients over 70 years of age. Neurochirurgie **43**: 15–20; 1997
17. Riffaud L, Mazzon A, Haegelen C, Hamlat A, Morandi X. Surgery for intracranial meningiomas in patients older than 80 years. Presse Med **36**: 197–202; 2007
18. Reinert M, Babey M, Curschmann J, Vajtai I, Seiler RW, Mariani L. Morbidity in 201 patients with small sized meningioma treated by microsurgery. Acta Neurochir **148**: 1257–1265; 2006
19. Yano S, Kuratsu J. Indications for surgery in patients with asymptomatic meningiomas based on an extensive experience. J Neurosurg **105(4)**: 538–543; 2006
20. Simpson D. Recurrence of intracranial meningiomas after surgical treatment. J Neurol Neurosurg Psychiatry **20**: 22–39; 1957
21. Chang JH, Chang JW, Choi JY, Park YG, Chung SS. Complications after gamma knife radiosurgery for benign meningiomas. J Neurol Neurosurg Psychiatry **74(2)**: 226–230; 2003
22. Chen CH, Shen CC, Sun MH, Ho WL, Huang CF, Kwan PC. Histopathology of radiation necrosis with severe peritumoral edema after gamma knife radiosurgery for parasagittal meningioma. A report of two cases. Stereotact Funct Neurosurg **85**: 292–295; 2007

23. Ganz JC, Schrottner O, Pendl G. Radiation-induced edema after gamma knife treatment for meningiomas. Stereotact Funct Neurosurg **66(Suppl 1)**: 129–133; 1996

24. Kalapurakal JA, Silverman CL, Akhtar N, Laske DW, Braitman LE, Boyko OB, Thomas PR. Intracranial meningiomas: factors that influence the development of cerebral edema after stereotactic radiosurgery and radiation therapy. Radiology **204(2)**: 461–465; 1997

25. Kan P, Liu JK, Wendland MM, Shrieve D, Jensen RL. Peritumoral edema after stereotactic radiosurgery for intracranial meningiomas and molecular factors that predict its development. J Neurooncol Epub 83(1): 33–38; 2007

26. Kim DG, Kim ChH, Chung HT, Paek SH, Jeong SS, Han DH, Jung HW. Gamma knife surgery of superficially located meningioma. J Neurosurg **102(Suppl 5)**: 255–258; 2005

27. Ma Z, Tang J, Qiu B, Hou Y, Peng Z, Liu Y. Gamma knife treatment of meningiomas. Hunan Yi Ke Da Xue Xue Bao 23(2): 161–163; 1998

28. Mindermann T, de Rougemont O. The significance of tumor location for Gamma Knife treatment of meningiomas. Stereotact Funct Neurosurg **82(4)**: 194–195; 2004

29. Pan DH, Guo WY, Chang YC, Chung WY, Shiau CY, Wang LW, Wu SM. The effectiveness and factors related to treatment results of gamma knife radiosurgery for meningiomas. Stereotact Funct Neurosurg **70(Suppl 1)**: 19–32; 1998

30. Singh VP, Kansai S, Vaishya S, Julka PK, Mehta VS. Early complications following gamma knife radiosurgery for intracranial meningiomas. J Neurosurg **93(Suppl 3)**: 57–61; 2000

31. Vermeulen S, Young R, Li F, Meier R, Raisis J, Klein S, Kohler E. A comparison of single fraction radiosurgery tumor control and toxicity in the treatment of basal and nonbasal meningiomas. Stereotact Funct Neurosurg **72(Suppl)**: 160–166; 1999

32. Lee JH, Sade B. The novel "CLASS" algorithmic scale for patient selection in meningioma surgery. In: Lee JH (ed) Meningiomas: Diagnosis, Treatment and Outcome. Springer Verlag London Limited, Godalming: pp 217–222; 2008

33. Abdel-Aziz KM, Froelich SC, Dagnew E, Jean W, Breneman JC, Zuccarello M, van Loveren HR, Tew JM Jr. Large sphenoid wing meningiomas involving the cavernous sinus: conservative surgical strategies for better functional outcomes. Neurosurgery **54(6)**: 1375–1383; 2004

34. Sindou M, Wydh E, Jouanneau E, Nebbal M, Lieutaud T. Long-term follow-up of meningiomas of the cavernous sinus after surgical treatment alone. J Neurosurg **107**: 937–944; 2007

35. Adegbite AB, Khan MI. The recurrence of intracranial meningiomas after surgical treatment. J Neurosurg **58**: 51–56; 1983

36. Al-Mefty O, Fox JL, Smith RR. Petrosal approach to petroclival meningiomas. Neurosurgery **22**: 510–517; 1988

37. Al-Mefty O, Holoubi A, Rifai A, Fox JL. Microsurgical removal of suprasellar meningiomas. Neurosurgery **16**: 364–372; 1985

38. Asgari S, Bassiouni H, Hunold A, Klassen D, Stolke D, Sandalcioglu IE. Extensive brain swelling with neurological deterioration after intracranial meningioma surgery – venous complication or 'unspecific' increase in tissue permeability. Zentralbl Neurochir **69(1)**: 22–29; 2008

39. Bambakidis NC, Kakarla UK, Kim LJ, Nakaji P, Porter RW, Daspit CP, Spetzler RF. Evolution of surgical approaches in the treatment of petroclival meningiomas: a retrospective review. Neurosurgery **61**: 202–209; 2007

40. Bassiouni H, Asgari S, Stolke D. Olfactory groove meningiomas: functional outcome in a series treated microsurgically. Acta Neurochir **149**: 109–121; 2007

41. Bassiouni H, Hunold A, Asgari S, Stolke D. Meningiomas of the posterior petrous bone: functional outcome after microsurgery. J Neurosurg **100**: 1014–1024; 2004

42. Bassiouni H, Hunold A, Asgari S, Stolke D. Tentorial meningiomas: clinical results in 81 patients treated microsurgically. Neurosurgery **55**: 108–116; 2004

43. Bassiouni H, Ntoukas V, Asgari S, Sandalcioglu EI, Stolke D, Seifert V. Foramen magnum meningiomas: clinical outcome after microsurgical resection via a posterolateral suboccipital retrocondylar approach. Neurosurgery **59**: 1177–1185; 2006

44. Borba LAB, Colli BO. Foramen magnum meningiomas. In: Lee JH (ed) Meningiomas: Diagnosis, Treatment and Outcome. Springer Verlag London Limited, Godalming: pp 449–456; 2008

45. Bricolo AP, Turazzi S, Talacchi A, Cristofori L. Microsurgical removal of petroclival meningiomas: a report of 33 patients. Neurosurgery 31: 813–828; 1992

46. Brihaye J, Brihaye van Geertruyden M. Management and surgical outcomes of suprasellar meningiomas. Acta Neurochir Suppl 42: 124–129; 1988

47. Colli BO, Assirati JA, Jr, Deriggi DJ, Neder L, dos Santos AC, Carlotti Jr CG. Tentorial meningiomas: follow-up review. Neurosurg Rev 31(4): 449–456; 2008

48. Cook SW, Smith Z, Kelly DF. Endonasal transsphenoidal removal of tuberculum sellae meningiomas: technical note. Neurosurgery 55: 239–244; 2004

49. Delfini R, Santoro A, Pichierri A. Cerebellar convexity meningiomas. In: Lee JH (ed) Meningiomas: Diagnosis, Treatment and Outcome. Springer Verlag London Limited, Godalming: pp 457–463; 2008

50. DeMonte F, Smith HK, al-Mefty O. Outcome of aggressive removal of cavernous sinus meningiomas. J Neurosurg 81(2): 245–251; 1994

51. Desgeorges M, Sterkers O, Poncet JL, Rey A, Sterkers JM. Surgery for meningioma of the posterior skull base. 135 cases. Choice of approach and results. Neurochirurgie 41: 265–290; 1995

52. DiBiase SJ, Kwok Y, Yovino S, Arena C, Naqvi S, Temple R, Regine WF, Amin P, Guo C, Chin LS. Factors predicting local tumor control after gamma knife stereotactic radiosurgery for benign intracranial meningiomas. Int J Radiat Oncol Biol Phys 60(5): 1515–1519; 2004

53. DiMeco F, Li KW, Casali C, Ciceri E, Giombini S, Filippini G, Broggi G, Solero CL. Meningiomas invading the superior sagittal sinus: surgical experience in 108 cases. Neurosurgery 55(6): 1263–1274; 2004

54. Dolenc V. Microsurgical removal of large sphenoidal bone meningiomas. Acta Neurochir Suppl 28: 391–396; 1979

55. Fahlbusch R, Schott W. Pterional surgery of meningiomas of the tuberculum sellae and planum sphenoidale: surgical results with special consideration of ophthalmological and endocrinological outcomes. J Neurosurg 96: 235–243; 2002

56. Gazzeri R, Galarza M, Gazzeri G. Giant olfactory groove meningioma: ophthalmological and cognitive outcome after bifrontal microsurgical approach. Acta Neurochir 150(11): 1117–1125; 2008

57. Guo HH, Zhou LF. Further experience in the diagnosis and treatment of sphenoidal ridge meningioma. Zhonghua Wai Ke Za Zhi 32: 740–742; 1994

58. Hassler W, Zentner J. Surgical treatment of olfactory groove meningiomas using the pterional approach. Acta Neurochir Suppl 53: 14–18; 1991

59. Hentschel SJ, DeMonte F. Olfactory groove meningiomas. Neurosurg Focus 14: e4; 2003

60. Hostalot C, Carrasco A, Bilbao G, Pomposo I, Garibi JM. Tentorial meningiomas. Report of our series. Neurocirugia Astur 15: 119–127; 2004

61. Jallo GI, Benjamin V. Tuberculum sellae meningiomas: microsurgical anatomy and surgical technique. Neurosurgery 51: 1432–1439; 2002

62. Javed T, Sekhar LN. Surgical management of clival meningiomas. Acta Neurochir Suppl 53: 171–182; 1991

63. Jiang YG, Xiang J, Wen F, Zhang LY. Microsurgical excision of the large or giant cerebellopontine angle meningioma. Minim Invasive Neurosurg 49: 43–48; 2006

64. Klink DF, Sampath P, Miller NR, Brem H, Long DM. Long-term visual outcome after nonradical microsurgery patients with parasellar and cavernous sinus meningiomas. Neurosurgery 47: 24–31; 2000

65. Lee JH, Sade B. Anterior clinoidal meningiomas. In: Lee JH (ed) Meningiomas: Diagnosis, Treatment and Outcome. Springer Verlag London Limited, Godalming: pp 347–362; 2008

66. Liu Y, Liu M, Chen Y, Li F, Wang H, Zhu S, Wu C. Microsurgical total removal of olfactory groove meningiomas and reconstruction of the invaded skull bases. Int Surg 92: 167–173; 2007

67. Lobato RD, Gonzaaez P, Alday R, Ramos A, Lagares A, Alen JF, Palomino JC, Miranda P, Perez-Nunez A, Arrese I. Meningiomas of the basal posterior fossa. Surgical experience in 80 cases. Neurocirugia (Astur) **15(6)**: 525–542; 2004

68. Mehdorn H, Buhl RM. Petrous meningiomas I: an overview. In: Lee JH (ed) Meningiomas: Diagnosis, Treatment and Outcome. Springer Verlag London Limited, Godalming: pp 433–441; 2008

69. Nakamura M, Roser F, Jacobs C, Vorkapic P, Samii M. Medial sphenoid wing meningiomas: clinical outcome and recurrence rate. Neurosurgery **58**: 626–639 discussion; 2006

70. Nakamura M, Roser F, Michel J et al. The natural history of incidental meningiomas. Neurosurgery **53**: 62–71; 2003

71. Nakamura M, Roser F, Mirzai S, Matthies C, Vorkapic P, Samii M. Meningiomas of the internal auditory canal. Neurosurgery **55**: 119–127; 2004

72. Nakamura M, Struck M, Roser F, Vorkapic P, Samii M. Olfactory groove meningiomas: clinical outcome and recurrence rates after tumor removal through the frontolateral and bifrontal approach. Neurosurgery **60**: 844–852; 2007

73. Nozaki K, Kikuta K, Takagi Y, Mineharu Y, Takahashi JA, Hashimoto N. Effect of early optic canal unroofing on the outcome of visual functions in surgery for meningiomas of the tuberculum sellae and planum sphenoidale. Neurosurgery **62(4)**: 839–844; 2008

74. Pamir MN, Ozduman K, Belirgen M, Kilic T, Ozek MM. Outcome determinants of pterional surgery for tuberculum sellae meningiomas. Acta Neurochir **147**: 1121–1130; 2005

75. Park CK, Jung HW, Yang SY, Seol HJ, Paek SH, Kim DG. Surgically treated tuberculum sellae and diaphragm sellae meningiomas: the importance of short-term visual outcome. Neurosurgery **59**: 238–243; 2006

76. Probst C. Possibilities and limitations of microsurgery in patients with meningiomas of the sellar region. Acta Neurochir **84**: 99–102; 1987

77. Puchner MJ, Fischer-Lampsatis RC, Herrmann HD, Freckmann N. Suprasellar meningiomas–neurological and visual outcome at long-term follow-up in a homogeneous series of patients treated microsurgically. Acta Neurochir **140**: 1231–1238; 1998

78. Radovanovic I, de Tribolet N. Falcotentorial and pineal reagion meningiomas. In: Lee JH (ed) Meningiomas: Diagnosis, Treatment and Outcome. Springer Verlag London Limited, Godalming: pp 485–494; 2008

79. Ramina R, Neto MC, Fernandes YB, Silva EB, Mattei TA, Aguiar PH. Surgical removal of small petroclival meningiomas. Acta Neurochir **150(5)**: 431–438; 2008

80. Ringel F, Cedzich C, Schramm J. Microsurgical technique and results of a series of 63 spheno-orbital meningiomas. Neurosurgery **60**: 214–221; 2007

81. Russell SM, Benjamin V. Medial sphenoid ridge meningiomas: classification, microsurgical anatomy, operative, nuances, and long-term surgical outcome in 35 consecutive patients. Neurosurgery **62 (3 Suppl 1)**: 38–50; 2008

82. Sade B, Lee JH. Petrous meningiomas II: ventral, posterior and superior subtypes. In: Lee JH (ed) Meningiomas: Diagnosis, Treatment and Outcome. Springer Verlag London Limited, Godalming: pp 443–447; 2008

83. Samii M, Ammirati M, Mahran A. Surgery of petroclival meningiomas: report of 24 cases. Neurosurgery **24(1)**: 12–17; 1989

84. Samii M, Carvalho GA, Tatagiba M, Matthies C. Surgical management of meningiomas originating in Mecke's cave. Neurosurgery **41**: 767–774; 1997

85. Sanna M, Flanagan S, DeDonato G, Bacciu A, Falcioni M. Jugular foramen meningiomas II. In: Lee JH (ed) Meningiomas: Diagnosis, Treatment and Outcome. Springer Verlag London Limited, Godalming: pp 521–528; 2008

86. Sasaki T, Kawahara N. Jugular foramen meningiomas I. In: Lee JH (ed) Meningiomas: Diagnosis, Treatment and Outcome. Springer Verlag London Limited, Godalming: pp 515–520; 2008

87. Schaller C, Meyer B, Jung A, Erkwoh A, Schramm J. Results for microsurgical removal of tentorial meningiomas. Zentralbl Neurochir **63**: 59–64; 2002

88. Sekhar LN, Jannetta PJ, Burkhart LE, Janosky JE. Meningiomas involving the clivus: a six-year experience with 41 patients. Neurosurgery **27(5)**: 764–781; 1990

89. Sekhar LN, Sen CN, Jho HD et al. Surgical treatment of intracavernous neoplasms: a four year experience. Neurosurgery **24**: 18–30; 1989
90. Solero CL, Giombini S, Morello G. Suprasellar and olfactory meningiomas. Report on a series of 153 personal cases. Acta Neurochir **67(3–4)**: 181–194; 1983
91. Tomasello F, de Divitiis O, Angileri FF, Salpietro FM, d'Avella D. Large sphenocavernous meningiomas: is there still a role for the intradural approach via the pterional-transsylvian route? Acta Neurochir **145**: 273–282; 2003
92. Turazzi S, Cristofori L, Gambin R, Bricolo A. The pterional approach for the microsurgical removal of olfactory groove meningiomas. Neurosurgery **45**: 821–825; 1999
93. Yan P, Wang S, Zhang H. Microsurgical treatment for meningioma of falco-tentorial junction. Zhonghua Wai Ke Za Zhi **37**: 245–247; 1999
94. Zevgaridis D, Medele RJ, Muller A, Hischa AC, Steiger HJ. Meningiomas of the sellar region presenting with visual impairment: impact of various prognostic factors on surgical outcome in 62 patients. Acta Neurochir **143**: 471–476; 2001
95. Zheng W, Qu X, Zhong M, Wu J, Zhuge Q, Lu X. Microsurgical treatment of cranial base meningioma. Zhonghua Wai Ke Za Zhi **38**: 429–431; 2000
96. Zhu W, Mao Y, Zhou LF, Zhang R, Chen L. Combined subtemporal and retrosigmoid keyhole approach for extensive petroclival meningiomas surgery: report of experience with 7 cases. Minim Invasive Neurosurg **51(2)**: 95–99; 2008
97. Sade B., Lee J.H., High incidence of optic canal involvement in clinoidal meningiomas: rationale for aggressive skull base approach. Acta Neurochir **150 (11)**: 1127–1132; 2008
98. Jacob M, Wydh E, Vighetto A, Sindou M. Visual outcome after surgery for cavernous sinus meningioma. Acta Neurochir **150(5)**: 421–429; 2008
99. Boulton MR, Cusimano MD. Foramen magnum meningiomas: concepts, classifications, and nuances. Neurosurg Focus **14(6)**: E10; 2003
100. Kawasawe T, Yoshida K, Uchida K. Petroclival meningiomas II. In: Lee JH (ed) Meningiomas: Diagnosis, Treatment and Outcome. Springer Verlag London Limited, Godalming: pp 415–423; 2008
101. Wu ZB, Yu CJ, Guan SS. Posterior petrous meningiomas: 82 cases. J Neurosurg **102**: 284–289; 2005
102. Chi JH, McDermott MW. Tuberculum sellae meningiomas. Neurosurg Focus **14(6)**: E6; 2003
103. Hasegawa T, Kida Y, Yoshimoto M, Koike J, Iizuka H, Ishii D. Long-term outcomes of gamma knife surgery for cavernous sinus meningioma. J Neurosurg **107(4)**: 745–751; 2007
104. Iwai Y, Yamanaka K, Ishiguro T. Gamma knife radiosurgery for the treatment of cavernous sinus meningiomas. Neurosurgery **52(3)**: 517–524; 2003
105. Lee JY, Niranjan A, McInerney J, Kondziolka D, Flickinger JC, Lunsford LD. Stereotactic radiosurgery providing long-term tumor control of cavernous sinus meningiomas. J Neurosurg **97(1)**: 65–72; 2002
106. Liscak R, Simonova G, Vymazal J, Janouskova L, Vladyka V. Gamma knife radiosurgery of meningiomas in the cavernous sinus region. Acta Neurochir **141(5)**: 473–480; 1999
107. Nicolato A, Foroni R, Alessandrini F, Bricolo A, Gerosa M. Radiosurgical treatment of cavernous sinus meningiomas: experience with 122 treated patients. Neurosurgery **51(5)**: 1153–1159; 2002
108. Nicolato A, Foroni R, Alessandrini F, Maluta S, Bricolo A, Gerosa M. The role of gamma knife radiosurgery in the management of cavernous sinus meningiomas. Int J Radiat Oncol Biol Phys **53(4)**: 992–1000; 2002
109. Pollock BE, Stafford SL. Results of stereotactic radiosurgery for patients with imaging defined cavernous sinus meningiomas. Int J Radiat Oncol Biol Phys **62(5)**: 1427–1431; 2005
110. Roche PH, Régis J, Dufour H, Fournier HD, Delsanti C, Pellet W, Grisoli F, Peragut JC. Gamma knife radiosurgery in the management of cavernous sinus meningiomas. J Neurosurg **93(Suppl 3)**: 68–73; 2000
111. Kondziolka D, Madhok R, Lunsford LD, Mathieu D, Martin JJ, Niranjan A, Flickinger JC. Stereotactic radiosurgery for convexity meningiomas. J Neurosurg **111(3)**: 458–463; 2009

112. Muthukumar N, Kondziolka D, Lunsford LD, Flickinger JC. Stereotactic radiosurgery for anterior foramen magnum meningiomas. Surg Neurol **51(3)**: 268–273; 1999

113. Kim IY, Kondziolka D, Niranjan A, Flickinger JC, Lunsford LD. Gamma knife radiosurgery for intraventricular meningiomas. Acta Neurochir (Wien) **151(5)**: 447–452; 2009

114. Bledsoe JM, Link MJ, Stafford SL, Park PJ, Pollock BE. Radiosurgery for large-volume (>10 cm^3) benign meningiomas. J Neurosurg **112(5)**: 951–956; 2009

115. Flickinger JC, Kondziolka D, Maitz AH, Lunsford LD. Gamma knife radiosurgery of imaging-diagnosed intracranial meningioma. Int J Radiat Oncol Biol Phys **56(3)**: 801–806; 2003

116. Ganz JC, Reda WA, Abdelkarim K. Gamma Knife surgery of large meningiomas: early response to treatment. Acta Neurochir (Wien) **151(1)**: 1–8; 2009

117. Haselsberger K, Maier T, Dominikus K, Holl E, Kurschel S, Ofner-Kopeinig P, Unger F. Staged gamma knife radiosurgery for large critically located benign meningiomas: evaluation of a series comprising 20 patients. J Neurol Neurosurg Psychiatry **80(10)**: 1172–1175; 2009

118. Kondziolka D, Levy EI, Niranjan A, Flickinger JC, Lunsford LD. Long-term outcomes after meningioma radiosurgery: physician and patient perspectives. J Neurosurg **91(1)**: 44–50; 1999

119. Iwai Y, Yamanaka K, Morikawa T. Adjuvant gamma knife radiosurgery after meningioma resection. J Clin Neurosci **11(7)**: 715–718; 2004

120. Malik I, Rowe JG, Walton L, Radatz MW, Kemeny AA. The use of stereotactic radiosurgery in the management of meningiomas. Br J Neurosurg **19(1)**: 13–20; 2005

121. Pollock BE. Stereotactic radiosurgery for intracranial meningiomas: indications and results. Neurosurg Focus **14(5)**: e4; 2003

122. Flannery TJ, Kano H, Lunsford LD, Sirin S, Tormenti M, Niranjan A, Flickinger JC, Kondziolka D. Long-term control of petroclival meningiomas through radiosurgery. J Neurosurg **112(5)**: 957–964; 2010

123. Roche PH, Pellet W, Fuentes S, Thomassin JM, Régis J. Gamma knife radiosurgical management of petroclival meningiomas results and indications. Acta Neurochir **145(10)**: 883–888; 2003

124. Aichholzer M, Bertalanffy A, Dietrich W, Roessler K, Pfisterer W, Ungersboeck K, Heimberger K, Kitz K. Gamma knife radiosurgery of skull base meningiomas. Acta Neurochir **142 (6)**: 647–652; 2000

125. Davidson L, Fishback D, Russin JJ, Weiss MH, Yu C, Pagnini PG, Zelman V, Apuzzo ML, Giannotta SL. Postoperative gamma Knife surgery for benign meningiomas of the cranial base. Neurosurg Focus **23(4)**: E6; 2007

126. Eustacchio S, Trummer M, Fuchs I, Schrottner O, Sutter B, Pendl G. Preservation of cranial nerve function following gamma knife radiosurgery for benign skull base meningiomas: experience in 121 patients with follow-up of 5 to 9.8 years. Acta Neurochir Suppl **84**: 71–76; 2002

127. Iwai Y, Yamanaka K, Nakajima H, Yasui T, Kishi H. Gamma knife radiosurgery for skull base meningiomas: the treatment results and patient satisfaction expressed in answers to a questionnaire. No Shinkei Geka **28(5)**: 411–415; 2000

128. Kreil W, Luggin J, Fuchs I, Weigl V, Eustacchio S, Papaefthymiou G. Long term experience of gamma knife radiosurgery for benign skull base meningiomas. J Neurol Neurosurg Psychiatry **76(10)**: 1425–1430; 2005

129. Nakaya K, Hayashi M, Nakamura S, Atsuchi S, Sato H, Ochiai T, Yamamoto M, Izawa M, Hori T, Takakura K. Low-dose radiosurgery for meningiomas. Stereotact Funct Neurosurg **72(Suppl 1)**: 67–72; 1999

130. Pendl G, Eustacchio S, Unger F. Radiosurgery as alternative treatment for skull base meningiomas. J Clin Neurosci **8(Suppl 1)**: 12–14; 2001

131. Pollock BE, Stafford SL, Utter A, Giannini C, Schreiner SA. Stereotactic radiosurgery provides equivalent tumor control to Simpson Grade 1 resection for patients with small- to medium-size meningiomas. Int J Radiat Oncol Biol Phys **55(4)**: 1000–1005; 2003

132. Zachenhofer I, Wolfsberger S, Aichholzer M, Bertalanffy A, Roessler K, Kitz K, Knosp E. Gamma-knife radiosurgery for cranial base meningiomas: experience of tumor control, clinical course, and morbidity in a follow-up of more than 8 years. Neurosurgery 58(1): 28–36; 2006
133. Chang HS. Peritumoral edema. In: Lee JH (ed) Meningiomas: Diagnosis, Treatment and Outcome. Springer Verlag London Limited, Godalming: pp 565–572; 2008
134. Black PM, Morokoff AP, Zauberman J. Surgery for extra-axial tumors of the cerebral convexity and midline. Neurosurgery 62(6 Suppl 3): 1115–1121; 2008
135. Couldwell WT, Kan P, Liu JK, Apfelbaum RI. Decompression of cavernous sinus meningioma for preservation and improvement of cranial nerve function. Technical note. J Neurosurg 105(1): 148–152; 2006
136. Iwai Y, Yamanaka K, Nakajima H. Two-staged gamma knife radiosurgery for the treatment of large petroclival and cavernous sinus meningiomas. Surg Neurol 56(5): 308–314; 2001
137. Ganz JC, Backlund EO, Thorsen FA. The results of gamma knife surgery of meningiomas, related to size of tumor and dose. Stereotact Funct Neurosurg 61(Suppl 1): 23–29; 1993
138. Ahn ES, Chin LS, Gyure KA, Hudes RS, Ragheb J, DiPatri AJ Jr. Long-term control after resection and gamma knife surgery of an intracranial clear cell meningioma: case report. J Neurosurg 102(3 Suppl): 303–306; 2005
139. Kondziolka D, Flickinger JC, Perez B. Judicious resection and/or radiosurgery for parasagittal meningiomas: outcomes from a multicenter review. Gamma Knife Meningioma Study Group. Neurosurgery 43(3): 405–413; 1998
140. Iwai Y, Yamanaka K, Ikeda H. Gamma knife radiosurgery for skull base meningioma: long-term results of low-dose treatment. J Neurosurg 109(5): 804–810; 2008
141. El Shehaby A, Ganz JC, Reda WA, Hafez A. Mechanisms of edema after gamma knife surgery for meningiomas. Report of two cases. J Neurosurg 102(Suppl): 1–3; 2005
142. Metellus P, Régis J, Muracciole X, Fuentes S, Dufour H, Nanni I, Chinot O, Martin PM, Grisoli F. Evaluation of fractionated radiotherapy and gamma knife radiosurgery in cavernous sinus meningiomas: treatment strategy. Neurosurgery 57(5): 873–886; 2005
143. Lim YJ, Leem W, Park JT, Rhee BA, Kim GJ. Cerebral infarction with ICA occlusion after gamma knife radiosurgery for pituitary adenoma: a case report. Stereotact Funct Neurosurg 72(Suppl 1): 132–139; 1999
144. Rowe JG, Walton L, Vaughan P, Malik I, Radatz M, Kemeny A. Radiosurgical planning of meningiomas: compromises with conformity. Stereotact Funct Neurosurg 82(4): 169–174; 2004
145. Ganz JC, El Shehaby A, Reda WA, Abdelkarim K. Protection of the anterior visual pathways during gamma knife treatment of meningiomas. Br J Neurosurg 24(3): 248–258; 2010
146. Roser F, Nakamura M, Martini-Thomas R, Samii M, Tatagiba M. The role of surgery in meningiomas involving the optic nerve sheath. Clin Neurol Neurosurg 108: 470–476; 2006
147. Schick U, Dott U, Hassler W. Surgical management of meningiomas involving the optic nerve sheath. J Neurosurg 101(6): 951–959; 2004
148. Al-Mefty O, Kadri PA, Pravdenkova JR, Sawyer JR, Stangeby. C, Hirsh M. Malignant progression in meningioma: documentation of a series and analysis of cytogenetic findings. J Neurosurg 101: 210–218; 2004
149. Jääskeläinen J, Haltia M, Laasonen E, Wahström T, Valtonen S. The growth rate of intracranial meningiomas and its relation to histology: an analysis of 43 patients. Surg Neurol 24: 165–172; 1985
150. Jääskeläinen J, Haltia M, Servo A. Atypical and Anaplastic meningiomas: radiology, surgery, radiotherapy, and outcome. Surg Neurol 25: 233–242; 1986

Chapter 15
Gamma Knife for Cerebral Metastases

Preamble About Problems

The study of the treatment of brain metastases (BMs) is fraught with problems. The tumours are the intracranial expression of a multifaceted series of complex systemic diseases. The expression of cerebral metastases is protean with great variety in size, number and tumour of origin. Clearly, no single treatment modality will be adequate is all cases. Once again, a multi-modal cooperation of varying expertise is needed. Moreover, the lethality of such tumours is so high that scientific evaluation of different forms of treatment is difficult. It should never be forgotten that the median survival of the untreated condition is 4–8 weeks. This makes randomisation of any treatment which seems effective a difficult proposition. The consequence is that very few of the many articles written on this subject can be claimed to provide level one evidence. Nonetheless, advances in knowledge and technology have now finally enabled the gradual publication of some level 1 studies, even though they remain a minority. These studies and their findings are necessarily important for evidence based treatment of BMs. However, before proceeding to the main text of this chapter it seems sensible to review some of the concepts, methods of patient assessment and relevant parameters which are used in this context. While much of what follows may be familiar in principle, it is easy to forget in detail. Moreover, the assembly of this information in one place is perhaps helpful. For those better informed please skip the current section and move on directly to the section on "Background".

To begin this section, there is the classification of clinical trials which lay the basis for acquiring knowledge of new treatments. These are summarised from the Institute of Cancer Research.

J.C. Ganz, *Gamma Knife Neurosurgery*,
DOI 10.1007/978-3-7091-0343-2_15, © Springer-Verlag/Wien 2011

Concepts Scales and Parameters for Evidence Based Treatment

Phases of Clinical Trials (Institute of Cancer Research)

Before a treatment can be given a license to treat patients on a day-to-day basis it needs to go through a series (or phases) of trials to test whether it is:

- Safe
- Has side effects (toxicity)
- Works better than the current standard treatment
- Helps people feel better (have an effect on quality of life)
- Is cost effective

A single clinical trial cannot answer all these questions at once. Therefore different aspects of a treatments effect are tested in the different phases.

Phase I

The aim of Phase I clinical trials is to test the safety of a new treatment. This will include looking at side effects (toxicity) of a treatment – for example, does it make people sick. If the treatment results in too many side effects it will not progress any further in development in that form. Phase I clinical trials involve only a small number of people (possibly as few as 15–20). Depending on the type of disease being studied, patients in phase I trials may be healthy volunteers or may be patients with advanced stages of a disease, such as cancer, where standard treatments are no longer considered to be of benefit. If the treatment is considered safe in a phase I trial, it will progress to a phase II clinical trial.

Phase II

In Phase II, clinical trials test the new treatment in a larger group of people who have the disease for which the treatment is to be used, to see whether the treatment is effective, at least in the short term. Effective in the case of cancer could mean that the treatment shrinks the size of a tumour in some of the patients with the disease. These studies are larger, possibly involving up to 200 people. Phase II clinical trials also collect information about safety in this larger group of people. Treatments only move into a phase III clinical trial if phase II is successful.

Phase III

The objective of Phase III clinical trials is to test the new treatment in an even larger group of people who have the disease for which the treatment is designed. Several hundred to a few thousand patients could be involved in a phase III clinical trial. Due to their large size this phase of trial could involve many hospitals and many countries. These clinical trials look at how well the new treatment works by comparing it with the best treatment currently in use, or occasionally with a placebo (a dummy drug, which looks like the drug being tested). In phase III trials, and sometimes in phase II trials, patients are allocated their treatment using randomisation.

The next scale refers to the assessment of the structure of a given study in relation to the reliability of the study's findings. This list is taken from the "Levels of Evidence and Grades of Recommendation" from the Oxford Centre for Evidence-Based Medicine.

Ranking of Evidence

1a:	Systematic reviews (with homogeneity) of randomized controlled trials
1a-:	Systematic review of randomized trials displaying worrisome heterogeneity
1b:	Individual randomized controlled trials (with narrow confidence interval)
1b-:	Individual randomized controlled trials (with a wide confidence interval)
1c:	All or none randomized controlled trials
2a:	Systematic reviews (with homogeneity) of cohort studies
2a-:	Systematic reviews of cohort studies displaying worrisome heterogeneity
2b:	Individual cohort study or low quality randomized controlled trials (<80% follow-up)
2b-:	Individual cohort study or low quality randomized controlled trials (<80% follow-up/ wide confidence interval)
2c:	Outcomes' Research; ecological studies
3a:	Systematic review (with homogeneity) of case–control studies
3a-:	Systematic review of case–control studies with worrisome heterogeneity
3b:	Individual case–control study
4:	Case-series (and poor quality cohort and case–control studies)
5:	Expert opinion without explicit critical appraisal, or based on physiology, bench research or "first principles"

In a group of systemic illnesses which can affect the functions of the patient in any number of ways the quality of life and daily function needs to be expressed. One of the more familiar methods for doing this is the Karnowsky Performance Scale outlined below.

Karnowsky Score

100%	Normal; no complaints; no evidence of disease
90%	Able to carry on normal activity; minor signs of disease
80%	Normal activity with effort, some signs or symptoms of disease
70%	Cares for self. Unable to carry on normal activity or to do active work
60%	Requires occasional assistance, but is able to care for most of own needs
50%	Requires considerable assistance and frequent medical care

(continued)

40%	Disabled, requires special care and assistance
30%	Severely disabled, hospitalisation is indicated although death not imminent
20%	Hospitalisation necessary, very sick, active supportive treatment necessary
10%	Moribund, fatal processes progressing rapidly
0%	Dead

The variability of expression and development of BMs is protean. To indicate the complexity of possible clinical patterns, a list of some major patient and treatment parameters which can affect results follows.

Parameters Concerned in the Management of BMs are Listed Below

Parameter	Possibilities and/or significance
Patient parameters	
Age and sex	Younger patients do better. Some tumours sex specific
Number of BMs	The prognosis is related to the number of BMs
Latency from primary diagnosis to diagnosis of BM	Synchronous – diagnosed at the same time primary tumour Metachronous – some time after diagnosis of the primary tumour – longer delay can mean better outlook
Tumour location(s)	Different locations include Supratentorial, Infratentorial, Superficial or Deep, Basal Ganglia, Cerebellum, BrainstemThese different locations affect management and result
Mental function	Affected by BMs and degree of functional loss affects QOL and survival
Neurological deficits	Affected by BMs and the degree of deficit affects QOL and survival
Extracranial disease	Both the Primary tumour growth and the spread of extracranial metastases
Tumour histology	Different tumours have different outlooks
Tumour volume	Bigger tumours are harder to control
KPS	Fitter patients do better
RPA	See below but fitter patients do better
Radiation treatment related parameters	
Dose	Dose relates to tumour control, complications and survival
Measure of success	Success may be measured by local control, distant control and survival
Possible complications	Radiation damage to brain, Tumour necrosis with swelling, Leukencephalopathy
Patterns of management	Whole Brain Radiotherapy (WBRT) alone WBRT + Radiosurgery Salvage WBRT + Surgery Salvage Surgery alone Surgery + Radiosurgery Radiosurgery alone Radiosurgery + WBRT Salvage

This is obviously complex. Thus, to bring some semblance of order into this abundance of measurable variables a number of prognostic scales have been devised, the idea of which is to enable evidence based assessment of a patient prior to treatment, to facilitate the choice of the optimal management. These scales are outlined below. The first was derived for the highly respected RTOG[1] in 1997 in the USA and is called Recursive Partitioning Analysis. It assesses 4 variables and has been seen to be reliable.

Recursive Partition Analysis (RPA) of the RTOG

RPA Class 1: Patients <65 years old with a Karnowsky Score ≥70, controlled primary tumour and no extracranial metastases
RPA Class 2: Patients intermediate between Class 1 and Class 3
RPA Class 3: Patients <65 years old with a Karnowsky Score <70 and systemic disease

The next scale was derived in Brazil and published in 1998. It is called the Score Index for Stereotactic Radiosurgery for Brain Metastases (SIR). After some initial redesigning it came into its current form published in 2001. It includes tumour volume and number of tumours in the assessment [1].

Score Index for Stereotactic Radiosurgery for Brain Metastases (SIR)

Variable	Score		
	0	1	2
Age	≥60	51–59	≤50
KPS	≤50 or less	60–70	80–100
Systemic disease status	Progressive	Stable	Complete remission or no evidence of disease
Number lesions	≥3	2	1
Largest lesion volume cm³	>13	5–13	<5

Its proponents claimed that it was a better predictor of outcome than the recursive partitioning analysis and simpler to use.

In 2004 the Brussels group came with a new protocol which they claim is even easier to use. This was the Basic Score for Brain Metastases (BS-BM) [2]

---

[1]Radiation Therapy Oncology Group.

Basic Score for Brain Metastases (BS-BM)

Variable	Score	
	0	1
KPS	50–70	80–100
Control of primary tumour	No	Yes
Extracranial metastases	Yes	No

Again the proponents claimed this was simpler and more reliable than other scores, but as can be seen ignores the intracranial parameters noted in the SIR.

Finally, in 2008 members of the RTOG group with access to their vast database came up with yet another prognostic assessment scale. They called it the Graded Prognostic Assessment Scale (GPA) [3].

Graded Prognostic Assessment (GPA)

Variable	Score		
	0	1	2
Age	>60	50–59	<50
KPS	<70	70–80	90–100
No. CNS Metastases	>3	2–3	1
Extra Cranial Metastases	Present	–	None

This includes the number of metastases as in the SIR but leaves out the tumour volume as they point out this parameter is not usually available until the day of treatment and is thus not helpful in deciding whether to treat or not.

It might be noted that each of the above scoring systems has its strengths. However, with the variability of reporting permitted today it is suggested that consistency of reporting is more important than small details of the method of reporting. In this context it is suggested that the RTOG RPA reporting should be obligatory for any author seeking to publish work on GKNS for BMs and that it would be an advantage if editors and reviewers were strict on this point.

It should be noted that unless otherwise stated, the references used in this chapter refer to papers reporting results with the Gamma Knife. There are numerous papers on the topic of metastases where different radiosurgery techniques have been used. However, since the technology and methodology used with non Gamma Knife "radiosurgery" is variable from site to site and user to user, it is suggested that clinical papers based on other techniques are not necessarily relevant to Gamma Knife users. On the other hand any report relating to non-clinical basic radiobiology or radiophysics would be of interest irrespective of the radiation technique used.

Background

The Size of the Problem

For those of us who were involved in the early days of Gamma Knife neurosurgery (GKNS) it is slightly odd to see how slowly the technique was used in the treatment of BMs from systemic tumours. All agree that metastases are the commonest intracerebral tumour but there remains a wide divergence of opinion as to the true incidence. In a recent book the incidence in the USA is stated to be 170,000 per year [4]. Other authors in the same book recount the difficulties of accurate assessment of the incidence of these tumours but in general quote a lower figure under 100/ million per year [5]. The RTOG group in their papers quote the 170,000 figure and claim on the other hand that 20–40% of cancer patients develop BMs. Other authors look at the matter in another way and state that 50% of all cancer patients get BMs. This figure is derived from autopsy studies [6, 7]. It is this 50% BM incidence for all cancers which provides the figure of 170,000 new cases per year quoted above. The CIA world Factbook states the estimated 2009 population of the USA to be 307,212,123. This would give a BM incidence roughly equivalent to 550 per million per year.

The Evolution of Imaging Techniques

The treatment of BMs was necessarily limited prior to the introduction of computed tomography (CT) in 1973. Prior to this metastases were largely invisible and there was no means of following the results of treatment. This made radiotherapy the only reasonable treatment with surgery limited to a minority of selected cases. The results of CT indicated that up to 50% of metastases were solitary. However, with the introduction of MRI in particular using T1 sequences with gadolinium, evidence has been acquired indicating that only 25–30% of metastases are solitary [8, 9].

Development of Treatment Methods

It is important for Gamma Knife users to remember that their method was intro-duced into a world which already had a treatment for BMs in the form of Whole Brain Radiotherapy (WBRT). In respected reviews of the treatment of brain metastases it is stated that the median survival of the untreated disease is 4 weeks [8] or less than 2 months with steroids [10]. Radiotherapy is claimed to increase survival to 3–6 months [8] or up to 6 months [10]. While radiotherapy clearly gave a benefit it was limited. A variety of radiation dose and fractionation schedules were attempted but there seems to have developed broad agreement that a treatment with 10 × 3 Gy fractions gives as good a result as any other.

Three level one publications assessed the consequences of adding surgery to the mix. These papers for obvious reasons were restricted to solitary metastases. Two groups found that surgery improved the survival [8, 11]. The third found no such benefit, but records that the patients died largely from extracranial disease, indicating this paper includes patients with a poorer general condition than the other two papers. The generally accepted conclusion from the results of this work is that surgery can improve the survival in patients who can tolerate an operation with a solitary easily accessible metastasis. This is clearly a minority of patients. Radiosurgery does not suffer the limitations of surgery but it was not until the 1990s that it received serious attention as a possible additional treatment to WBRT. However, the frequency of BMs and the desperate situation of the patients with these tumours led to a rapid, indeed almost explosive growth in the use of this new method.

The Introduction of Radiosurgery

Stockholm Studies

The group in Stockholm were the first to treat metastases in the Gamma Knife and they published a review of their work in 1993 on a material which dated back to 1975. Only five patients were treated between 1975 and 1986. This pattern reflects Leksell's dislike of treating malignant disease. The reason was the judgement that radiosurgery required more publications recording long term survival of treated patients in order to increase the acceptance of the method. This guiding principle rather fell into desuetude following his death in 1986. The Stockholm group were aware of the high incidence of cerebral metastases as quoted above [6]. They also quote early work from the radiation therapy oncology group (RTOG) which found that more than 50% of patients die from progression of their cerebral metastases when treated with conventional fractionated radiotherapy [12]. This led them to the view that conventional radiotherapy was not particularly useful. They presented a material of 160 patients with 235 metastases treated from 1975. They achieved tumour control in 94% of cases [13] using a mean margin dose of 27 Gy (range 10–56 Gy). This local control was not related to histology.

Adverse radiation effects (AREs) were found in 13% of treated tumours. In most this was limited to a temporary steroid responsive oedema. However, in a few there was a more chronic reaction. The findings in these cases simulated tumour recurrence and this could only be distinguished from true recurrence in their material by the use of a low 18-FDG glucose uptake PET scan. They also found that the incidence of new distant metastases varied with the number of metastases at the initial treatment. With one tumour the incidence was 13%, with 2 or 3 it was 34% and for those with more tumours at the initial treatment the incidence of a new distal metastasis was 100%. They also found a mean survival of 7 months. Of the 62 deaths in the material, only two were the result of uncontrolled intracranial disease.

The point is made that while the control of BMs was very effective this had little effect on survival. Thus it was suggested that the appropriate endpoint for treatment would be tumour control rather than survival. They suggest their findings indicate that patients presenting with many metastases have a more aggressive disease in view of the higher incidence of distant metastases in these patients. They acknowledge that WBRT improves the local control of surgically treated patients. However, this in effect applies only to solitary tumours, which represent about 25% of cases. They also query the evidence for prophylactic radiation reducing the incidence of distal metastases. They mention the risks of dementia following WBRT and query the value of using WBRT at all. They conclude that GKNS alone would seem to be an adequate treatment method for controlling small intracerebral metastases.

Boston Studies

There were groups using linear accelerators who had published early work; including the Cologne group [14], the Heidelberg group [15] and the Stanford group [16]. In the late 1980s and early 1990s the clinical material was based on small numbers. On the other hand, the Boston Group had treated larger numbers like the Stockholm group and their findings and conclusions were in keeping with the results of other users of linear accelerator stereotactic single session radiotherapy. These findings were summed up in a book published in 1993 [17]. They reported a reasonably large material of 196 patients with 282 metastases. Selection factors for acceptance for treatment were a Karnowsky Performance Score (KPS) was 60 or more, absence of systemic disease and failed prior radiotherapy. Again 94% of tumours were controlled. Moreover, as with the Gamma Knife histology was not a predictor of tumour control. Tumour volume was noted to have a negative correlation with tumour control. There were in principle no differences between the Boston and Stockholm results in terms of response to treatment. The Boston group also observed similar complications. The major difference between the two studies relates to the use of WBRT. The Boston group claimed that the use of WBRT increased the tumour control and reduced the chance of developing future metastases. They quote a paper from Stanford in support of this notion [18].

End Point of Treatment

Local Tumour Control

In their 1993 paper Kihlström et al [13]. noted that tumour control might be a more reliable treatment endpoint. They argued that since GKNS only affects one limited aspect of the systemic illness it could not reliably be expected to affect survival, which in many patients could be decided by the progress of the extracranial disease. This view was incorporated into one of the level one studies of the effects of radiosurgery on BMs [19]. There are now a substantial number of articles recording the control of cerebral metastases treated by the Gamma Knife [2, 20–77].

As the experience of treating metastases with radiosurgery expanded and deepened it was natural for the question to arise as to whether radiosurgery alone was as effective for tumour control as using a radiosurgery boost to WBRT. Some groups report that there is a significant increase in tumour control if WBRT is added to GKNS [24, 28, 49, 55, 70, 78–84]. However, there are also a number of papers which conclude that WBRT has little or no effect on the local control rate [26, 35, 39, 40, 61, 63, 64, 85–87]. This disagreement may well reflect the fact that the great majority of the published material relates to retrospective non-randomised studies; in other words Class 3 or at best Class 2 evidence.

Findings of Level 1 Evidence Studies

In a number of early studies the primary treatment was WBRT and authors compared the effects of adding radiosurgery to patients who had received WBRT [10, 19, 80, 88]. In all instances the addition of radiosurgery improved the local control achieved with WBRT alone. In other papers attempts were made to assess the effect of a WBRT on the local control achieved by a radiosurgery treatment. In one study radiosurgery with or without WBRT was superior to WBRT alone [19]. However, the frequency of distal metastases was reduced with WBRT. In two other papers the local control was improved if WBRT was added to the radiosurgery treatment [70, 89].

Patient Survival

A number of papers have failed to demonstrate any advantage in survival for patients receiving WBRT in addition to radiosurgery [28, 55, 56, 59, 63, 69, 78, 83, 87, 89–100]. A single well constructed level one paper shows a survival advantage when WBRT is added to radiosurgery in the special situation of a solitary metastasis. Thus it may be seen that the great majority of writers believe that WBRT does not improve survival. This is widely accepted but is challenged by one prominent and distinguished group.

Findings of Level 1 Evidence Studies

The workers from Kentucky have discussed this matter in a review article [9]. They discount the results in two other studies [19, 80]. They state for one level one study from Pittsburgh [80] *"This study . . . . . . used nonstandard end-points. As a result this trial was uninterpretable"*. It may be noted that the endpoint used was '*imaging-defined control of brain disease*'. Referring to a published abstract from a level one study from Brown University Rhode Island [19] the same paper states "*A second study . . . . . . contained methodological problems that made it impossible to draw firm conclusions from the data*". In neither of these cases do the authors enlarge, justify, specify, or explain their specific objections to these studies, which are usually accepted as excellent. It is perhaps almost ironic that this review was written 2 years before the eminent Aoyama paper published in JAMA, which also finds no relationship between WBRT and survival. The point in mentioning the above is that this is an area of dispute and the published opinions on occasion seem to be coloured more by passion than evidence. As far as one can judge at present WBRT does not improve survival except perhaps with solitary metastases. The reader should please note that the author is not expressing an isolated personal opinion. In 2008 a paper was written with the very title "Adjuvant Whole Brain Radiotherapy. Strong emotions decide but rational studies are needed" [24].

Treatment-Related Complications Principles

Acute Adverse Effects After WBRT

Toxicity is sometimes reported as early ($\leq$3months after treatment) or late or delayed (>3 months after treatment) [101]. The early complications are fairly non-specific consisting of headache, nausea, vomiting, vertigo, alopecia and in some cases epilepsy. These are seldom severe and no good correlation exists of their relationship to imaging changes.

Adverse Radiation Effects and Radionecrosis

Shaw et al. described a table for the grading of complications by the RTOG. These are delayed focal complications occurring at the location of the tumour(s) treated.

Radiation Therapy Oncology Group central nervous system toxicity criteria	
Grade	Definition
1	No toxicity, mild neurologic symptoms, no medication required
2	Moderate neurologic symptoms, outpatient medications[a] required
3	Severe neurologic symptoms; outpatient or inpatient medications[a] required
4	Life-threatening neurologic symptoms, including status epilepticus, paralysis, coma, or radionecrosis requiring operation
5	Fatal toxicity

[a]e.g., Corticosteroids

In Shaw et al's work [102] the toxicity concerned is associated with subjective symptomatic changes accompanied by adverse radiation reactions visible on the imaging. The imaging can show AREs of different kinds including tumour necrosis, radionecrosis and radiation induced oedema. In Shaw et al's work this can occur at

1 month or 15 months so the division into early and late may not seem to fit. However, perhaps the right approach is consider the early effects seen in this context are "accelerated late effects" as discussed in Chap. 7.

Severe delayed complications can provide a diagnostic dilemma. The complications here considered are focal and relate to the region/regions of the tumour/ tumours which has/have been treated. They can amongst other things cause a tumour to swell and be associated with a new peritumoural oedema. This can mimic treatment failure with tumour growth. An 18 FDG PET scan is among the better methods for sorting out the difference [13]. Until recently MRI was considered not so useful. However, very recent work has indicated a simple method to make this distinction. If the size of the contrast enhancing lesion on MR T1 series matches the lesion seen on T2 images, it is most likely that the volume increase is due to tumour growth. If there is no such correspondence then the tumour swelling is most likely radiation damage [103]. In addition if an increased T2 signal follows the anatomy of the gyri it is most probably a tumour [104].

Most patients with AREs respond well to corticosteroid treatment given together with antacid medication. A tiny minority may require surgical decompression. If the increase in tumour volume is a genuine treatment failure, then a retreatment will be required.

Radiation Induced Dementia and Leukoencephalopathy

There is another problem associated with radiation to the brain, specifically to WBRT. This is a diffuse effect associated with loss of tissue on imaging and a clinical dementia called radiation induced leukoencephalopathy. The loss of tissue is considered due to demyelination secondary to vascular damage to small blood vessels. It is seen most often when high doses of intracranial irradiation are associated with the use of chemotherapeutic agents such as methotrexate. Large fractions are also considered to increase the risk of this condition. Al-Mefty et al. published a paper on this topic in relation to the long term side-effects of radiation therapy for benign brain tumours [105]. That is to say the paper dealt with long term survival in adults and with benign tumours. There were 17 patients who suffered "delayed parenchymal changes attributed to radiation treatment". In all but 2 cases the latent interval from treatment to the development of symptoms was more than 2.5 years. The median and mean latent intervals were 10 years. This indicates that the chance of developing these changes in a population of patients with BMs, where the median survival is about 9 months is not high. Nonetheless, recent studies have demonstrated that some form of reduction in neurocognitive function does occur following the use of WBRT [78, 106]. The effects were so clear cut in one of the studies, which was prospective in design, that the relevant ethics committee stopped the trial after 56 of the planned 80 patients had been treated, since the cognitive damage due WBRT was shown to be both statistically significant in terms of incidence and undesirable in terms of quality of life.

Treatment Strategies for BMs

Should Up Front WBRT Be Used in All Patients?

The literature on this topic is passionate, controversial and not entirely clear. There is now broad agreement that WBRT improves the results of surgery for solitary tumours and that it improves the survival in non-operated patients. However, the improvements are not impressive so that for multiple tumours it is tempting to combine it with other treatment measures and the commonest measure in use today is RS. There has been broad agreement that RS and WBRT give better tumour control and survival than WBRT alone. The question then arises, to what extent is WBRT necessary?

The underlying principle propagated by those who believe WBRT is essential is that it will treat the invisible micro-metastases at the same time as it treats the visible tumours. There is however a fallacy in that argument. A question arises. How effective is WBRT for the metastasis arising the day after WBRT is over? This possible phenomenon has received scant if any attention in the literature.

Another issue is that GKNS for metastases was originally conceived as a multiple session treatment [13]. New metastases were expected after the first treatment and a follow up system was devised to catch them early and to treat them as required. Yet this notion has been largely ignored in the literature with one particular exception [107].

The Arguments for and Against Using WBRT

1. WBRT with RS increases the local control rate and distant control rate of metastases and therefore should be used [10, 87, 89, 93, 100, 107–111].

   There is sufficient evidence both pro- and retrospective to support this notion that it is considered in this book that combined RS and WBRT does result in a higher local and distant control rate than either method used alone. **NB This applies to a RS used only once and the need for WBRT instead of repeated RS receives scant attention in the literature.**

2. WBRT with RS improves the survival of patients with metastases compared with RS alone [10, 88].

   There is a single level one evidence paper indicating [10] that for RPA Group 1 patients with solitary metastases survival with combined WBRT and RS is greater than with either method used alone.

3. Neurological deterioration in patients with BMs is usually due to uncontrolled tumour growth not radiation toxicity therefore WBRT with its effect on improving local and distal tumour control is needed for maintaining quality of life [110, 112]

   This may be true but as yet the evidence is not clear.

4. Neurological Improvement is seen in the absence of WBRT [106]
5. WBRT is not associated with an increased radiation related toxicity [24]

   There is evidence to support this notion. It should be noted that clinically important radiation toxicity is expected to affect the quality of life (QOL)

6. WBRT is associated with an increased radiation related toxicity [89, 106, 109, 113, 114]

   There is also evidence to support this notion. It should be noted that clinically important radiation toxicity is expected to affect the quality of life (QOL). **One particularly important recent paper suggests that for patients with 1–3 metastases and in classes RPA 1–3 that WBRT increases the chances of mental deterioration. This is a prospective Class 1 study from the MC Anderson Center, which was broken off because the results were so clear cut. This series used a high frequency of surgical salvage but demonstrated an increased survival in the patients who did NOT receive WBRT** [106]

7. There is at present inadequate data concerning quality of life after WBRT [88, 106, 115].

   This would seem to be the point of view of most serious unbiased workers at the present.

8. Dementia is less common than imaging changes indicating radiation toxicity [89, 112, 114]

   This is an important concept. The incidence of radiation induced imaging change can be up to 30% in WBRT treated patients but the clinical expression of this radiation damage is much lower.

9. Dementia requires a more thorough battery of tests than provided by MMSE [89, 112, 116]

   While this may be true, there is an impression that this is an argument used by those who really want to retain WBRT as an up front treatment modality when the results of papers concerning radiation toxicity indicate that maybe WBRT should be avoided.

Additional Considerations

The above list doesn't make it easy to decide whether WBRT should or should not be used. The following list of factors might be considered important when deciding on the best treatment for a given patient.

The key issues are as follows
Survival in most series is not improved by WBRT added to RS
There is little useful information of QOL with and without WBRT

(continued)

Healthier patients do better (RPA 1 AND 2 or high KPS score and young age)

The principle of expecting to need multiple GKNS treatments as part of the planned management has received too little attention. These multiple treatments were part of the original concept of GKNS for metastases but are often referred to with the rather pejorative and inaccurate term salvage therapy.

In a group of patients with an expected prognosis of between 6 and 12 months spending 2–3 weeks receiving a treatment of uncertain benefit does not seem altogether sensible

The temporary effects of alopecia nausea and vomiting may be temporary but in the context of expected survival and patient comfort they are still not negligible.

There will always be patients where metastasis numbers preclude RS

There are still centres where the primary treatment of solitary tumours is both surgery and radiosurgery [38].

What About Salvage Treatments?

There are a few papers covering the subject of salvage treatments. This refers to retreatment following a failure of the original treatment. This sounds very negative when expressed in this way, but from the earliest experience of the Stockholm group, retreatment with the Gamma Knife has been considered a part of the management of metastases [13]. As mentioned above it was called re-treatment and not salvage treatment. It is clearly a part of the concept that new metastases can occur after a GKNS treatment. The control arrangements are designed to catch and treat these new tumours.

In the literature there are papers concerned with various kinds of salvage as follows:

Primary treatment	Salvage treatment
Gamma Knife	Gamma Knife [13, 50, 51]
Gamma Knife	WBRT [87, 89, 100, 117, 118]
WBRT	Gamma Knife [119]

One of the great weaknesses in the current knowledge of whether to use WBRT or not is that there is no first class literature on management based on the principle that Gamma Knife treatment will often have to be repeated because of the nature of the disease.

Advice to Gamma Knife Users About WBRT

Every user has to decide for him/herself. The evidence simply is not complete enough for making a simple decision applicable for all situations. The treatments have to be decided on a case by case basis at the present time. All readers are advised to read the excellent article mentioned above "Whole Brain Radiotherapy: Strong emotions decide but rational studies are needed" [115]. It is full of good sense and the very title underlines the less than scientific influences which are present in the current milieu. However, the new paper from the MC Anderson group [106] does lend support to the notion of NOT using WBRT as a primary treatment in patients with 1–3 metastases and an RPA of 1 or 2.

The Effect of Dose on Results and Complications

The recorded range of local tumour control varies between 71% and 100% for Gamma Knife surgery used alone. This variation may be related to the doses used in different centres [2, 21, 23, 28, 30, 32–36, 38, 40, 42, 45, 52–58, 63, 64, 67, 70–72, 82–84, 108, 120]. The application of statistical methods to data derived from a metanalysis is not the most reliable source of information. Nonetheless the mean control rate for tumours receiving a prescription dose of less than 18 Gy was 83.6% and for those receiving 18 Gy or more the rate was 91.1%.

There are a surprisingly few papers which discuss the most effective dose. Some workers suggest that a prescription dose in excess of 18 Gy is necessary for adequate local control [2, 71, 121, 122]. Others consider that 20 Gy is consistent with effective local control [70, 88]. Some point out that prescription doses over 20 Gy are associated with an increased frequency of radiation toxicity [70, 88, 101]. In addition to the above mentioned papers there are the papers from Shaw et al [102, 111]. They used a dose escalation technique to define the optimal dose. However, the study design is not without problems in respect of the matter under discussion; the correct dose to a cerebral metastasis. To begin with both studies examined the effects of radiation on both gliomas and metastases and not just metastases. It is not clear to what extent the results on gliomas could be considered relevant for patients with metastases. The second problem with the studies is that the treatments given were given both by LINAC and Gamma Knife and with the varying dosimetric characteristics of the two technologies it is not clear how much their results can be intermingled in a study specifically aimed at defining GKNS dose . Finally, the clinical material used in both studies consisted of patients who had already received WBRT. Thus, the findings are not necessarily relevant for deciding the prescription dose for a first time metastasis treatment.

This brings us to the core of the problem. The doses stated in all the studies mentioned above are either mean dose or median dose in a series. This means that a varying number of patients will have received what would appear to be an inadequate dose. The choice of dose would appear to be made first and foremost to avoid the occurrence of complications. It might be considered illogical to treat a tumour with a dose which is not certain to be adequate just because the tumour volume may be large and thus the risk of complications higher. If the studies mentioned above give an indication as to the correct dose, then it might be sensible to give all metastases a prescription dose between 18 and 20 Gy. This has not been done so that the complication rate is uncertain. However, from the Shaw work with previously irradiated patients, with tumours between 3 and 4 cm in diameter a prescription dose of 15 Gy was used. These patients suffered a 2 year radio-toxicity incidence of 11%. Few metastases treated with GKNS are this large. This might suggest that using a dose of 18–20 Gy in even bigger BMs appropriate for GKNS could be effective with acceptable toxicity in what is an extremely lethal disease. The study to determine if this is the case would seem to be worth doing. To date nobody has done it.

As stated in an earlier chapter, the tendency to gear prescription dose more to toxicity risk than effective dose makes the interpretation of results difficult.

Practical Treatment

Referral

The assessment of whether or not a patient is suitable for GKNS requires that the following information is available.

- Clinical Information adequate to give the patient an RPA score
- Histology where possible
- A radiological report confirming the diagnosis of metastasis
- An MR examination of the brain with at the least T2 images and T1 images with and without gadolinium and taken within 4 weeks of the planned treatment date. It is often necessary to specify these requirements to referring colleagues in order to keep the service efficient. Ideally a volume series with contrast gives the best chance of detecting metastases

Acceptance

As indicated above the rules for acceptance vary from centre to centre and there is also considerable variation in practice among referring physicians. The author would accept up to 5 metastases at the time of referral and would of course treat any more that turned up on the day of treatment. Other colleagues might prefer different criteria. As far as is known the world record for number of metastases treated in the Gamma Knife in single session is 42 [123]. This is perhaps a record which should be allowed to stand unchallenged. Most workers consider 1–5 as suitable. In two recent level 1 studies the maximum number treated were 4 [89] and 3 [10]. These are guidelines not rules.

In addition to the number of metastases the volume must be considered. Roughly speaking the total volume of tumours should not exceed 20 cm^3.

Admission

The patients are received and managed in the same way as other patients as described in Chap. 12. They are made aware of the assessed chances of local control based on the given departments results. They are told of potential complications. It is emphasised that the radiosurgery is only a component of a greater total

treatment which is in the hands of their oncologist. They are informed that sometimes a retreatment may be necessary. They are made aware of the necessity of
frequent follow up MR examinations. For claustrophobic patients an open MR can
be used as CT is a relatively poor substitute for MR in showing the effects of GK
treatment on metastases.

Day of Treatment

Frame Application

Perfexion

There is no particular skill involved in applying the frame if the patient is to be
treated with Gamma Knife "Perfexion". However, it is wise to measure the posts of
the frame and the screws in addition to checking that the plastic helmet cap fits. It
may often be necessary to check these values at the time of treatment before the
machine will accept the patient.

Gamma Knife 4C

Metastases are the condition which requires the greatest skill on the part of the
surgeon. The reader is referred to the chapter on frame application. It will often be
necessary with different rotations of the frame to enable all tumours to be treated. It
may be necessary to retreat the patient when a single frame application is not
compatible with the treatment of all the tumours. In the author's experience it is
extremely unusual to require more than two treatments. Figure 8.9 taken from a
patient treated in the Gamma Knife 4 B (same geometry as the 4 C) exemplifies this.

Imaging

A 3D T1 MRI series is taken with contrast. This is reviewed, if necessary with a
neuroradiologist to ensure that all the tumours are identified. An axial reconstruction of the volume series is sent to GammaPlan. This seems to be the safest way of
identifying all the metastases present.

Dose Plan

With solitary tumours there is no particular problem. With multiple tumours it will
be necessary to use multiple matrices and multiple targets. The process is made
much simpler if each tumour is given a name relating to its anatomical location.

In the event of two tumours being in say the frontal lobe they can be referred to as frontal upper or lower, or again as frontal anterior and posterior. The matrix for every tumour should have the same name as the tumour being treated.

In the author's practice a dose of 18–20 Gy is given if the patient has not received previous radiation treatments. If the patient is being treated after previous radiation the dose is reduced according to the best judgement of the physician. The 12 Gy volume as indicated by the Pittsburgh Group is recorded [124] and the dose adjusted to keep this volume down. The current difficulty is that nobody really knows the tolerable 12 Gy volume. In the same work from Pittsburgh the 12 Gy volume of 1 cm^3 did not correlate with either imaging changes or with new persisting neurological deficit. This study pertained to the brainstem and while the notion of the study was of interest, it did not really provide any guidelines. In the present context it is interesting to note that this study recorded new neurological deficit for the most part with cavernous haemangiomas. However, the study explicitly excluded malignant lesions so the significance of its findings for metastases is not clear. Lesions in particular locations such as the brainstem may be treated with slightly lower doses. However, if the dose has to be reduced much below 18 Gy for the first treatment it would be this author's view that the patient is not suitable for radiosurgery and he/she would not be accepted.

Follow up

Routines

There are various routines. It is suggested that a neurological status and RPA assessment together with an MR of the whole brain with 3D T1 with contrast should be taken at 4 weeks, 3, 6, 9 and 12 months after treatment. A thin slice T2 MR series should be taken at the same time. Thereafter the frequency can be relaxed or not according to the course of the illness in the particular patient. MMSE examinations may be performed but it is suggested this is quite an onerous examination and should only be used if a scientific investigation is being performed. Otherwise the MR examinations will permit the observation of the changing size of the treated tumour(s), the presence of AREs and the development of new metastases. New tumours can be treated as they arise.

Complications

Complications have been mentioned in outline above as a matter of principle. Here they are mentioned in more detail since it is during follow up that they appear and need to be managed. GKNS is a powerful treatment in this instance being aimed at a lethal disease. Some degree of complications is unavoidable. Understand it is hoped will keep the number to a minimum. Many papers refer to complications as minor and temporary and this is true. Thus, temporary headache or a 2 inch temporary patch of alopecia and the like are not recorded here. The comments below refer only to complications which can significantly affect function and quality of life.

1. Radiation damage to the brain surrounding a tumour
   (a) The tumour size is unchanged or smaller but there is an increase in peritumoural oedema which may or may not be associated with a clinical deterioration. If associated with symptoms it is treated with steroids and the steroid dose is adjusted to the individual needs of the patient.
2. Radiation damage to the tumour causing swelling associated with secondary oedema and BBB breakdown
   (a) This is an underrated complication occurring between 10 and 13% of cases [13, 125]. It is again managed with steroids in most occasions. In certain cases it will require surgery but this is very rare.
   (b) The real problem is to distinguish between radiation induced tumour swelling and treatment failure with tumour growth. There is no sure fire way of achieving this but However, FDG-18 PET scans [13, 125], SPECT [126] and MR Perfusion imaging [22] all have been used to help in the diagnosis of these two conditions and recently new MR practice have proved most helpful as indicated below.
3. Treatment failure with tumour growth
   (a) Inevitably a few tumours will resist treatment either because they are unusually resistant or more often because size, location or previous radiation treatment have resulted in a lower than usual prescription dose. There is no easy answer as to what to do in this situation. Each patient has to be managed on a case by case basis.
   Very recent work has indicated a simple method to make this distinction. If the size of the contrast enhancing lesion on MR T1 series matches the lesion seen on T2 images, it is most likely that the volume increase is due to tumour growth. If there is no such correspondence then the tumour swelling is most likely radiation damage [103]. In addition if an increased T2 signal follows the anatomy of the gyri it is most probably a tumour [104].
4. In some patients both necrosis and tumour regrowth may occur
   The important point is that referring physicians should be adequately informed about the difficulty of distinguishing between radiation damage and treatment failure so that unnecessary extra treatments are avoided. This implies that for this particular sub category of patients there should be close regular contact between the Gamma Knife Centre and the referring physician. There may well be a period when MR as often as once a month may be necessary until the lesion shows either progression or regression.
5. Development of new tumours
   (a) Since GKNS is a focal treatment and since an uncontrolled systemic cancer can fire off new metastases at any time, it is not surprising new metastases

appear after a primary treatment. In this case the patient may be retreated for the new tumour. The extremely focal nature of GKNS means that the total brain radiation load is minimised with this approach. It is again emphasised that re-treatment does not imply "salvage" therapy but merely is an expression of a planned staged treatment. Moreover, it is a treatment which minimises the patient's time away from home.

(b) There is evidence that the chances of suffering new distant metastases are related to the number of metastases at the initial presentation [13].

Conclusions

1. GKNS seems to be an excellent palliative treatment for suitable BMs
2. The treatment is simple, safe and has been shown to be effective in obtaining tumour control of treated tumours
3. It is suggested that the correct end point for GKNS of BMs remains tumour control and not survival, since GKNS has no effect on extracranial disease
4. The treatment involves intensive follow up and includes the possibility of retreatment in a proportion of patients mostly for distant metastases but occasionally for failed control of a treated lesion
5. It is suggested that all papers should include RTOG RPA scores in the results both before and after treatment. It may be possible to devise newer and better scores but what is needed now is consistency of reporting which includes the effect of the systemic disease. It would be pleasant if editors and reviewers were stricter on this point
6. The arguments about which other supplementary treatments should be associated with GKNS for BMs remain unresolved. The author cannot state what is the correct management paradigm, in the face of such varied opinion from so many distinguished colleagues. However, it is fair to say he himself would advise against WBRT for those patients where GKNS is a suitable treatment

References

1. Weltman E, Salvajoli JV, Brandt RA, de Morais Hanriot R, Prisco FE, Cruz JC, de Oliveira Borges S, Lagatta M, Ballas Wajsbrot D. Radiosurgery for brain metastases: who may not benefit? Int J Radiat Oncol Biol Phys 51(5): 1320–1327; 2001
2. Lorenzoni J, Devriendt D, Massager N, David P, Ruiz S, Vanderlinden B, Van Houtte P, Brotchi J, Levivier M. Radiosurgery for treatment of brain metastases: estimation of patient eligibility using three stratification systems. Int J Radiat Oncol Biol Phys 60(1): 218–224; 2004
3. Sperduto PW, Berkey B, Gaspar LE, Mehta M, Curran W. A new prognostic index and comparison to three other indices for patients with brain metastases: an analysis of 1,960 patients in the RTOG database. Int J Radiat Oncol Biol Phys 70(2): 510–514; 2008

4. Walker MT, Kapoor V. Neuroimaging of parenchymal brain metastases. In: Brain metastses, eds. Razier JJ, Abrey LE. Springer Verlag Vienna. p 31; 2007
5. Sul J, Posner JB. Brain metastases: epidemiology and pathophysiology. In: Brain Metastses. eds. Razier JJ, Abrey LE. Springer Verlag Vienna. pp 1–3; 2007
6. Pickren JW, Lopez G, Tzuduka Y. Brain Metastases. An autopsy study. Cancer Treat Symp **2**: 295–313; 1982
7. Posner J. Management of central nervous system metastases. Semin Oncol **4**: 81–91; 1977
8. Patchell RA, Tibbs PA, Regine WF, Dempsey RJ, Mohiuddin M, Kryscio RJ, Markesbery WR, Foon KA, Young B. Postoperative radiotherapy in the treatmnet of single metastases to the brain. JAMA **280(17)**: 1485–1489; 1998
9. Patchell RA. The management of brain metastases. Cancer Treat Rev **29(6)**: 533–540; 2003
10. Andrews DW, Scott CB, Sperduto PW, Flanders AE, Gaspar LE, Schell MC, Werner-Wasir M, Demas W, Ryu J, Bahary J-P, Southami L, Rotman M, Mehta MP. Whole brain radiation therapy with or without stereotactic radiosurgery boost for patients with one to three brain metastases: phase III results of the RTOG 9508 randomised trial. Lancet **363**: 1665–1672; 2004
11. Vecht CJ, Haaxma-Reiche H, Noordijk EM, Padberg GW, Voormolen JH, Hoekstra FH, Tans JT, Lambooij N, Metsaars JA, Wattendorff AR. Treatment of single brain metastasis: radiotherapy alone or combined with neurosurgery? Ann Neurol **33(6)**: 583–590; 1993
12. Borgelt B, Gelber R, Kramer S, Brady LW, Chang CH, Davis LW, Perez CA, Hendrickson FR. The palliation of brain metastases. The final results of the first two studies by the radiation therapy oncology group. Int J Radiat Oncol Biol Phys **6**: 1–9; 1980
13. Kihlström L, Karlsson B, Lindquist C. Gamma Knife surgery for cerebral metastases: implications for survival based on 16 years experience. Stereotact Funct Neurosurg **61 (Suppl 1)**: 45–50; 1992
14. Sturm V, Kober B, Hover KH, Schlegel W, Boesecke R, Pastyr O, Hartmann GH, Schabbert S, zum Winkel K, Kunze S. Stereotactic percutaneous single dose irradiation of brain metastases with a linear accelerator. Int J Radiat Oncol Biol Phys **13(2)**: 279–282; 1987
15. Engehart R, Romahn J, Gademann G, Muller-Schimpfle M, Hover K-H, Kimmig BN, Wannemacher M. Indications for radiosurgery in treatment of brain metastases. In: Stereotactic Radiosurgery Update, ed. Lunsford LD. Elsevier, New York. pp 393–399; 1992
16. Adler JR, Cox RS, Kaplan I, Martin DP. Stereotactic radiosurgical treatment of brain metastases. J Neurosurg **76(3)**: 444–449; 1992
17. Loeffler JS, Alexander III E. Radiosurgery for the treatment of intracranial metastases. In: Stereotactic Radiosurgery, eds. Alexander III E, Loeffler JS, Lunsford LD McGraw Hill, New York. pp 197–206; 1993
18. Fuller BG, Kaplan ID, Adler JR et al. Stereotaxic radiosurgery for brain metastases: the importance of adjuvant whole brain radiation. Int J Radiat Oncol Biol Phys **23(2)**: 413–418; 1992
19. Chougule PB, Burton-Williams M, Zheng Z, Ponte B, Noren G, Alderson L, Friehs G, Wazer D, Epstein M. Randomized treatment of brain metastasis with gamma knife radiosurgery whole brain radiotherapy or both. Int J Radiat Oncol Biol Phys **48(Suppl 1)**: 114; 2000
20. Amendola BE, Wolf AL, Coy SR, Amendola M, Bloch L. Brain metastases in renal cell carcinoma: management with gamma knife radiosurgery. Cancer J **6(6)**: 372–376; 2000
21. Baardsen R, Larsen JL, Wester K, Pedersen PH. Cerebral metastases treated with stereotaxic gamma radiation. 6-year experience with the "gamma knife" at the Haukeland hospital. Tidsskr Nor Laegeforen **117(11)** 1591–1595; 1997
22. Barajas RF, Chang JS, Sneed PK, Segal MR, McDermott MW, Cha S. Distinguishing recurrent intra-axial metastatic tumor from radiation necrosis following gamma knife radiosurgery using dynamic susceptibility-weighted contrast-enhanced perfusion MR imaging. Am J Neuroradiol **30(2)**: 367–372; 2009
23. Bhatnagar AK, Flickinger JC, Kondziolka D, Lunsford LD. Stereotactic radiosurgery for four or more intracranial metastases. Int J Radiat Oncol Biol Phys **64(3)**: 898–903; 2006

24. Brown PD, Brown CA, Pollock BE, Gorman DA, Foote RL. Stereotactic radiosurgery for patients with "radioresistant" brain metastases. Neurosurgery **62(Suppl 2)**: 790–801; 2008
25. DiBiase SJ, Chin LS, Ma L. Influence of gamma knife radiosurgery on the quality of life in patients with brain metastases. Am J Clin Oncol **25(2)**: 131–134; 2002
26. Fernandez-Vicioso E, Suh JH, Kupelian PA, Sohn JW, Barnett GH. Analysis of prognostic factors for patients with single brain metastasis treated with stereotactic radiosurgery. Radiat Oncol Investig **5(1)**: 31–37; 1997
27. Firlik KS, Kondziolka D, Flickinger JC, Lunsford LD. Stereotactic radiosurgery for brain metastases from breast cancer. Ann Surg Oncol **7(5)**: 333–338; 2000
28. Flickinger JC, Kondziolka D, Lunsford LD, Coffey RJ, Goodman ML, Shaw EG, Hudgins WR, Weiner R, Harsh GR, Sneed PK. A multi-institutional experience with stereotactic radiosurgery for solitary brain metastasis. Int J Radiat Oncol Biol Phys **28(4)**: 797–802; 1994
29. Friehs GM, Legat J, Zheng Z, Pendl G, Noren GC. Outcomes in patients treated with gamma knife radiosurgery for brain metastases from malignant melanoma. Neurosurg Focus **4(6)**: e1; 1998
30. Fuentes S, Delsanti C, Metellus P, Peragut JC, Grisoli F, Régis J. Brainstem metastases: management using gamma knife radiosurgery. Neurosurgery **58(1)**: 37–42; 2006
31. Gaudy-Marqueste C, Régis JM, Muracciole X, Laurans R, Richard MA, Bonerandi JJ, Grob JJ. Gamma-Knife radiosurgery in the management of melanoma patients with brain metastases: a series of 106 patients without whole-brain Radiotherapy. Int J Radiat Oncol Biol Phys **65(3)**: 809–816; 2006
32. Gerosa M, Nicolato A, Foroni R, Tomazzoli L, Bricolo A. Analysis of long-term outcomes and prognostic factors in patients with non-small cell lung cancer brain metastases treated by gamma knife radiosurgery. J Neurosurg Suppl **102**: 75–80; 2005
33. Gerosa M, Nicolato A, Foroni R, Zanotti B, Tomazzoli L, Miscusi M, Alessandrini F, Bricolo A (2002) Gamma knife radiosurgery for brain metastases: a primary therapeutic option. J Neurosurg **97(5 Suppl)**: 515–524
34. Gerosa M, Nicolato A, Severi F, Ferraresi P, Masotto B, Barone G, Foroni R, Piovan E, Pasoli A, Bricolo A. Gamma Knife radiosurgery for intracranial metastases: from local tumor control to increased survival. Stereotact Funct Neurosurg **66(Suppl 1)**: 184–192; 1996
35. Hasegawa T, Kondziolka D, Flickinger JC, Germanwala A, Lunsford LD. Brain metastases treated with radiosurgery alone: an alternative to whole brain radiotherapy? Neurosurgery **52** **(6)**: 1318–1326; 2003
36. Huang CF, Kondziolka D, Flickinger JC, Lunsford LD. Stereotactic radiosurgery for brain-stem metastases. J Neurosurg **91(4)** 563–568; 1999
37. Hussain A, Brown PD, Stafford SL, Pollock BE. Stereotactic radiosurgery for brainstem metastases: survival, tumor control, and patient outcomes. Int J Radiat Oncol Biol Phys **67** **(2)**: 521–524; 2007
38. Iwai Y, Yamanaka K, Yasui T. Boost radiosurgery for treatment of brain metastases after surgical resections. Surg Neurol **69**: 181–186; 2008
39. Jawahar A, Matthew RE, Minagar A, Shukla D, Zhang JH, Willis BK, Ampil F, Nanda A. Gamma knife surgery in the management of brain metastases from lung carcinoma: a retrospective analysis of survival, local control, and freedom from new brain metastasis. J Neurosurg **100(5)**: 842–847; 2004
40. Jawahar A, Willis BK, Smith DR, Ampil F, Datta R, Nanda A. Gamma knife radiosurgery for brain metastases: do patients benefit from adjuvant external-beam radiotherapy? An 18-month comparative analysis. Stereotact Funct Neurosurg **79(3–4)**: 262–271; 2002
41. Kano H, Kondziolka D, Zorro O, Lobato-Polo J, Flickinger JC, Lunsford LD. The results of resection after stereotactic radiosurgery for brain metastases. J Neurosurg **111(4)**: 825–831; 2009
42. Kida Y, Kobayashi T, Tanaka T. Radiosurgery of the metastatic brain tumours with gamma-knife. Acta Neurochir **89**: 89–94; 1995

43. Kida Y, Kobayashi T, Tanaka T, Oyama H, Iwakoshi T. Gamma-radiosurgery of metastatic brain tumors. No Shinkei Geka **21(11)**: 991–997; 1993
44. Kihlstrom L, Karlsson B, Lindquist C, Noren G, Rahn T. Gamma knife surgery for cerebral metastasis. Acta Neurochir Suppl **52**: 87–89; 1991
45. Kim CH, Im YS, Nam DH, Park K, Kim JH, Lee JI. Gamma knife radiosurgery for ten or more brain metastases. J Korean Neurosurg Soc **44(6)**: 358–363; 2008
46. Kim SH, Chao ST, Toms SA, Vogelbaum MA, Barnett GH, Suh JH, Weil RJ. Stereotactic radiosurgical treatment of parenchymal brain metastases from prostate adenocarcinoma. Surg Neurol **69**: 641–646; 2008
47. Kim YS, Kondziolka D, Flickinger JC, Lunsford LD. Stereotactic radiosurgery for patients with nonsmall cell lung carcinoma metastatic to the brain. Cancer **80(11)**: 2075–2083; 1997
48. Kondziolka D, Martin JJ, Flickinger JC, Friedland DM, Brufsky AM, Baar J, Agarwala S, Kirkwood JM, Lunsford LD. Long-term survivors after gamma knife radiosurgery for brain metastases. Cancer **104(12)**: 2784–2791; 2005
49. Kondziolka D, Patel A, Lunsford LD, Flickinger JC. Decision making for patients with Multiple brain metastases: radiosurgery, Radiotherapy, or resection? Neurosurg Focus **9(2)**: e4; 2000
50. Kwon KY, Kong DS, Lee JI, Nam DH, Park K, Kim JH. Outcome of repeated radiosurgery for recurrent metastatic brain tumors. Clin Neurol Neurosurg **109(2)**: 132–137; 2006
51. Lavine SD, Petrovich Z, Cohen-Gadol AA, Masri LS, Morton DL, O'Day SJ, Essner R, Zelman V, Yu C, Luxton G, Apuzzo ML. Gamma knife radiosurgery for metastatic melanoma: an analysis of survival, outcome, and complications. Neurosurgery **44(1)**: 59–64; 1999
52. Maesawa S, Kondziolka D, Thompson TP, Flickinger JC, Lunsford LD. Brain metastases in patients with no known primary tumor. Cancer **89(5)**: 1095–1101; 2000
53. Mathieu D, Kondziolka D, Flickinger JC, Fortin D, Kenny B, Michaud K, Mongia S, Niranjan A, Lunsford LD. Tumor bed radiosurgery after resection of cerebral metastases. Neurosurgery **62(4)**: 817–823; 2008
54. Monaco E, III, Kondziolka D, Mongia S, Niranjan A, Flickinger JC, Lunsford LD. Management of brain metastases from ovarian and endometrial carcinoma with stereotactic radiosurgery. Cancer **113(9)**: 2610–2614; 2008
55. Mori Y, Kondziolka D, Flickinger JC, Logan T, Lunsford LD. Stereotactic radiosurgery for brain metastasis from renal cell carcinoma. Cancer **83(2)**: 344–353; 1998
56. Muacevic A, Kreth FW, Horstmann GA, Schmid-Elsaesser R, Wowra B, Steiger HJ, Reulen HJ. Surgery and Radiotherapy compared with gamma knife radiosurgery in the treatment of Solitary cerebral metastases of small diameter. J Neurosurg **91(1)**: 35–43; 1999
57. Muacevic A, Kreth FW, Mack A, Tonn JC, Wowra B. Stereotactic radiosurgery without radiation therapy providing high local tumor control of Multiple brain metastases from renal cell carcinoma. Minim Invasive Neurosurg **47(4)**: 203–208; 2004
58. Muacevic A, Kreth FW, Tonn JC, Wowra B. Stereotactic radiosurgery for multiple brain metastases from breast carcinoma. Cancer **100(8)**: 1705–1711; 2004
59. Pan HC, Sheehan J, Stroila M, Steiner M, Steiner L. Gamma knife surgery for brain metastases from lung cancer. J Neurosurg Suppl **102**: 128–133; 2005
60. Payne BR, Prasad D, Szeifert G, Steiner M, Steiner L. Gamma surgery for intracranial metastases from renal cell carcinoma. J Neurosurg **92(5)**: 760–765; 2000
61. Radbill AE, Fiveash JF, Falkenberg ET, Guthrie BL, Young PE, Meleth S, Markert JM. Initial treatment of melanoma brain metastases using gamma knife radiosurgery: an evaluation of efficacy and toxicity. Cancer **101(4)**: 825–833; 2004
62. Sansur CA, Chin LS, Ames JW, Banegura AT, Aggarwal S, Ballesteros M, Amin P, Simard JM, Eisenberg H. Gamma knife radiosurgery for the treatment of brain metastases. Stereotact Funct Neurosurg **74(1)**: 37–51; 2000
63. Schoeggl A, Kitz K, Ertl A, Dieckmann K, Saringer W, Koos WT. Gamma-knife radiosurgery for brain metastases of renal cell carcinoma: results in 23 patients. Acta Neurochir **140 (6)**: 549–555; 1998

64. Schoeggl A, Kitz K, Ertl A, Reddy M, Bavinzski G, Schneider B. Prognostic factor analysis for multiple brain metastases after gamma knife radiosurgery: results in 97 patients. J Neurooncol **42(2)**: 169–175; 1999

65. Serizawa T, Ono J, Iichi T, Matsuda S, Sato M, Odaki M, Hirai S, Osato K, Saeki N, Yamaura A. Gamma knife radiosurgery for metastatic brain tumors from lung cancer: a comparison between small cell and non-small cell carcinoma. J Neurosurg **97(5 Suppl)**: 484–488; 2002

66. Serizawa T, Yamamoto M, Nagano O, Higuchi Y, Matsuda S, Ono J, Iwadate Y, Saeki N. Gamma Knife surgery for metastatic brain tumors. J Neurosurg Suppl **109**:118–121; 2008

67. Seung SK, Sneed PK, McDermott MW, Shu HK, Leong SP, Chang S, Petti PL, Smith V, Verhey LJ, Wara WM, Phillips TL, Larson DA. Gamma knife radiosurgery for malignant melanoma brain metastases. Cancer J Sci Am **4(2)**: 103–109; 1998

68. Sheehan J, Kondziolka D, Flickinger J, Lunsford LD. Radiosurgery for patients with recurrent small cell lung carcinoma metastatic to the brain: outcomes and prognostic factors. J Neurosurg Suppl **102**: 247–254; 2005

69. Sheehan JP, Sun MH, Kondziolka D, Flickinger J, Lunsford LD. Radiosurgery for non-small cell lung carcinoma metastatic to the brain: long-term outcomes and prognostic factors influencing patient survival time and local tumor control. J Neurosurg **97(6)**: 1276–1281; 2002

70. Shehata MK, Young B, Reid B, Patchell RA, St Clair W, Sims J, Sanders M, Meigooni A, Mohiuddin M, Regine WF. Stereotatic radiosurgery of 468 brain metastases < or =2 cm: implications for SRS and whole brain radiation therapy. Int J Radiat Oncol Biol Phys **59(1)**: 87–93; 2004

71. Shiau CY, Sneed PK, Shu HK, Lamborn KR, McDermott MW, Chang S, Nowak P, Petti PL, Smith V, Verhey LJ, Ho M, Park E, Wara WM, Gutin PH, Larson DA. Radiosurgery for brain metastases: relationship of Dose and pattern of enhancement to local control. Int J Radiat Oncol Biol Phys **37(2)**: 375–383; 1997

72. Shuto T, Inomori S, Fujino H, Nagano H. Gamma knife surgery for metastatic brain tumors from renal cell carcinoma. J Neurosurg **105(4)**: 555–560; 2006

73. Siebels M, Oberneder R, Buchner A, Zaak D, Mack A, Petrides PE, Hofstetter A, Wowra B. Ambulatory radiosurgery in cerebral metastatic renal cell carcinoma. 5-year outcome in 58 patients. Urologe A **41(5)**: 482–488; 2002

74. Simonova G, Liscak R, Novotny JJr, Novotny J. Radiosurgery with the Leksell gamma knife in the treatment of solitary brain metastasis – 5-year results. Vnitr Lek **45(5)**: 284–290; 1999

75. Simonova G, Liscak R, Novotny J Jr, Novotny J. Solitary brain metastases treated with the Leksell gamma knife: prognostic factors for patients. Radiother Oncol **57(2)**: 207–213; 2000

76. Vesagas TS, Aguilar JA, Mercado ER, Mariano MM. Gamma knife radiosurgery and brain metastases: local control, survival, and quality of life. J Neurosurg **97(5 Suppl)**: 507–510; 2002

77. Wowra B, Siebels M, Muacevic A, Kreth FW, Mack A, Hofstetter A. Repeated gamma knife surgery for multiple brain metastases from renal cell carcinoma. J Neurosurg **97(4)**: 785–793; 2002

78. Chang EL, Wefel JS, Rees KR, Allen PK, Lang FF, Kornguth DG, Arbuckle RB, Swint JM, Shiu AS, Maor, MH, Meyers CA. A pilot study of neurocognitive function in patients with one to three new brain metastases initially treated with stereotactic radiosurgery alone. Neurosurgery **60(2)**: 277–283; 2009

79. Hoffman R, Sneed PK, McDermott MW, Chang S, Lamborn KR, Park E, Wara WM, Larson DA. Radiosurgery for brain metastases from primary lung carcinoma. Cancer J **7(2)**: 121–131; 2001

80. Kondziolka D, Patel A, Lunsford LD, Kassam A, Flickinger JC. Stereotactic radiosurgery plus whole brain radiotherapy versus radiotherapy alone for patients with multiple brain metastases. Int J Radiat Oncol Biol Phys **45(2)**: 427–434; 1999

81. Shirato H, Takamura A, Tomia M, Suzuki K, Nishioka T, Isu T, Kato T, Sawamura Y, Miyamachi K, Abe H, MIyasaka K. Stereotactic irradiation without whole-brain irradiation for single brain metastasis. Int J Radiat Oncol Biophys **37**(2): 385–391; 1997

82. Somaza S, Kondziolka D, Lunsford LD, Kirkwood JM, Flickinger JC. Stereotactic radiosurgery for cerebral metastatic melanoma. J Neurosurg **79**(5): 661–666; 1993

83. Varlotto JM, Flickinger JC, Niranjan A, Bhatnagar A, Kondziolka D, Lunsford LD. The impact of whole-brain radiation therapy on the long-term control and morbidity of patients surviving more than one year after gamma knife radiosurgery for brain metastases. Int J Radiat Oncol Biol Phys **62**(4): 1125–1132; 2005

84. Varlotto JM, Flickinger JC, Niranjan A, Bhatnagar AK, Kondziolka D, Lunsford LD. Analysis of tumor control and toxicity in patients who have survived at least one year after radiosurgery for brain metastases. Int J Radiat Oncol Biol Phys **57**(2): 452–464; 2003

85. Goyal S, Prasad D, Harrell FJr, Matsumoto J, Rich T, Steiner L. Gamma knife surgery for the treatment of intracranial metastases from Breast cancer. J Neurosurg **103**(2): 218–223; 2005

86. Mingione V, Oliveira M, Prasad D, Steiner M, Steiner L. Gamma surgery for melanoma metastases in the brain. J Neurosurg **96**(3): 544–551; 2002

87. Sneed PK, Lamborn KR, Forstner JM, McDermott MW, Chang S, Park E, Gutin PH, Phillips TL, Wara WM, Larson DA. Radiosurgery for brain metastases: is whole brain radiotherapy necessary? Int J Radiat Oncol Biol Phys **43**(3): 549–558; 1999

88. Hazard LJ, Jensen RL, Shrieve SC. Role of stereotactic radiosurgery in the treatment of brain metastases. J Clin Oncol **28**(4): 403–410; 2005

89. Aoyama H, Shirato H, Tago M, Nakagawa K, Toyoda T, Hatano K, Kenjyo M, Oya N, Hirota S, Shioura H, Kunieda E, Inomata T, Hayakawa K, Kazuhige H, Katoh N, Kobashi G. Stereotactic radiosurgery plus whole-brain radiation therapy vs stereotactic radiosurgery alone for treatment of brain metastases. JAMA **295**(21): 2483–2491; 2006

90. Chen JC, Petrovich Z, O'Day S, Morton D, Essner R, Giannotta SL, Yu C, Apuzzo ML. Stereotactic radiosurgery in the treatment of metastatic disease to the brain. Neurosurgery **47**(2): 268–279; 2000

91. Chidel MA, Suh JH, Reddy CA, Chao ST, Lundbeck MF, Barnett GH. Application of recursive partitioning analysis and evaluation of the use of whole brain radiation among patients treated with stereotactic radiosurgery for newly diagnosed brain metastases. Int J Radiat Oncol Biol Phys **47**(4): 993–999; 2000

92. Golden DW, Lamborn KR, McDermott MW, Kunwar S, Wara WM, Nakamura JL, Sneed PK. Prognostic factors and grading systems for overall survival in patients treated with radiosurgery for brain metastases: variation by primary site. J Neurosurg **109(Suppl)**: 77–86; 2008

93. Gonzalez-Martinez J, Hernandez L, Zamorano L, Sloan A, Levin K, Lo S, Li Q, Diaz F. Gamma knife radiosurgery for intracranial metastatic melanoma: a 6-year experience. J Neurosurg **97**(5 **Suppl**): 494–498; 2002

94. Mori Y, Kondziolka D, Flickinger JC, Kirkwood JM, Agarwala S, Lunsford LD. Stereotactic radiosurgery for cerebral metastatic melanoma: factors affecting local disease control and survival. Int J Radiat Oncol Biol Phys **42**(3): 581–589; 1998

95. Petrovich Z, Yu C, Giannotta SL, O'Day S, Apuzzo ML. Survival and pattern of failure in brain metastasis treated with stereotactic gamma knife radiosurgery. J Neurosurg **97**(5 **Suppl**): 499–506; 2002

96. Schoeggl A, Kitz K, Reddy M, Zauner C. Stereotactic radiosurgery for brain metastases from colorectal cancer. Int J Colorectal Dis **17**(3): 150–155; 2002

97. Sheehan JP, Sun MH, Kondziolka D, Flickinger J, Lunsford LD. Radiosurgery in patients with renal cell carcinoma metastasis to the brain: long-term outcomes and prognostic factors influencing survival and local tumor control. J Neurosurg **98**(2): 342–349; 2003

98. Shu HK, Sneed PK, Shiau CY, McDermott MW, Lamborn KR, Park E, Ho M, Petti PL, Smith V, Verhey LJ, Wara WM, Gutin PH, Larson DA. Factors influencing survival after

gamma knife radiosurgery for patients with single and multiple brain metastases. Cancer J Sci Am **2(6)**: 335–342; 1996

99. Shuto T, Fujino H, Inomori S, Nagano H. Repeated gamma knife radiosurgery for Multiple metastatic brain tumours. Acta Neurochir **146(9)**: 989–993; 2004

100. Sneed PK, Suh JH, Goetsch SJ, Sanghavi SN, Chappell R, Buatti JM, Regine WF, Weltman E, King VJ, Breneman JC, Sperduto PW, Mehta MP. A multi-institutional review of radiosurgery alone vs. radiosurgery with whole brain Radiotherapy as the initial management of brain metastases. Int J Radiat Oncol Biol Phys **53(3)**: 519–526; 2002

101. Majhail NS, Chander S, Mehta VS, Juika PJ, Ganesh T, Rath GK. Factors influencing early complications following Gamma Knife surgery: a prospective study. Stereotact Funct Neurosurge **76(1)**: 36–46; 2001

102. Shaw E, Scott C, Souhami L, Dinapoli R, Bahary JP, Kline R, Wharam M, Schultz C, Davey P, Loeffler J, Del Rowe J, Marks L, Fisher B, Shin K. Radiosurgery for the treatment of previously irradiated recurrent primary brain tumors and brain metastases: initial report of radiation therapy oncology group protocol (90-05). Int J Radiat Oncol Biol Phys **34(2)**: 647–654; 1996

103. Kano H, Kondziolka D, Lobato-Polo J, Zorro O, Flickinger JC, Lunsford LD. T1/T2 matching to differentiate tumor growth from radiation effects after stereotactic radiosurgery. Neurosurgery **66(3)**: 486–492; 2010

104. Dequesada IM, Quisling RG, Yachnis A, Friedman WA. Can standard magnetic resonance imaging reliably distinguish recurrent tumor from radiation necrosis after radiosurgery for brain metastases? A radiographic-pathological study. Neurosurgery **63(5)**: 898–903; 2008

105. al-Mefty O, Kersh JE, Routh A, Smith RR. The long-term side effects of radiation therapy for benign brain tumors in adults. J Neurosurg **73(4)**: 502–512; 1990

106. Chang EL, Wefel JS, Maor MH, Hassenbusch SJ 3rd, Mahajan A, Lang FF, Woo SY, Mathews LA, Allen PK, Shiu AS, Meyers CA. Neurocognition in patients with brain metastases treated with radiosurgery for radiosurgery plus whole-brain irradiation: a randomised controlled trial. Lancet Oncol **5**: e1–e8; 2009

107. Larson D, Sahgal S. Adjuvant whole brain radiotherapy; strong emotions decide but rational studies are needed: in regard to Brown et al. Int J Radiat Oncol Biol Phys 70(5): 1305-1309; 2008. Int J Radiat Oncol Biol Phys **72(3)**: 959; 2008

108. Amendola BE, Wolf AL, Coy SR, Amendola M, Bloch L. Gamma knife radiosurgery in the treatment of patients with single and multiple brain metastases from carcinoma of the breast. Cancer J **6(2)**: 88–92; 2000

109. Nakagawa K, Tago M, Terahara A, Aoki Y, Sasaki T, Kurita H, Shin M, Kawamoto S, Kirino T, Otomo K. A Single institutional outcome analysis of Gamma Knife radiosurgery for single or multiple brain metastases. Clin Neurol Neurosurg **102(4)**: 227–232; 2000

110. Regine WF, Huhn JL, Patchell RA, St Clair WH, Strottmann J, Meigooni A, Sanders M, Young AB. Risk of symptomatic brain tumor recurrence and neurologic deficit after radiosurgery alone in patients with newly diagnosed brain metastases: results and implications. Int J Radiat Oncol Biol Phys **52(2)**: 333–338; 2002

111. Shaw E, Scott C, Souhami L, Dinapoli R, Kline R, Loeffler J, Farnan N. Single dose radiosurgical treatment of recurrent previously irradiated primary brain tumors and brain metastases: final report of RTOG protocol 90-05. Int J Radiat Oncol Biol Phys **47(2)**: 291–298; 2000

112. Aoyama H, Tago M, Kato N, Toyoda T, Kenjyo M, Hirota S, Shioura H, Inomata T, Kunieda E, Hayakawa K, Nakagawa K, Kobashi G, Shirato H. Neurocognitive function of patients with brain metastasis who received either whole brain radiotherapy plus stereotactic radiosurgery or radiosurgery alone. Int J Radiat Oncol Biophys **68(5)**: 1388–1395; 2007

113. Huang F, Alrefae M, Langleben A, Roberge D. Prophylactic cranial irradiation in advanced breast cancer: a case for caution. Int J Radiat Oncol Biol Phys **73(3)**: 752–758; 2009

114. Shibamoto Y, Baba F, Oda K, Hayashi S, Kokubo M, Ishihara S, Itoh Y, Ogion H, Koizumi M. Incidence of brain atrophy and decline in mini-mental state examination score after

whole-brain radiotherapy in patients with brain metastase. Int J Radiat Oncol Biophys **72(4)**: 1168–1173; 2008

115. Brown PD, Asherm AL, Farace E. Adjuvant whole brain radiotherapy. Strong emotions decide but rational studies are needed. Int J Radiat Oncol Biol Phys **70(5)**: 1305–1309; 2008

116. Regine WF, Schmitt FA, Scott CB, Dearth C, Patchell RA, Nichols RC Jr, Gore EM, Franklin RL 3rd, Suh JH, Mehta MP. Feasibility of neurocognitive outcome evaluations in patients with brain metastases in a multi-institutional cooperative group setting: results of Radiation Therapy Oncology Group trial BR-0018. Int J Radiat Oncol Biol Phys **58(5)**: 1346–1352; 2004

117. Levin KJ, Youssef EF, Sloan AE, Patel R, Zabad RK, Zamorano L. Gamma knife radiosurgery in patients with advanced Breast cancer undergoing bone marrow transplant. J Neurosurg **97(5 Suppl)**: 663–665; 2002

118. Limbrick DD, Lusis EA, Chicoine MR, Rich KM, Dacey RG, Dowling JL, Grubb RL, Filiput EA, Drzymala RE, Mansur DB, Simpson JR. Combined surgical resection and stereotactic radiosurgery for treatment of cerebral metastases. Surg Neurol **71(3)**: 280–288; 2008

119. Chao ST, Barnett GH, Vogelbaum MA, Angelov L, Weil RJ, Neyman G, Reuther AM, Suh JH. Salvage stereotactic radiosurgery effectively treats recurrences from whole-brain radiation therapy. Cancer **113 (8)**: 2198–2204; 2008

120. Iwai Y, Yamanaka K. Gamma Knife radiosurgery for skull base metastasis and invasion. Stereotact Funct Neurosurg **72(Suppl 1)**: 81–87; 1999

121. Lorenzoni JG, Devriendt D, Massager N, Desmedt F, Simon S, Van Houtte P, Brotchi J, Levivier M. Brain stem metastases treated with radiosurgery: prognostic factors of survival and life expectancy estimation. Surg Neurol **71(2)**: 188–195; 2008

122. Pan HC, Sun MH, Chen CC, Chen CJ, Lee CH, Sheehan J. Neuroimaging and quality-of-life outcomes in patients with brain metastasis and peritumoral edema who undergo Gamma Knife surgery. J Neurosurg Suppl **109**: 90–98; 2008

123. Yamamoto M, Ide M, Jimbo M, Aiba M, Ito M, Hirai T, Usukua M. Gamma knife radiosurgery with numerous target points for intracranially disseminated metastases. In: Radiosurgery 1997, ed. Kondziolka D. Radiosurgery. Basel, Karger **2**: 94–109; 1998

124. Sharma MS, Kondziolka D, Khan A, Kano H, Niranjan A, Flickinger JC, Lunsford LD. Radiation tolerance limits of the brainstem. Neurosurg **63(4)**: 728–732; 2008

125. Lippitz BE, Kraepelien T, Hautanen K, Ritzling M, Rahn T, Ulfarsson E, Boethius J. Gamma knife radiosurgery for patients with multiple cerebral metastases. Acta Neurochir Suppl **71**: 79–87; 2004

126. Serizawa T, Saeki N, Higuchi Y, Ono J, Matsuda S, Sato M, Yanagisawa M, Iuchi T, Nagano O, Yamaura A. Diagnostic Value of thallium-201 chloride single-photon emission computerized tomography in differentiating tumor recurrence from radiation injury after gamma knife surgery for metastatic brain tumors. J Neurosurg Suppl **102**: 266–271; 2005

Chapter 16
Intraparenchymal Intrinsic Brain Tumours

Introduction

This chapter deals with tumours whose origin is from intracerebral cells. They include a whole family of tumours of which the commonest are the gliomas. However, the list includes ependymomas, haemangioblastomas and others. The chapter sections will be grouped according to the cell of origin of the tumours being considered. Clinical presentations will not be presented since they are to be found in any standard neurosurgery textbook. The questions to be examined here are the suitability of GKNS as a treatment once the diagnosis is established. Since the role of the treatment is in fact in debate for all the indications mentioned in this chapter, the subject matter will be limited to the commoner disease processes concerning which there is some degree of useful documentation. Moreover, it should be mentioned that stereotactic fractionated treatments are in use and their role is being assessed. They are however not included in this chapter being considered outside the scope of this book.

The importance of selection skewing results cannot be overestimated. In a very sensible paper from the London regional cancer centre, the authors analysed 101 consecutive patients with gliomas. Twenty seven percent of these were deemed eligible for radiosurgery. Their median survival was 23.4 months compared with 8.6 months for patients deemed unsuitable. It follows that the reader must be very careful when interpreting material presented below, based as it is on retrospective studies. Selection can outweigh all other factors.

This chapter is also contributed by Paal-Henning Pedersen.

J.C. Ganz, *Gamma Knife Neurosurgery*,
DOI 10.1007/978-3-7091-0343-2_16, © Springer-Verlag/Wien 2011

Gliomas

Classification

These tumours arise from the connective tissue cells of the brain or glial cells. "Glia" is a word deriving from the Greek for glue. The main kinds of glial cells are the astrocytes and the oligodendroglia, giving rise to astrocytomas and oligodendrogliomas. There a number of variants and mixed tumour types, but the above grouping is sufficient for the current purpose. The astrocytomas are considered as grades one to four where the most usual grade one tumour is the pilocytic astrocytomas and grade four is synonymous with glioblastoma multiforme. Grades 1 and 2 are called low grade gliomas and grades 3 and 4 high grade gliomas [1].

Low Grade Gliomas

Grade 1: Pilocytic Astrocytomas

This is a somewhat circumscribed, often macrocystic astrocytic tumor composed in varying proportions of compact tissue consisting of bipolar, hair like (piloid), heavily fibrillated astrocytes accompanied by Rosenthal fibers or loose-textured, microcyst-rich tissue made up of poorly fibrillated astrocytes associated with eosinophilic granular bodies and/or protein droplets. Degenerative nuclear atypia is common, but mitoses are rare or lacking. Their mean 20 year survival is 80%.[1] Characteristically they occur near the midline though this is not an exclusive characteristic. They often occur in younger people. Treatment is ideally total surgical removal. Prognosis depends on localisation. They tend to enhance on MRI with gadolinium. They are typically the focal gliomas found in the brainstem.

Grade 2: Diffuse Astrocytomas

This is a diffusely infiltrative tumor composed of astrocytic cells showing nuclear atypia (nucleomegaly, hyperchromasia and pleomorphism). The finding of a solitary mitosis is acceptable only in large specimens. Endothelial proliferation and necrosis are lacking. The predominant cell type can vary including gemistocytic, fibrillary and protoplasmic types. They are intimately infiltrative often over large volumes, with surprisingly few clinical symptoms. They are found mostly above the tentorium or in the brain stem. They do not usually enhance with contrast on MR examination. Most brainstem gliomas are fibrillary astrocytomas. Surgery is seldom

---

[1]The information on tumour type and pathology for all groups is taken from http://www.icdns.org/, the website of the International Classification of Diseases of the Nervous System.

an option for these tumours, unless a lobectomy can be performed to gain space for raised intracranial pressure symptoms.

Grade 2: Oligodendrogliomas

These are less common slow-growing gliomas characterized by numerous small, round or ovoid oligodendroglial cells uniformly distributed in a sparse fibrillary stroma. They are usually supratentorial and often apparently focal and localised. They thus would seem to make excellent objects for surgical removal, although as with other gliomas, total surgical removal is an illusion. They have an indolent course in most instances, though WHO does distinguish a grade 3 oligodendroglioma. This account will be restricted to the commoner grade 2.

High Grade Gliomas

Grade 3: Anaplastic Astrocytomas

This is a diffusely infiltrative tumor composed of astrocytic cells also showing nuclear atypia (nucleomegaly, hyperchromasia, pleomorphism) and mitotic activity (one mitosis in a small eg. stereotactic specimen, or more in a large specimen). On MRI partial contrast enhancement is common.

Grade 4: Glioblastoma Multiforme

This is a diffusely infiltrative tumor composed of astrocytic cells featuring nuclear atypia (nucleomegaly, hyperchromasia, pleomorphism), mitotic activity, and either or both endothelial proliferation or necrosis with or without palisading. The tumor varies greatly in cytology and may be widely infiltrative or relatively circumscribed. This is the commonest of the gliomas.

Gamma Knife Treatment of Glioma

Low Grade Gliomas

Low grade glioma is an unsatisfactory term as it lumps together some very different pathological entities. These are the pilocytic astrocytomas, diffuse grade 2 astrocytomas and the oligodendroglioma. However, the latter has its own particular characteristics and will be considered separately. Thus, while there are a much greater variety of WHO grade 1 and grade 2 glial tumours than the two mentioned here, it is these two which account for all the significant literature about low grade glial tumours which are treated by the Gamma Knife so attention will be restricted to these two. They will however, be treated separately and not bunched together under the blanket term "low grade gliomas". The justifications for this are as follows. Firstly, there is the definition given above. Secondly there is the statement made by the Guidelines and Outcomes Committee of the American Association of Neurological Surgeons, in their advisory document on low grade gliomas. "There is little controversy related to the management of pilocytic astrocytomas. They are generally curable by means of gross-total resection. This report will focus on supratentorial nonoptic pathway non pilocytic LGG" (low grade gliomas) [2].

For reasons that will become clear below, it is considered sensible not to consider LGG as a useful grouping but to keep to the specific tumour type when recounting what can be expected of GKNS.

Grade 1: Pilocytic Astrocytomas

While pilocytic astrocytomas may be treated by total removal as stated above, their location does not always permit this. This is where alternative therapies may play a part. The earliest reports using GKNS suffered from small numbers and short control, but at relatively low doses between 12 and 14 Gy gave the impression of ease of control for the duration of follow up [3, 4]. In both these series the GKNS was applied as a primary treatment, or following biopsy or subtotal resection. No other radiation was used. The GKNS could be considered the definitive treatment in these cases. Another early paper from Pittsburgh also recorded encouraging early results [5].

Subsequently, the Karolinska group reported 19 patients with a confirmed histological diagnosis [6]. This was from biopsy in to patients and partial resection in 17. Two patients had received conventional radiotherapy and one was treated with brachytherapy. The median radiological follow up time was 4.7 years. In 18 of 19 tumours there was control. The 19th tumour required a GKNS retreatment which was successful. Two serious complications occurred. In one patient who had received previous fractionated radiotherapy an operation was necessary because of radionecrosis. Another patient developed a radiation induced hemiparesis. Two patients developed cysts, one of which required multiple drainage procedures and one of which was asymptomatic and subsequently shrank. This series is mentioned in some detail because of the relatively large number of tumours followed for over 4 years with all the classical characteristics of pilocytic astrocytomas.

More recent evidence is not so clear cut. Firstly, let us consider a paper dedicated to pilocytic astrocytomas per se [7]. The report to be considered comes from Pittsburgh. The case material of 37 patients is similar to the Stockholm material with 20 patients treated for recurrence, 11 for residual tumour and six after biopsy. Nine patients had received previous radiotherapy or cyst drainage. However, the findings and results are different. The median follow up after radiosurgery was no more than 28 months. The dosimetry was similar to that in previous reports. What is unusual is the mention of four multifocal diffuse tumours. The overall tumour control was only 68% of patients. On the other hand the tumour control of solid circumscribed tumours was 84%. Local progression was noted in four circumscribed tumours, three out of four diffuse tumours and in five of eight cystic tumours there was an increase in cyst size. Factors associated with a poor outcome were high age, location, tumour volume, previous failed fractionated radiotherapy, cystic tumours and diffuse tumours. The dose threshold for consistent success in this series was 15 Gy. In the discussion the authors mention that these lesions rarely undergo progression to anaplasia mentioning a single case in the literature of a cerebellar tumour which did exactly that, going malignant 39 years after treatment [8]. The patient had been operated and received radiotherapy in 1932 at the age of 16. There is in fact a similar and historically somewhat more interesting reference to the same phenomenon. In this case the patient had survived 48 years after the primary surgery for a cerebellar astrocytoma and the original surgeon had been Harvey Cushing [9]. This patient had received radiotherapy following an inadequate craniotomy in 1928 followed by radiotherapy for a "pontine glioma". Shortly afterwards she was seen and operated on by Cushing and the operation was followed by another course of radiotherapy. The paper mentions five patients in all with malignant deterioration 20 or more years after initial surgery. Four received radiotherapy and one did not. Thus, this is a rare occurrence for pilocytic cerebellar astrocytomas of children but not unknown.

There remain two papers on pilocytic astrocytomas that may be considered together. They are recently published and again come from the Pittsburgh group [10, 11]. One is concerned with pilocytic astrocytomas in children [11] and one in the same tumour in adults [10]. There were 50 children reported with a median follow up of 55 months. In this series there was a 97.4% 10 year survival. The only death was in a child with Down's syndrome who succumbed to pneumonia. However, there was failure of tumour control in 2 and cyst enlargement in 10. The two solid tumours were retreated with GKNS and controlled. Thus, the findings of this paper are very much in keeping with the Karolinska paper but at odds with the earlier paper from their own department. Nonetheless, while only one patient died from non tumour related causes, there was some radiological progression, associated with certain factors on univariate analysis, including brain stem involvement, tumour volume, the presence of a cyst and the timing of treatment. The timing of treatment refers to the finding that early treatment of residual tumour after surgery resulted in a better tumour control than treatment for recurrent tumour following earlier treatment modalities including, surgery and radiotherapy. There is no information about why the brainstem tumours had a shorter progression free interval. It could be that they receive a lower dose, but this is not mentioned.

The explanation for this discrepancy between the earlier and later Pittsburgh papers is to be found in the paper on pilocytic astrocytomas in adults [10]. This is a rarer tumour and the series consists of 14 patient, nine with solid and five with cystic tumours. Two patients died from tumour progression and one from tumour dissemination across the subarachnoid space. Since all tumours were biopsy confirmed pilocytic astrocytomas this series provides a powerful indication that the tumour behaves differently in adults and children. Since the earlier paper [12]

Fig. 16.1 Pilocytic
astrocytoma – biopsy
confirmed – volume 2.7 cm^3
with prescription dose 12 Gy.
The tumour shrank slightly
over 3 years. Otherwise the
boy was doing as well at
school as his efforts would
permit. Leading a normal
active life 3 years after
treatment

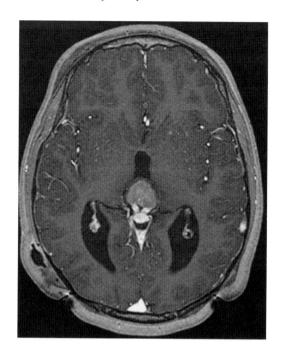

Fig. 16.2 Pilocytic
astrocytoma – operated.
Incidental finding after CT
following a head injury which
caused vomiting. Was
operated. Came for GKNS for
residual tumour. Seven years
old with prescription dose
12 Gy to 8.7 cm^3 tumour. Has
an internal ophthalmoplegias
with course nystagmus. After
1 year was fit and eye
symptoms had disappeared.
Marked shrinkage of the
tumour and no loss of vision

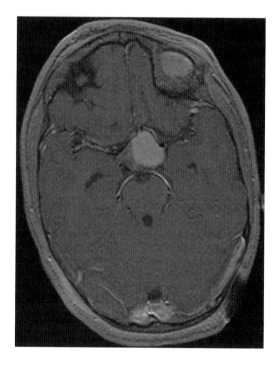

included both adults and children, this could be the reason why its results were inferior to other reports. Figs. 16.1 and 16.2 illustrate typical paediatric cases with pilocytic astrocyctoma.

The relationship of GKNS to previous radiotherapy is of interest. In this paper on adults the time from surgery to tumour progression was prolonged in the group in which radiotherapy had been given. However, by the same token the radiotherapy had not been adequate or GKNS would not have been necessary. In the paper on children there was better 5 and 10 year progression free survival for GKNS given up front after subtotal surgery than when it was given for a recurrence after previously failed treatment including radiotherapy.

Thus, the principles of treatment for pilocytic astrocytomas would seem to be radical microsurgery where possible. If this cannot be achieved GKNS may be offered. From the information shown above, there is some indication that GKNS in children is to be preferred if it is given early after partial treatment rather than late for recurrent tumour. This regimen would also reduce the total radiation to the developing brain. Adverse radiation effects are minimal.

It should be born in mind that the adult tumours are seemingly more aggressive than the commoner children's tumours. The other major negative factor is the presence of a cyst. Repeated stereotactic aspiration for symptoms would seem to be the best option. It is the senior author's experience that Ommaya reservoirs are disappointing in this context as the fluid coagulates so easily that the reservoirs most often become blocked.

In conclusion, it may be mentioned that there have been reported instances of pilocytic astrocytomas regressing, but these are almost always associated with the visual pathway or occur in patients with neurofibromatosis type I. A single case of regression of a temporal lobe tumour has recently been reported. This is at present such a rare occurrence it cannot be used as a guide to management [13].

Grade 2: Diffuse Astrocytomas

The tumour to be considered here is the diffuse fibrillary astrocytoma, defined as quoted above [2]. The first paper on this came from Stockholm in 1994 with a mean follow up of 6 years (range 2–15 years) This group used some higher doses at first but came down to recommend a 12–14 Gy prescription dose. All six patients had tumour control for the duration of the study. Half the patients were children and half were adults. Further mention of this paper will be made in the section on pineal region tumours.

The next step was a paper from Kida et al. in 2000 with 51 patients with a mean follow up of 27.6 months [14]. Twelve of these patients had pilocytic astrocytomas and a mean age of 9.8 years. The remaining 39 had grade 2 astrocytomas with a mean age of 30.9. The tumour control rate was 91% for grade 1 tumours which received a mean margin dose of 12.5 Gy. The control rate was 87.2% for the Grade 2 tumours which received a mean margin dose of 15.7 Gy. The higher margin dose may have contributed to the relatively high control rate of grade 2 tumours in this series. However, in the grade 2 tumours 41% suffered radiation induced oedema and half of these patients suffered symptoms and deficits.

The groups in Pittsburgh and Charlottesville have followed their patients over a number of years now and it seems appropriate to comment on the most recent papers from these two centres. The Pittsburgh group followed 12 patients presenting in the period between 1987 and 2000 [15]. There were four children and eight adults. The patients had received a variety of prior procedures before GKNS including surgery, biopsy, cyst drainage, ventriculoperitoneal shunt and radiotherapy. The diagnosis was confirmed by stereotactic biopsy. A mean prescription dose of 16 Gy was used. Median follow up after radiosurgery was 52 months (range 12–159 months). No patients died. In eight patients the tumour was controlled. In three there was cyst enlargement and in one true tumour progression. Subsequent surgery on this patient revealed anaplasia. The major imaging modality in this series was MRI with T1 enhancement which does raise a question of the true grade of the tumour at the time of GKNS, no matter what grade it had had at the time of primary treatment. The results would seem to be commendable.

The recent paper to consider from the Charlottesville group is a bit more difficult to understand at first sight. First published in 2005 it was republished in 2008 [16, 17]. The paper discusses the findings in 63 patients followed for a median radiological follow up of 59 months (range 2–180 months). The patients were reviewed retrospectively. The indications for treatment were location in an eloquent area, residual tumour after surgery or recurrence following surgery. Only five patients had previous radiotherapy. The median age was 27 (range 2–70 years). Eight patients died and of these seven died from tumour progression. The eight had shown tumour progression but definitive information was not available. The median tumour volume was 2.4 cm^3 and the median dose was 15 Gy so the dosimetry was in keeping with the other studies mentioned. The tumour control rate was 73% which is reasonable for grade 2 tumours. The difficulty is that 21 of the 49 tumours were pilocytic astrocytomas and uniquely, histology had no effect on the result. From what has been written above it seems reasonable to assume the poor results with grade 1 patients may relate to the fact that many wear adult, although this is not specified as such. Another recent paper with a long follow up described a 10-year progression free survival of 65% [18]

In conclusion, all the papers noted above indicate a place for GKNS in the treatment of pilocytic astrocytomas which cannot be removed totally. It is probable that earlier treatment is advantageous but this is still not demonstrated beyond doubt. The results with Grade 2 tumours are less good as one might expect. The same is true of adult grade 1 tumours, for which GKNS will always be a limited option. For the Grade 2 tumour it seems reasonable to advocate the use for small tumour remnants that have begun to grow or clear cut enhancing nodules. However, the existence of such enhancing nodules may indicate that the tumour is beginning to become more aggressive. On the other hand it should also be noted that the occurrence of contrast enhancement after GKNS may just be a part of the response to radiation and not indicate deterioration [19, 20]. More information is needed in particular more series with a greater number of patients stratified by tumour grade and age are required before it is possible to say more about the management of these lesions.

Grade 2: Oligodendrogliomas

There is much less information about GKNS and these tumours. A lengthy review of over 200 patients published from the University in Bergen [21] reported on over 200 patients with oligodendrogliomas. A combined therapy of as radical surgery as possible with subsequent radiotherapy was advised as optimal treatment. This gave a substantially longer median survival time. A curiosity of this paper was the finding that the blood group A was observed as a negative prognostic factor although no reason was found for this. Back in 1985 when that paper was published it was thought that oligodedrogliomas accounted for 5% of all primary brain tumours. In more recent papers the range of 4.2–18% is quoted [22, 23]. The Mayo Clinic described a series of 18 patients with 21 tumours. Ten of the tumours were Grade 2. All of these were recurrent tumours following surgery, and or radiotherapy. They had a median survival of 28 months. Two patients had repeated surgery and one had chemotherapy.

A recent paper comes from Pittsburgh and describes 30 patients with oligodendrogliomas. The mean follow up was 39.2 months (range 12–133 months). Twelve of these lesions were grade 2 tumours and 18 were grade 3. It is the grade 2 lesions which are our concern. All of these tumours were recurrences after previous surgery and or radiotherapy and in some cases chemotherapy. Grade 2 tumours had an 81.5% progress free survival at 5 years. Within this material, tumour grade and target volume were the only two parameters to correlate significantly with prolonged survival.

Thus it would seem that patients with recurrent grade 2 oligodendrogliomas can experience a benefit from GKNS at the time of recurrence.

Follow up of Patients with Gliomas Grades 1 and 2

It is suggested that a 3D T1 MR with and without Gadolinium together with fine slice axial T2 series through the lesion should be performed every 3 months for a year. Thereafter, the frequency could be reduced to every 6 months for 4 years and after that to every 5 years. In the event of clinical deterioration that could be due to the tumour a new MR should be taken at once and the follow up and management reviewed.

High Grade Gliomas

The grades 3 and 4 gliomas are regarded as impossible to remove in toto because of size, location and the impossibility of removing invisible microscopic invasion around the visible tumour seen at surgery. Following attempts at surgery the residual tissue will produce a recurrent tumour, most commonly adjacent to the resection cavity. With grade 4 tumours this will happen quicker than with the grade 3. Thus while the aim of treatment is the same as for any tumour, total removal, the reality of surgical treatment is frustration.

There is a splendid review of this topic from McGill University and every interested person is strongly advised to read it [24]. Their conclusions are that there is no decent evidence for the use of stereotactic radiosurgery for the definitive treatment of high grade gliomas. They suggest that in selected cases that radiosurgery can be useful as a palliative treatment of recurrent tumours. In this context one should mention a recent paper which supplies retrospective evidence that the right time to use GKNS is not up front but at the time of recurrence [25]. Thus, treatment is assessed on a case by case basis. In view of limitations of space this matter will not be pursued in more detail here and the interested reader is referred to the References to be found at Springer's website.

The same MR follow-up technique is suggested as for the grade 1 and 2 tumours with the difference that an extra MR should be taken 4 weeks after treatment. With these patients the treatment will also have to be timed carefully so as not to interfere with the more modern more effective chemotherapy used in these patients such as Temozolomide.

Special Gliomas

Anterior Optic Pathway Gliomas

Optic chiasm gliomas are rare. Two patients with optic nerve gliomas treated with GKNS have been reported [26]. While surgery will remove the tumour the obvious price will be loss of vision. In the 2 cases described the tumours shrank and the vision improved over a follow up period of 24 months in one case and 43 months in the other. This report has not been followed up but seems an interesting area for application for GKNS. Otherwise in association with NF1 optic nerve tumours are observed and if bilateral are more or less pathognomonic for NF1. They are indolent, slowly growing lesions and are only operated upon if there is severe loss of vision, problematic proptosis or posterior extension into and expanding the optic canal.

Brain Stem Gliomas

These are partly considered in the section on tumours of the pineal region. However, the usual diffuse brainstem glioma consists of a mixture of neoplastic and functioning neural tissue. It cannot in principle be a suitable object for treatment by GKNS which spares normal tissue by geometric definition between the pathological and normal tissue. However, focal brainstem low grade gliomas do occur in the brainstem as recorded by the Charlottesville group with encouraging results [27].

Gliomas Conclusions

GKNS has little part to play in the primary treatment of gliomas in the light of current knowledge. However, they seem to have a useful palliative effect at the time of recurrence. This benefit applies for all types and grades of tumour about which there is information. More studies with properly structured and stratified trials are needed to assess the role of the method more precisely.

Other Tumours Arising from Cerebral Tissue

Choroid Plexus Papillomas

These are vascular mainly benign tumours with a characteristic histology. They are also rare. Total removal is usually associated with cure. However, a substantial proportion of them arise in locations which make radical surgery impossible, such as the third and fourth ventricles. In a major recent paper from the Mayo Clinic only 56% of 41 patients had a radical resection [28]. Of the partially resected tumours around half remained stable and half proceeded to relapse and grow. At this time another partial resection was done followed by radiotherapy. Second relapses were treated with radiation alone. The authors did not develop a clear cut philosophy in respect of radiation treatment. This is the largest series in existence. The median follow up was 6.5 years

A second paper concerning GKNS for treatment resistant tumours was published in 2008. It concerns six patients with 11 tumours which had proved treatment resistant. These are the most aggressive tumours presenting a considerable contrast to the tumours reported in the previous paper. Two patients died. Four survived for periods from 39 to 120 months. Thus, for this the rare aggressive forms of this tumour which have resisted all other forms of treatment there might be a place for GKNS on a case by case basis in an attempt to achieve life prolonging palliation. There is to date no firm evidence that the Gamma Knife can be curative for these lesions.

Ependymomas

Intracranial ependymomas comprise about 5% of all intracranial neoplasms and about 30% of those occurring in children under 3 [29]. The role of radiosurgery is marginal but unlike most of the tumours in this chapter the opinions are somewhat divided. Nearly all the series on which to base an opinion are small: something which makes selection issues more important and which also makes the interpretation of Kaplan Meier graphs difficult. Most workers regard the treatment as of possible use for recurrent disease after surgery and radiotherapy [29–35]. However, one group considers that it is possible that radiosurgery as a boost together with the primary radiotherapy may give better tumour control [29]. Krieger et al. who performed a metanalysis of altogether of 28 articles selected as relevant from a much greater number came to no firm conclusion [36].

Just to make life a bit more confusing there is a recent paper from Pittsburgh where they found that tumour control and progression free intervals were not related to either dose or tumour grade but were related to tumour volume [37]. They still found GKNS useful palliation in the face of treatment failure.

Thus, it would seem thus that despite some varied opinions, this tumour remains a formidable disease for which radiosurgery might have a role to play but at present that role remains undetermined. Thus, again most Gamma Knife users will find themselves treating a few cases of treatment resistant tumours where the volume is not too great.

Medulloblastomas

Medullblastomas represent about 25% of all brain tumours in children and 2–5% in adults. The diseases are different in adults and children [38]. This paper also agrees with an earlier publication, that the majority of recurrences occur in or close to the original tumour site [39]. This opens the possibility of boosting conventional radiotherapy with a radiosurgery boost as part of the primary tumour. Increasingly the term medulloblastoma is being replaced by primitive neuroectodermal tumour or PNET. The Pittsburgh group reported 12 adult patients with PNETs, of which six were recurrent and six were residual. The patients received one to three treatments with GKNS following conventional treatment failure. Once again, this tumour would seem to provide occasional examples of tumour resistant to treatment being controlled at least for a while by GKNS. Once again, the use of GKNS will necessarily be on an ad hoc case by case basis. Not enough is known to have a consistent treatment policy.

Pineal Region Tumours

This is a complex region because of the range and rarity of the different tumours which occur there. Moreover, it is a region which is relatively inaccessible to the surgeon, which historically made surgery dangerous. Modern microsurgery technique has improved the results and reduced the complications. The majority of these tumours occur in childhood.

Not only are these tumours rare but there is a whole family of them as illustrated in the table below. To make it even more complicated, it is common for any given tumour to contain more than one cell type, resulting in tumours of mixed cells of origin or mixed regions of aggression with the same histology. Added to all of the above there is a risk of the seeding of tumour cells under surgery which increases the technical problems of treatment. Not surprisingly therefore there are a range of opinions on how best to treat these lesions. The current state of knowledge is admirably summed up in three recent reviews [40–42]. It is of interest that none of these reviews can perceive a clear cut role for radiosurgery, even though one of the papers is a chapter from a book on radiosurgery [42]. The list of possible diagnoses is shown in the aforementioned table. While there are a considerable number of different possibilities, the distribution of tumour types is uneven with only a few tumour types covering most of the cases seen. In general the papers present either tumours of pineal parenchyma [43–48] or tumours of the pineal region [40, 42, 49–57], The former are traditionally radioresistant while some of the germ cell tumours are very radiosensitive.

Tumour type	Subdivision
Germ cell tumours	Germinoma
(Germinomatous)	
(Non-germinomatous)	Teratoma (mature and immature)
	Embryonal Carcinoma
	Yolk Sac Tumours
	Choriocarcinoma
Pineal parenchymal tumours	Pineocytoma
	Pineoblastoma
	Pineal parenchymal tumours of intermediate determination
Others	Gliomas
	Tectal
	Thalamic
	Pineal
	Meningiomas
	Ependymomas
	Metastases
	Lymphoma

Tumours Arising from the Pineal Gland

Type of Biopsy

All serious authors insist that biopsy is essential [40, 42, 43, 45, 48, 49, 51, 54, 55], In the past there has been a view that biopsy can be avoided and a GKNS performed on the basis of the image as a sort of therapeutic trial [50]. This is not acceptable in view of the variety of possible diagnoses and the individual cellular variety within a given tumour. Moreover, MRI or CT alone do not with current technique permit certainty of histological diagnosis. Since the different tumour types behave very differently biopsy remains essential. Some authors insist that open biopsy is mandatory because it ensures that adequate tissue is taken, opens the way for tumour removal [40–43]. Other authors insist that stereotactic biopsy is adequate [41, 45–48, 51, 52, 55, 57]. The papers to which reference is made here are the work of very distinguished authors and it is not possible at the present time to know which method is to be preferred.

GKNS and Pineal Parenchymal Tumours

The Marseille group have published on the subject of a collection of 13 pine-ocytomas and pineoblastomas. With a mean follow up of 34 months all the pine-ocytomas are alive and under control while 2 of 5 pineoblastomas are dead [48]. Another GKNS series from Miami, treating 20 patients collected over 10 years [49]. A Kaplan Meier graph extending for 6 years showed three patients had died. One died of unrelated causes with a controlled tumour. One died of an uncontrolled pineoblastoma. One patient was in a desperate condition at the time of treatment with GKNS and survived only a few weeks. This series contained a greater variety of diagnoses the majority of whom were germinomatous germinomas.

The most consistent and long lasting follow up of this condition has been performed by the group in Pittsburgh who by 2009 had accumulated 20 patients with pineocytomas, pineoblastomas and mixed pineocytic tumours. At an average follow up of 54.1 months six patients were dead and 14 were living. Overall survival after GKNS was 95, 68.6 and 51.4% at 1 5 and 10 years respectively. It is emphasised that these results concern only tumours originating from pineocytes. For other kinds of pineal region tumours the Pittsburgh group has constructed a complex algorithm of varied treatments which has evolved over the years but reflects a well thought out approach to a disparate group of diseases. Their results with GKNS in their limited material are at least as good as those with surgery with or without radiotherapy [40, 41].

There is one paper from Japan which recounts the treatment of 33 pineal region tumours with a mean follow up of 23.3 months. All patients had been received surgery and or shunting so all cases were treatment resistant tumours. There was tumour control in 73.3% of patients available to follow up. There was tumour progression in eight patients of whom seven died. As might be expected the deaths occurred in the more aggressive tumours including 5 cases of malignant germinoma, one pineoblastoma and one germinoma with syncytiotrophoblastic cells [53].

Reviews of Pineal Parenchymal Tumours

Firstly, let us consider the primary treatment. The two reviews regard microsurgery as the gold standard treatment with conventional fractionated radiotherapy added where required [40–42]. In a comment to an article proposing a stereotactic approach to pineocytomas it is suggested that primary radiosurgery be limited to elderly and infirm patients with smaller non infiltrative tumours. With larger infiltrating tumours, partial resection and radiotherapy is to be preferred [58]. These review articles are all agreed on the paradigm of maximal removal where possible through open surgery and fractionated radiotherapy. They are not clear about the role of radiosurgery but indicate that it may well have a role, especially in the presence of failed conventional therapy. This is fair comment, since a great number of the patients described in the papers on radiosurgery for pineal tumours have received previous treatment in the form of surgery and or radiotherapy. No paper using GKNS alone as a primary treatment of these tumours exists at the time of writing.

Hydrocephalus

Hydrocephalus is an almost constant accompaniment of these tumours and there is broad agreement that endoscopic ventriculostomy from the third ventricle to the subarachnoid cisterns is to be preferred to shunting procedures [40–42], provided the tumour does not extend anteriorly across the floor of the third ventricle behind the mamillary bodies [41].

Germ Cell Tumours

These are the commonest tumours arising from the pineal gland itself accounting for about 30–80% of the lesions [59]. There is no clear cut role for the use of GKNS for these tumours. They are much commoner in Japan where the standard treatment today in many centres remains shunting and radiotherapy without biopsy. It is hard to justify this practice today, given the uncertainty of diagnosis even when a biopsy is available. Moreover, there is a risk of endocrinological and intellectual damage to the usually young patients who will be subjected to high volume radiation aimed at including the pineal region and the ventricles. The success rate with the most radiosensitive lesions, the germinomatous germinomas varies between 60 and 100%. Thus, new tumours arise either from failed treatment, undetected pre-radiotherapy seedlings or the development of new tumours at a distance. There is a fairly recent and somewhat unsatisfactory paper from Sendai which describes a technique aimed at reducing the volume of irradiated tissue with germinomas while not limiting it to visible tumour. Three cases are described with GKNS to visible pineal tumour tissue and an extra dose limited to the ventricles. The technique of this ventricular dose is regrettably not described. In addition the follow up is short.

Tumours Arising in the Pineal Region

These are listed in the table above and each tumour is treated in accordance with the principles which apply for the same tumour elsewhere in the body. However, a little notice should be addressed to the gliomas. While these may be the same sort of glioma with every grade from I–IV, there is one tumour which deserves special mention. This is the so called tectal glioma. These have the following character-istics. They are usually described histologically as grade 2 [60, 61]. They run however an unusually indolent course. They are quite distinct from the other brainstem gliomas which are mainly diffuse [62, 63], though a few may be focal and pilocytic. These tectal gliomas are so indolent the main burden of treatment is resolution of hydrocephalus by endoscopic third ventriculostomy. This procedure can then be followed by observation [61]. If there is sign of growth GKNS can be a useful therapeutic approach [4].

Concluding Remarks About Pineal Region Tumours

It would seem nobody has the answer to these difficult lesions at this time. However, the authors can commend a comment and recommend a reference. The comment is made by Manfred Westfal [64]. He makes the point that the rarity, complexity, technical difficulty and variety of these tumours should result in their referral to and treatment at centres specially equipped to do so. These are not lesions to be managed by regional neurosurgical departments. The recommendation is to read the review by Bruce and Ogden. This paper is well informed, balanced, academic and includes information of the interaction between surgeons during the development of the treatment of pineal tumours. The article is a gem [41].

Neurocytoma

Neurocytomas are a reasonably recent addition to the nosology of intracranial neoplasia. They were first described in 1982 by Hassoun and reviewed in detail in 1992 [65]. From 2001 on an interest grew in the possibility of using GKNS in certain circumstances. The tumour was known to be radioresponsive and to be associated with lengthy survival. This made the side effects of whole brain radiation unattractive. They are also known to have an indolent tendency to recurrence even after a long time [66]. There were first a number of case reports with good control of the tumour with follow up periods varying between 12 and 83 months [67–70]. Subsequently a few series with small numbers have been published [31, 66, 71, 72]. This is after all a rare tumour. Bertalanaffy [66] and Yen et al. [72] recorded good control of residual or recurrent tumours. Kim et al. went a step further reporting also good control in both primary and secondary treatments. Thirteen patients in this series were treated with control of all tumours at a mean follow up of 61 months although two patients required two treatments.

The information above suggests that for these tumours GKNS may well have a role, but because of the late nature of recurrence even after apparent total removal of these albeit rare tumours, it will be some years before the precise role of GKNS can be asserted with any degree of certainty.

Haemangioblastoma

Haemangioblastomas arise in two very different contexts. There are the isolated tumours and there the tumours which are part of the von Hippel Lindau (VHL) diathesis. Around 80% are solitary and 20% are VHL cases. The management and prognosis varies with these two groups. Solitary lesions are restricted to the brain, almost always in the posterior fossa. VHL patients have intracerebral haemangio-blastomas, but also have lesions in the spinal cord, the retina, a tendency to renal cell carcinoma and phaeochromocytomas. Moreover, the variability of manage-ment of the intracranial targets is compounded by two further factors. Sometimes the major mass of a lesion is solid and sometimes it is due to a tumour associated cyst. A further problem in predicting the results of treatment is the well documented intermittent growth of these lesions over long periods even exceeding 10 years [73, 74]. This makes it very difficult to interpret the results of treatments where the end point is unchanged tumour volume.

Despite these difficulties there are a number of papers advocating the treatment of these lesions with GKNS given that certain conditions are met [75–82]. The treatments recorded in these papers are almost invariably palliative following failed surgery or other management. There is a broad agreement that a higher prescription dose (18–20 Gy) and a smaller tumour were positive prognostic findings. Moreover, there is evidence to suggest that cystic tumours should not be treated. Post treatment adverse radiation effects have tended to be mild and temporary. Mortality in the reported series has been rather high for a benign tumour. A most recent review concerned 32 patients [76]. There were 74 intracerebral tumours and 13 of the 32 had VHL. At a median of 50 months seven patients had died from disease progres-sion and one from heart failure. Interestingly, sporadic tumours had a bigger chance of progressive growth after GKNS than VHL tumours. Other factors associated with disease control otherwise were tumour volume, prescription dose and the presence of a cyst. The authors of the paper concluded that cystic tumours were unsuitable for treatment with GKNS. It may be mentioned that in other papers after GKNS a new cyst sometimes arose [77]. These cysts might require intervention though this was not universal.

Thus, the current position of GKNS for haemangioblastomas is that it may be used as palliation for residual or recurrent tumours where other treatments have failed. Its use should be limited to tumours of less than 3 cm in diameter and a prescription dose between 15 and 20 Gy is preferred. However, the tumours are known to recur late after a long intermission [73, 74], and not all radiologically demonstrated tumours require treatment [74]. It is likely that a deal of time must pass before a definitive decision can be reached concerning the role of GKNS for intracerebral haemangioblastomas.

References

1. Irish WD, Macdonald DR, Cairncross JG. Measuring bias in uncontrolled brain tumor trials – to randomize or not to randomize? Can J Neurol Sci **24(4)**: 307–312; 1997
2. Low-Grade Glioma Guidelines Team in Association with the Guidelines and Outcomes Committee of the American Association of Neurological Surgeons. Practice parameters in adults with suspected or known supratentorial nonoptic pathway low-grade glioma. Neurosurgical Focus **4(6)**: e10; 1998

3. Ganz JC, Smievoll AI, Thorsen F. Radiosurgical treatment of gliomas of the diencephalon. Acta Neurochir Suppl **62**: 62–66; 1994
4. Kihlstrom L, Lindquist C, Lindquist M, Karlsson B. Stereotactic radiosurgery for tectal low-grade gliomas. Acta Neurochir Suppl **62**: 55–57; 1994
5. Somaza SC, Kondziolka D, Lunsford LD, Flickinger JC, Bissonette DJ, Albright AL. Early outcomes after stereotactic radiosurgery for growing pilocytic astrocytomas in children. Pediatr Neurosurg **25(3)**: 109–115; 1996
6. Boethius J, Ulfarsson E, Rahn T, Lippittz B. Gamma knife radiosurgery for pilocytic astrocytomas. J Neurosurg **97(5 Suppl)**: 677–680; 2002
7. Hadjipanayis CG, Kondziolka D, Gardner P, Niranjan A, Dagam S, Flickinger JC, Lunsford LD. Stereotactic radiosurgery for pilocytic astrocytomas when multimodal therapy is necessary. J Neurosurg **97(1)**: 56–64; 2002
8. Scott RM, Ballantine HT. Cerebellar astrocytoma: malignant recurrence after prolonged postoperative survival. Case report. J Neurosurg **39(6)**: 777–779; 1973
9. Kleinman GM, Schoene WC, Walshe TM, Richardson EP. Malignant transformation in benign cerebellar astrocytoma. Case report. J Neurosurg **49(1)**: 111–118; 1978
10. Kano H, Kondziolka D, Niranjan A, Flickinger JC, Lunsford LD. Stereotactic radiosurgery for pilocytic astrocytomas part 1: outcomes in adult patients. J Neurooncol **95(2)**: 211–218; 2009
11. Kano H, Niranjan A, Kondziolka D, Flickinger JC, Pollack IF, Jakacki RI, Lunsford LD. Stereotactic radiosurgery for pilocytic astrocytomas part 2: outcomes in pediatric patients. J Neurooncol **95(2)**: 219–229; 2009
12. Hadjipanayis CG, Kondziolka D, Flickinger JC, Lunsford LD. The role of stereotactic radiosurgery for low-grade astrocytomas. Neurosurg Focus **14(5)**: e15; 2003
13. Rozen WM, Joseph S, Lo PA. Spontaneous regression of low-grade gliomas in pediatric patients without neurofibromatosis. Pediatr Neurosurg **44(4)**: 324–328; 2008
14. Kida Y, Kobayashi T, Mori Y. Gamma knife radiosurgery for low-grade astrocytomas: results of long-term follow up. J Neurosurg **93(Suppl 3)**: 42–46; 2000
15. Hadjipanayis CG, Niranjan A, Tyler-Kabara E, Kondziolka D, Flickinger JC, Lunsford LD. Stereotactic radiosurgery for well-circumscribed fibrillary grade II astrocytomas: an initial experience. Stereotact Funct Neurosurg **79(1)**: 13–24; 2002
16. Heppner PA, Sheehan JP, Steiner LE. Gamma knife surgery for low-grade gliomas. Neurosurgery **62(Suppl 2)**: 755–762; 2008
17. Heppner PA, Sheehan JP, Steiner LE. Gamma knife surgery for low-grade gliomas. Neurosurgery **57(6)**: 1132–1139; 2005
18. Wang LW, Shiau CY, Chung WY, Wu HM, Guo WY, Liu KD, Ho DM, Wong TT, Pan DH. Gamma knife surgery for low-grade astrocytomas: evaluation of long-term outcome based on a 10-year experience. J Neurosurg **105(Suppl)**: 127–132; 2006
19. Kondziolka D, Comment on Heppner PA, Sheehan JP, Steiner LE. Gamma knife surgery for low-grade gliomas. Neurosurgery **57(6)**: 1138; 2005
20. Pollock BE, Comment on Heppner PA, Sheehan JP, Steiner LE Gamma knife surgery for low-grade gliomas. Neurosurgery **57(6)**: 1138; 2005
21. Mørk SJ, Lindegaard KF, Halvorsen TB, Lehmann EH, Solgaard T, Hatlevoll R, Harvei S, Ganz J. Oligodendroglioma: incidence and biological behavior in a defined population. J Neurosurg **63(6)**: 881–889; 1985
22. Kano H, Niranjan A, Khan A, Flickinger JC, Kondziolka D, Lieberman F, Lunsford LD. Does radiosurgery have a role in the management of oligodendrogliomas? J Neurosurg **110(3)**: 564–571; 2009
23. Sarkar A, Pollock BE, Brown PD, Gorman DA. Evaluation of gamma knife radiosurgery in the treatment of oligodendrogliomas and mixed oligodendroastrocytomas. J Neurosurg **97(5 Suppl)**: 653–656; 2002
24. Roberge D, Souhami L. High-grade gliomas. in (eds) Chin LS, Regine WF: Principles and Practice of Stereotactic Radiosurgery. Springer Science + Business Media LLC, New York: pp 207–222; 2008

25. Hsieh PC, Bhangoo S, Panagiotopoulos K, Kalapurakal JA, Marymont MH, Cozzens. JW, Levy RM. Adjuvant gamma knife stereotactic radiosurgery at the time of tumor progression potentially improves survival for patients with glioblastoma. Neurosurgery 57: 684–692; 2005

26. Lim YJ, Leem W. Two cases of gamma knife radiosurgery for low-grade optic chiasm glioma. Stereotact Funct Neurosurg **66(Suppl 1)**: 174–183; 1996

27. Yen CP, Sheehan J, Steiner M, Patterson G, Steiner L. Gamma knife surgery for focal brainstem gliomas. J Neurosurg **106(1)**: 8–17; 2007

28. Krishnan S, Brown PD, Scheithauer BW, Ebersold MJ, Hammack JE, Buckner JC. Choroid plexus papillomas: a single institutional experience. J Neurooncol **68(1)**: 49–55; 2004

29. Mansur DB, Drzymala RE, Rich KM, Klein EE, Simpson JR. The efficacy of stereotactic radiosurgery in the management of intracranial ependymoma. J Neurooncol **66(1–2)**: 187–190; 2004

30. Applegate GL, Marymont MH. Intracranial ependymomas: a review. Cancer Invest **16(8)**: 588–593; 1998

31. Bertalanffy A, Roessler K, Koperek O, Gelpi E, Prayer D, Knosp E. Recurrent central neurocytomas. Cancer **104(1)**: 135–142; 2005

32. Endo H, Kumabe T, Jokura H, Shirane R, Tominaga T. Stereotactic radiosurgery for nodular dissemination of anaplastic ependymoma. Acta Neurochir **146(3)**: 291–298; 2004

33. Jawahar A, Kondziolka D, Flickinger JC, Lunsford LD. Adjuvant stereotactic radiosurgery for anaplastic ependymoma. Stereotact Funct Neurosurg **73(1–4)**: 23–30; 1999

34. Lo SS, Abdulrahman R, Desrosiers PM, Fakiris AJ, Witt TC, Worth RM, Dittmer PH, Desrosiers CM, Frost S, Timmerman RD. The role of gamma knife radiosurgery in the management of unresectable gross disease or gross residual disease after surgery in ependymoma. J Neurooncol **79(1)**: 51–56; 2006

35. Stafford SL, Pollock BE, Foote RL, Gorman DA, Nelson DF, Schomberg PJ. Stereotactic radiosurgery for recurrent ependymoma. Cancer **88(4)**: 870–875; 2000

36. Krieger MD, McComb JG. The role of stereotactic radiotherapy in the management of ependymomas. Childs Nerv Syst **25(10)**: 1269–1273; 2009

37. Kano H, Niranjan A, Kondziolka D, Flickinger JC, Lunsford LD. Outcome Predictors for intracranial ependymoma radiosurgery. Neurosurgery **64(2)**: 279–288; 2009

38. Woo C, Stea B, Lulu B, Hamilton A, Cassady JR. The use of stereotactic radiosurgical boost in the treatment of medulloblastomas. Int J Radiat Oncol Biol Phys **37(4)**: 761–764; 1997

39. Inoue HK, Nakamura M, Ono N, Kawashima Y, Hirato M, Ohye C. Long-term clinical effects of radiation therapy for primitive gliomas and medulloblastomas: a role for radiosurgery. Stereotact Funct Neurosurg **61(Suppl 1)**: 51–58; 1993

40. Blakeley JO, Grossman SA. Management of pineal region tumors. Curr Treat Options Oncol 7 **(6)**: 505–516; 2006

41. Bruce JN, Ogden AT. Surgical strategies for treating patients with pineal region tumors. J Neurooncol **69(1–3)**: 221–236; 2004

42. Lekovic GP, Shetter AG. Pineal region tumours. in (eds) Chin LS, Regine WF: Principles and Practice of Stereotactic Radiosurgery. Springer Science + Business Media LLC, New York: pp 355–364; 2008

43. Deshmukh VR, Smith KA, Rekate HL, Coons S, Spetzler RF. Diagnosis and management of pineocytomas. Neurosurgery **55(2)**: 349–355; 2004

44. Endo H, Kumabe T, Jokura H, Tominaga T. Stereotactic radiosurgery followed by whole ventricular irradiation for primary intracranial germinoma of the pineal region. Minim Invasive Neurosurg **48(3)**: 186–190; 2005

45. Hasegawa T, Kondziolka D, Hadjipanayis CG, Flickinger JC, Lunsford LD. Stereotactic radiosurgery for CNS nongerminomatous germ cell tumors. Report of four cases. Pediatr Neurosurg **38(6)**: 329–333; 2003

46. Hasegawa T, Kondziolka D, Hadjipanayis CG, Flickinger JC, Lunsford LD. The role of radiosurgery for the treatment of pineal parenchymal tumors. Neurosurgery **51(4)**: 880–889; 2002

47. Kano H, Niranjan A, Kondziolka D, Flickinger JC, Lunsford D. Role of stereotactic radiosurgery in the management of pineal parenchymal tumors. Prog Neurol Surg **23**: 44–58; 2009

48. Reyns N, Hayashi M, Chinot O, Manera L, Peragut JC, Blond S, Régis J. The role of gamma knife radiosurgery in the treatment of pineal parenchymal tumours. Acta Neurochir **148(1)**: 5–11; 2006

49. Amendola BE, Wolf A, Coy SR, Amendola MA, Eber D. Pineal tumors: analysis of treatment results in 20 patients. J Neurosurg **102(Suppl)**: 175–179; 2005

50. Chasan CB, Goetsch S, Ott K. Radiosurgery for pineal tumors: is biopsy indicated? Stereotact Funct Neurosurg **66(Suppl 1)**: 157–163; 1996

51. Dempsey PK, Kondziolka D, Lunsford LD. Stereotactic diagnosis and treatment of pineal region tumours and vascular malformations. Acta Neurochir **116(1)**: 14–22; 1992

52. Dempsey PK, Lunsford LD. Stereotactic radiosurgery for pineal region tumors. Neurosurg Clin N Am **3(1)**: 245–253; 1992

53. Kobayashi T, Kida Y, Mori Y. Stereotactic gamma radiosurgery for pineal and related tumors. J Neurooncol **54(3)**: 301–309; 2001

54. Lekovic GP, Gonzalez LF, Shetter AG, Porter RW, Smith KA, Brachman D, Spetzler RF. Role of gamma knife surgery in the management of pineal region tumors. Neurosurg Focus **23**: E12; 2007

55. Manera L, Régis J, Chinot O, Porcheron D, Levrier O, Farnarier P, Peragut JC. Pineal region tumors: the role of stereotactic radiosurgery. Stereotact Funct Neurosurg **66(Suppl 1)**: 164–173; 1996

56. Mori Y, Kobayashi T, Hasegawa T, Yoshida K, Kida Y. Stereotactic radiosurgery for pineal and related tumors. Prog Neurol Surg **23**: 106–118; 2009

57. Subach BR, Lunsford LD, Kondziolka D. Stereotactic radiosurgery in the treatment of pineal regions tumours. in (eds) Lunsford LD, Kondziolka D, Flickinger JC: Gamma Knife Brain Surgery. Proc Neurol Surg Basel, Karger **14**: 175–194; 1998

58. Levivier M, Brotchi J. Comment on 'Hasegawa T, Kondziolka D, Hadjipanayis CG, Flickinger JC, Lunsford LD. The role of radiosurgery for the treatment of pineal parenchymal tumors. Neurosurgery **51(4)**: 880–889; 2002' Neurosurgery **51(4)**: 887–888

59. Germanwala AV, Mai JC, Tomycz ND, Niranjan A, Flickinger JC, Kondziolka D, Lunsford LD. Boost gamma knife surgery during multimodality management of adult medulloblastoma. J Neurosurg **108**: 204–209; 2008

60. Bowers DC, Georgiades C, Aronson LJ, Carson BS, Weingart JD, Wharam MD, Melhem ER, Burger PC, Cohen KJ. Tectal gliomas: natural history of an indolent lesion in pediatric patients. Pediatr Neurosurg **32(1)**: 24–29; 2000

61. Stark AM, Fritsch MJ, Claviez A, Dörner L, Mehdorn HM. Management of tectal glioma in childhood. Pediatr Neurol **33(1)**: 33–38; 2005

62. Guillamo JS, Monjour A, Taillandier L, Devaux B, Varlet P, Haie-Meder C, Defer GL, Maison P, Mazeron JJ, Cornu P, Delattre JY, Association des Neuro-Oncologues d'Expression Française (ANOCEF). Brainstem gliomas in adults: prognostic factors and classification. Brain **124(Pt 12)**: 2528–2539; 2001

63. Hargrave D, Bartels U, Bouffet E. Diffuse brainstem glioma in children: critical review of clinical trials. Lancet Oncol **7(3)**: 241–248; 2006

64. Westphal M. Comment on 'Deshmukh VR, Smith KA, Rekate HL, Coons S, Spetzler RF. Diagnosis and management of pineocytomas. Neurosurgery **55(2)**: 349–355; 2004' Neurosurgery **55(2)**: 356; 2004

65. Figarella-Branger D, Pellissier JF, Daumas-Duport C, Delisle MB, Pasquier B, Parent M, Gambarelli D, Rougon G, Hassoun J. Central neurocytomas. Critical evaluation of a small-cell neuronal tumor. Am J Surg Pathol **16(2)**: 97–109; 1992

66. Bertalanffy A, Roessler K, Dietrich W, Aichholzer M, Prayer D, Ertl A, Kitz K. Gamma knife radiosurgery of recurrent central neurocytomas: a preliminary report. J Neurol Neurosurg Psychiatry **70(4)**: 489–493; 2001

67. Anderson RC, Elder JB, Parsa AT, Issacson SR, Sisti MB. Radiosurgery for the treatment of recurrent central neurocytomas. Neurosurgery **48(6)**: 1231–1237; 2001
68. Hara M, Aoyagi M, Yamamoto M, Maehara T, Takada Y, Nojiri T, Ohno K. Rapid shrinkage of remnant central neurocytoma after gamma knife radiosurgery: a case report. J Neurooncol **62(3)**: 269–273; 2003
69. Pollock BE, Stafford SL. Stereotactic radiosurgery for recurrent central neurocytoma: case report. Neurosurgery **48(2)**: 441–443; 2001
70. Tyler-Kabara E, Kondziolka D, Flickinger JC, Lunsford LD. Stereotactic radiosurgery for residual neurocytoma. Report of four cases. J Neurosurg **95(5)**: 879–882; 2001
71. Kim CY, Paek SH, Jeong SS, Chung HT, Han JH, Park CK, Jung HW, Kim DG. Gamma knife radiosurgery for central neurocytoma: primary and secondary treatment. Cancer **110**: 2276–2284; 2007
72. Yen CP, Sheehan J, Patterson G, Steiner L. Gamma knife surgery for neurocytoma. J Neurosurg **107**: 7–12; 2007
73. Ammerman JM, Lonser RR, Dambrosia J, Butman JA, Oldfield EH. Long-term natural history of hemangioblastomas in patients with von Hippel-Lindau disease: implications for treatment. J Neurosurg **105**: 248–255; 2006
74. Jagannathan J, Lonser RR, Smith R, DeVroom HL, Oldfield EH. Surgical management of cerebellar hemangioblastomas in patients with von Hippel-Lindau disease. J Neurosurg **108** (2): 210–222; 2008
75. Jawahar A, Kondziolka D, Garces YI, Flickinger JC, Pollock BE, Lunsford LD. Stereotactic radiosurgery for hemangioblastomas of the brain. Acta Neurochir **142(6)**: 641–644; 2000
76. Kano H, Niranjan A, Mongia S, Kondziolka D, Flickinger JC, Lunsford LD. The role of stereotactic radiosurgery for intracranial haemangioblastomas. Neurosurgery **63(3)**: 443–450; 2008
77. Matsunaga S, Shuto T, Inomori S, Fujino H, Yamamoto I. Gamma knife radiosurgery for intracranial haemangioblastomas. Acta Neurochir **149**: 1007–1013; 2007
78. Niemela M, Lim YJ, Soderman M, Jaaskelainen J, Lindquist C. Gamma knife radiosurgery in 11 hemangioblastomas. J Neurosurg **85(4)**: 591–596; 1996
79. Park YS, Chang JH, Chang JW, Chung SS, Park YG. Gamma knife surgery for multiple hemangioblastomas. J Neurosurg **102(Suppl)**: 97–101; 2005
80. Rajaraman C, Rowe JG, Walton L, Malik I, Radatz M, Kemeny AA. Treatment options for von Hippel-Lindau's haemangioblastomatosis: the role of gamma knife stereotactic radiosurgery. Br J Neurosurg **18(4)**: 338–342; 2004
81. Tago M, Terahara A, Shin M, Maruyama K, Kurita H, Nakagawa K, Ohtomo K. Gamma knife surgery for hemangioblastomas. J Neurosurg **102(Suppl)**: 171–174; 2005
82. Wang EM, Pan L, Wang BJ, Zhang N, Zhou LF, Dong YF, Dai JZ, Cai PW, Chen H. The long-term results of gamma knife radiosurgery for hemangioblastomas of the brain. J Neurosurg **102(Suppl)**: 225–229; 2005

Chapter 17
Tumours of the Pituitary Region

Pituitary Adenomas

Introduction and a Little Surgical History

Those interested in a more detailed account of the history of the development of the treatment of pituitary tumours are referred to the excellent chapter of Professor Landolt [1]. A more succinct account may be found in another chapter by Professor Takakura et al. [2]. For the present purpose it is enough to illustrate the canvas of history with broad brush strokes. Horsley is credited with the first successful craniotomy for a pituitary macroadenoma in 1889 [3]. Cushing famous for his work on pituitary adenomas performed 338 operations of which only 107 were undertaken via a craniotomy approach. It is of perhaps only academic interest but his approach was entirely extradural until the level of the sphenoid ridge was reached [4]. His operative mortality was 6.2% and as late as 1959 Krayenbűhl reported an operative mortality of 8.4% [1]. This persistent high mortality led to increased interest in the use of radiotherapy for the treatment of pituitary Macro-adenomas, the symptoms of which were due to mass effects.

The other sorts of pituitary tumours were of course those presenting with a hormonal disturbance which are commonly excess production of growth hormone (GH) adedenocorticotrophic hormone (ACTH) or prolactin (PRL). GH excess is associated with gigantism rarely and more commonly acromegaly. ACTH excess is called Cushings disease or (CD) to distinguish it from the much commoner Cushing's syndrome which can be the result of drugs or adrenal disease. Hyperprolacti-naemia gives rise to amenorrhoea, galactorrhea and infertility in women and impotence in men. It is the commonest of the oversecretion syndromes. In general terms tumour volume is smallest with CD, largest with prolactinomas and interme-diate for acromegaly, though these are just rough guidelines.

J.C. Ganz, *Gamma Knife Neurosurgery*,
DOI 10.1007/978-3-7091-0343-2_17, © Springer-Verlag/Wien 2011

The modern surgery of pituitary adenomas derived from technical improvements in 3 areas. The introduction of the binocular internally illuminated operating microscope made all forms of microsurgery easier, whether the approach was from below or above. The introduction of radioimmunoassay for GH and ACTH in the late 1960s and PRL in 1971 made the assessment of endocrinopathies before and after surgery far more precise. Jules Hardy reintroduced transsphenoidal microsurgery revolutionised management and resulted in a much reduced morbidity and mortality. A useful subclassification was microadenoma for tumours with a diameter of 1 cm or less. Surgical results could be related to this size. Then in 1973 CT was introduced and around 10 years later MRI came into use enabling the surgeon to better plan what he could do before surgery and what he had done afterwards. In the following paragraphs the abbreviations will be used; non functioning adenoma (NFA) functioning adenoma (FA)

GKNS Reminiscences

The original Gamma Unit was as stated earlier in this book designed for use in functional diseases. By chance, referrals to neurosurgeons of these indications for a variety reasons decreased. The Gamma Unit was soon in use for the treatment of AVMs because of their visibility on available images in the late 1960s and early 1970s. The only tumours that could be located were those made visible on skull X-rays or cisternograms, in other words vestibular schwannomas and tumours of the pituitary region. ACTH producing tumours were chosen as suitable targets for the new method of GKNS and thus form the first group of tumours to be considered.

At the time in question the treatment of Cushing's Disease was fraught with difficulties. The tumour could not be seen. Adrenalectomy had been favoured with a mortality in one series of 16% and with a recurrence rate of 16.4% from a series of 116 patients treated at the Mayo Clinic [5]. Radiation therapy at the time carried a risk of around 50% hypopituitarism as of course would hypophysectomy [6]. Since ACTH producing tumours were known to be small and mostly limited to the pituitary fossa, they could be treated using the imaging technology of the day. Thus, Gamma Knife experience with the pituitary region began with Cushing's Disease. The dose used was 70–100 Gy to a maximum point, since it would have been impossible to outline a margin to map out for a particular isodose [7]. Treatment was mostly once but was repeated in some cases up to 4 times. It was possible to record a late follow up of 18 of the original 89 patients with a mean follow up of 17 years. None of the patients who had died in the intervening years had died as a result of the treatment. In this group of long term follow up patients there was normal corticosteroid function (measured by 24 h urine cortisol examinations) in 83% of patients. However, two thirds of the patients had varying degrees of hypopituitarism [8]. No damage to vision was noted. So this was the first use of GKNS with pituitary tumours.

Some General Principles

What follows is by necessity selective as there are many ways to treat pituitary adenomas and GKNS is only one of them and every attempt will be made to keep to this point.

Primary or Secondary Treatment Option

Today there is broad agreement that microsurgery is the primary treatment of pituitary tumours while GKNS is an adjunctive treatment [9–32]. There is also broad agreement that primary treatment may be considered when a patient for whatever reason is not fit enough to undergo surgery or in a few cases simply refuses an operation [33–38]. There remain papers where GKNS was chosen as the primary treatment. Most of these are reporting early material [7, 8, 39, 40] but a few represent the inevitable variability of medical opinion [41–44]. Tumours sitting in the cavernous sinus, with their relatively low location are poor targets for surgery but attractive targets for GKNS.

Comparison with Fractionated External Beam Radiotherapy

There is also a fair body of opinion that GKNS is superior to external beam conventional fractionated radiotherapy both in terms of endocrinopathy correction, tumour control, speed of result and number of complications [27, 31, 34, 35, 38, 45–51].

Visual Fields Complications

There is broad agreement that any radiation treatment for a pituitary adenoma should avoid damage to the visual pathways at all costs. This has been achieved in nearly every recorded series. In the few instances where visual field damage has occurred it has been permanent in two patients in a two papers where the tumours were large and required subsequent debulking [29, 52]. It is probable these patients are the same people reported in two different analyses from the same source. It has occurred in single patient in one paper where the dose was increased to achieve better control of CD [53]. This too is a paper published later with long term review of earlier work. There is a single report of a partial quadrantinopsia developing after treatment for CD but no information is given about the tumour volume, dose or prior treatments [19]. There is a single case of a deterioration of vision in the early days with less efficient dose planning software and imaging equipment than is currently available [54]. There is also a report of a single case of deterioration of visual field in a patient with acromegaly, but in this case the deterioration was due to continued tumour growth, not radiation damage.

The majority of papers which report visual field defects report none [1, 7, 8, 27, 33, 42, 55–61]. There are any number of papers suggesting the correct dose. However, many suffer defects of assessment of the dose or other technical problems. For further detail the reader is referred to the following references which permit a consistent and reproducible well functioning method for protecting the anterior visual pathway in the presence of pituitary adenomas [62–64].

Tumour Location

Tumours sitting in the cavernous sinus, with their relatively low location are poor targets for surgery but attractive targets for GKNS. The same may be said of recurrent or even residual tumour sitting in the base of an enlarged pituitary fossa, since recurrent surgery has a considerably lower chance of success than a primary operation. It is then attractive to consider the notion that the tumour may be killed rather than re-operated. The position of the visual pathway, especially downward descent of the chiasm into an empty sella must be taken into account when making decisions about treatment. With most NFAs this is not a problem but with FAs it can be.

Radiation Induced Hormone Deficiencies After GKNS

These are not uncommon and vary between 10 and 50% depending on pre-treatment function, tumour dose and tumour volume [7, 8, 11, 12, 19, 27, 28, 30, 32, 33, 36, 37, 41, 43, 47, 49, 53, 54, 58, 65–76]. While unwanted these are treatable conditions and may be a necessary price to pay for normalising hypersecretion of a particular enzyme.

Radiation Induced Carotid Ischaemia

In an early case treating a patient whose tumour was too large for conventional GKNS and with a high dose for an NFA post GKNS infarction in the territory of the carotid artery enclosed within the high dose region was reported [77]. It is only a single case but it suggests one should try to spare the carotids from over dosage and also to avoid too high a dose on patients with NFAs.

Prescription Dose

This parameter has varied widely between different series. As stated above it is the constant aim to avoid damage to the visual pathway and in general this aim is achieved in almost every case. There is a tendency for the dose to non functioning adenomas to be lower since here the only concern is control of growth. The mean/median doses in the literature range between 12 and 20 Gy [8, 26, 27, 29, 37, 49, 51, 52, 55, 67, 78].

The prescription dose for tumours associated with an endocrinopathy will tend to be higher since a higher dose is required to close down this over production, even in the presence of demonstrated tumour shrinkage [79]. The dose and volumes will be mentioned further under the individual tumours.

Variation in Reporting

The reporting of pituitary adenomas is not an easy topic to follow. There has been an evolving opinion about what does and does not constitute a measure of endocrine cure for all the patients with endocrinopathies. Moreover, within the individual endocrinopathies there are histological variations which have prognostic significance and to which more mention will be made in respect of acromegaly. There has also been a tendency with in the radiation therapy community to report a reduction in excess hormone production as a therapeutic success. Endocrinologists in this author's experience demand normalisation of an endocrinopathy to be the only true measure of success and the only certain measure that the hormone excess no longer poses a threat to the patient.

We shall now move on to the individual endocrinopathies.

Cushing's Disease

Aims of Treatment

The aims of treatment in Cushing's disease to normalise the increased secretion of adrenal corticosteroid hormones and where this is due to a pituitary adenoma this requires removal of the adenoma. Every effort is made to avoid the complications mentioned above. The mainstay of treatment is microsurgery but a fair number of cases are not cured by this means. The details of surgical management and its successes is outside the range of this book. It must be remembered that prior to the development of synthetic adrenal corticosteroids which permitted the operation of adrenalectomy, the mortality of untreated Cushing's disease over 5 years was 100% [80]. This is mentioned to underline the danger of this condition.

Figure 17.1 illustrates the problem with microadenomas producing an endocrinopathy. The figure shows the successful effect on tumour volume but the effect on the endocrinopathy was essentially nothing. After transsphenoidal surgery the patient was cured. This patient was one of a group of four whose course persuaded our group to stop using the Gamma Knife as a primary treatment modality. The success rate of GKNS is generally taken to mean the normalisation of 24 h urine

Fig. 17.1 This patient had
Cushing's disease due to a
visible right sided
microadenoma. This received
25 Gy to the margin. On the
left the stalk is dislocated to
the *left* and the adenoma can
be seen as a swelling. On the
right the stalk has
straightened and the adenoma
is barely visible. Nonetheless,
the urinary cortisol remained
markedly raised. The patient
was operated and her
Cushing's disease normalised

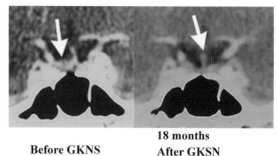

Before GKNS

**18 months
After GKSN
Prior to Microsurgery**

cortisol measurements. While ACTH can be measured in the serum it has, for
technical reasons proven to be a less reliable measure of therapeutic success. The
highest success rate is found in the material from Stockholm which has been
followed for the longest period. In 1986 the success rate was 76% [7] and in 2001
it was 83% [8]. The group in Prague also quoted a success rate of 85% [53] after
2 years follow up. This group like the Stockholm group used high doses. The
Charlottesville group reported 73% of patients with normal 24 h urine cortisol after
a mean latency of 16 months. Unfortunately, in this paper the specific dosimetry
and tumour volume is not recorded [19]. The majority of other reported papers
quote a success rate of between 40 and around 60% [10, 65, 75, 81–83]. It seems
reasonable to assume that the success rate increases with the passage of time and
bears a relationship with the dose used.

The major complication is increasing pituitary deficiencies which also increase
with the passage of time reaching over 60% in the paper with the longest follow up
[8]. The dose to aim for is 35 Gy to the tumour margin but this will not always be
achievable, depending on the tumour's size, location and relationship to the visual
pathways.

Acromegaly

The aim of treatment is again hormonal normalisation. This may be measured in
terms of serum GH level, serum IGF or the effects of the oral glucose tolerance test
in suppressing GH. The normal values are found in standard texts. This is because
the normal GH remains a subject of debate and IGF has to be age modified. Again, it
is emphasised that reduction in pathological elevation of a serum GH or IGF cannot

count as therapeutic success. For comparison with surgical series only normalisation of these values is acceptable. It may be helpful to remember that it can take 3–4 months for an IGF to normalise. As with Cushing's disease the mainstay of treatment is transsphenoidal microsurgery. GKNS has for the most part a secondary role. This was underlined for this author who treated a pair of identical twins with acromegaly. The one because of his heart condition could not tolerate microsurgery and was treated in the Gamma Knife. The other was treated with transsphenoidal microsurgery. The GKNS patient did not normalise his GH while the operated patient did.

The disease has been stated to shorten life by about 10 years [84]. The mortality is mainly related to the cardiovascular side effects and the secondary diabetes. The association of acromegaly with an increased incidence of neoplasia remains unconfirmed. Nonetheless, the documented shortening of life associated with the disease illustrates the importance of trying to correct the endocrinopathy.

The success rate following GKNS has varied between 19% [85] and 93% [44]. The success rate does seem to be dependent on dose, volume and duration of follow up. Two papers have artificially raised success rates. In one the rate of 93% is due to the use of a normal GH value far higher than is normally accepted. Another with a success rate of 65% after only 18 months is due to the same reason [86]. The low value of 19% [85] is due to the use of consistently low doses. The more usual normalisation values using internationally accepted measures of normal function vary between around 40 and 60% [17, 18, 21, 33, 36, 53, 58, 66]. Landolt et al. found normalisation in 67.7% of patients after a mean follow up of less than 2 years. However, again a rather high normal value of GH (<10 IU/ml) [87] was used. Landolt in another paper related improvement in control of GH excess secretion to stopping octreotide prior to treatment [88]. However, in another paper using the more generally accepted normal GH value of 2 mg/l and age adjusted IGF, octreotide use had no effect on the results [12]. In this paper 3 years after treatment, 25% of patients had normal hormonal values without further treatment and a further 23% of patients could normalise their endocrinopathy using octreotide, which had been impossible before GK treatment.

Even allowing for the variation in reporting of normalisation there is still a very wide variation in the success rates reported. Kobayashi et al. [85] and Castinetti et al. [12] achieved similar long term results where the mean dose in the Japanese material was 18.9 Gy and the range is not stated, while in the French material the range is 10–40 Gy but the mean is not stated. However, the French paper makes the important point that dose varies in relation to tumour location, volume and previous variability.

There is one other factor which will affect the results. It is known that acromegaly may arise from tumours with varied cellular morphology [89]. According to this paper [89] the prognosis of therapeutic success varies with the different cell types responsible for the excess secretion of GH. Thus, yet another variable should be added to those previously mentioned to provide a basis for understanding the variability of results in this condition. Only a large series systematically reporting previous radiation treatment in detail, tumour volume, tumour dose, length of follow up and histological subtype could provide an improved level of understanding. For practical reasons in the management of this uncommon tumour, it seems unlikely that such a paper will be written any time soon.

The major complication of GKNS in this disease was also hypopituitarism [11, 12, 19, 33, 36, 53, 66, 68, 71–73, 76]. The reported rates vary between 8 and 36%.

Prolactinomas

Prolactinomas are in general best treated with dopamine agonists, of which bromocriptine was the original but today its popularity has waned in favour of carbergoline which is better tolerated by most patients. They are the most frequently used medicaments to control prolactinomas at present. However, some patients tolerate medical treatment badly and they can reasonably be treated with radiosurgery. These are the commonest pituitary adenomas comprising at least 50%. While there are microadenomas common in women macroadenomas are also common equally distributed between women and men [90]. The larger tumours may invade the cavernous sinus where they may be followed though this is at best an uncertain procedure, because the region is necessarily difficult to visualize at operation and because of the importance of not damaging the nerves and vessels. Thus, it is the most likely place for residual tumour to be found, following surgery. In terms of danger, the smaller tumours threaten function rather than life, as compared with Cushing's disease and acromegaly. However, the functions concerned are hypogonadism in men and infertility in women which results in the patients being most eager to be cured. The risk to life with prolactinomas concerns the larger tumours and the few biologically aggressive variants.

Results with Microprolactinomas

It is the author's opinion that GKNS should only be offered to women with prolactinomas and infertility if they have been operated without success, cannot tolerate an effective dose of dopamine agonist and want to have a baby. The success rate in normalising hyperprolactinaemia with the GKNS is not that good, with one exception [53] where the success rate was 67%. This is a Czech paper but one assumes from the abstract and the doses quoted that the tumours treated were unusually small. Two papers report success in more than 40% of cases, but one is a series of only four patients and the other comes from a centre where the criteria of normality are not well defined. In general one can expect a success rate of 25–35% in terms of normalising PRL [74, 91–93]. In addition there is a possibility of hypopituitarism in [41, 71, 74]. Since FSH and LH are the hormones most likely to be affected by hypopituitarism this makes the use of GKNS something to use only with care and on smaller tumours where all other possibilities have run out.

There is further comment to be made here. Let us assume that a woman with prolactinoma really wants a baby and all other alternatives have been used up. Let us further assume that she cannot tolerate dopamine agonists at an effective dose. It is suggested that a very successful result of GKNS would not necessarily to normalise the PRL. It could be to reduce the PRL production sufficiently that the patient could thereafter tolerate an effective dose of dopamine agonist. The author has seen this in individual anecdotal cases lead to a successful pregnancy.

Having mentioned pregnancy, it is important to also mention the three possible effects of successful treatment of a prolactinoma irrespective of the technique. The easiest success to achieve is the normalisation of a raised PRL. The next easiest is the restoration of menstruation. The most difficult is a treatment resulting in the possibility of a pregnancy. The patient needs to be informed of this.

There is another aspect of the management of prolactinomas which bears mention. Based on a single article from a most distinguished author it has become widely believed that stopping dopamine agonists prior to treatment will increase the chance of therapeutic success. This is similar to the notion that ocretotide should be stopped prior to GKNS for acromegaly about which the ambivalent documentation has already been noted. With the greatest respect the author would wish to question this assumption which it can be stated with some certainty is known about amongst endocrinologists who themselves are not convinced of its validity. The reasons for doubting the argument are twofold. The table classifying results in respect of octreotide contains small numbers and no significances. The significance achieved using Kaplan Meier showed a significance of <0.03 but the use of Kaplan Meier with the small numbers and varied sub classes involved might be considered inappropriate. This article contains no reference to the effect of volume on the dose delivered but only on the dose to the median eminence. The current author has again an anecdotal case with a small tumour (ca. 4 cm^3) where the bromocriptine has not been prescribed. The PRL was more than 1,000 ng/ml. He was started on bromocriptine and 4 weeks later the tumour was 2.7 cm^3. It was possible to give him a full dose of 35 Gy. Over the next 12 months his PRL normalised and he was able do discontinue bromocriptine and retain a normal PRL. It would not have been possible to deliver such a high dose if the tumour volume had not been decreased with the dopamine agonist.

Macroadenomas

These will be mostly prolactinomas but 30% of macroadenomas are NFA [94]. Some of these tumours will also be producers of growth hormone. Many are located in the cavernous sinus or at the base of the sella turcica where they lie far away from the visual pathway, unless the chiasm has descended into an empty sella in which case special care will be required.

It is taken as indisputable that microsurgery is the treatment of choice. A macroadenoma with elevation of the visual pathway is not suitable for GKNS

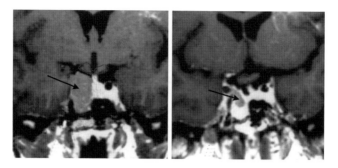

Fig. 17.2 The *black arrow* indicates the surgically inaccessible tumour component in the right cavernous sinus. Please note the visual pathway is outlined. The image on the left is prior GKNS but after surgery. The image on the right is 3 years after GKNS. Clear shrinkage has occurred following a dose of 12 Gy

even as a secondary treatment except in cases where further surgery is not possible. If the visual pathway is not visible of if the visual field exceeds a bitemporal hemianopsia then if surgical decompression is not possible it will be possible to deliver a higher effective radiation dose using external beam fractionated radiotherapy than can be achieved by GKNS. The required therapeutic prescription dose in this situation cannot be delivered without risking loss of vision. Since endocrinopathies require a higher dose than NFAs fractionated radiotherapy is even more clearly indicated for macroadenomas with the anatomical characteristics outlined above.

On the other hand for low lying tumours in the base of the pituitary fossa or in the cavernous sinus the Gamma Knife can be a very useful and effective alternative (Fig. 17.2). Tumour growth control may be achieved in 90–100% of cases using doses mainly between 16 and 20 Gy [8, 26, 27, 37, 38, 43, 47, 48, 52, 55, 57, 60, 67, 69, 78, 81, 95–98]. The current author has yet to see a macroadenoma grow in volume following treatment using a prescription dose of 12 Gy.

Thus, GKNS may be used for macroadenomas provided judgement common sense and an appreciation of the biology of the tumours, the limitations of the method are born in mind when assessing a given patient for treatment.

Nelson's Syndrome

Here again the Gamma Knife has been described as producing a reduction of serum ACTH in a proportion of patients. In Charlottesville the success rate was 14.3% with a 37% increase in hypopituitarism. Two patients died of progressive disease [19]. The quoted paper states that the usual margin dose was 15 Gy for a group of pituitary adenomas of all types without specifying what it was for the patients with Nelson's syndrome. Tumour volume is not mentioned in the paper. At the Mayo

Clinic 78% of the patients achieved growth control. Two large tumours were inadequately covered. No patient achieved a normal ACTH though the blood level fell in most. One patient died from progressive disease. All complications occurred in patients who had received prior radiotherapy. The mean tumour volume approximated to 2.4 cm^3. The median margin dose was 20 Gy. Median follow up was just over 3 years. In Bergen a group of ten patients were treated with a mean follow up of 7 years. ACTH fell in eight normalized in one and presumably was unchanged in one though this is not stated. No tumour grew further. The prescription dose was 25 Gy in seven patients 20 Gy in two and 12 Gy in one. The mean tumour volume was 1.076 cm^3 and the median volume was 0.81 cm^3. Four patients developed new hormone deficiencies while three patients could have their pretreatment hormone substitution stopped.

The results of these papers are consistent in recording a low frequency of normalisation of ACTH. However, the variation in growth control between the Mayo Clinic and Bergen results presumably is related to the larger tumour volume and related lower dose used at the Mayo Clinic. An increased requirement for hormone substitution was reported in all the papers. Thus, one must conclude that while GKNS is an efficient method for controlling the growth of small Nelson's tumours it is inefficient in correcting the hypersecretion of ACTH and is frequently associated with increases in hypopituitarism, particularly if the patient has received previous radiotherapy.

Craniopharyngiomas

Introduction

When considering GKNS and the management of craniopharyngiomas certain basic factors must be born in mind. To being with length of follow up is essential. Backlund documented the importance of long term follow up in a paper where the **minimum** follow up was 10 years [99]. The ability of these tumours to recur even after long periods is a major problem. Backlund was also a proponent of the use of multimodality treatment for these tumours. This is a view shared by a variety of authors [100–103].

Another feature that must be born in mind is that the tumours behave differently in adults and children with children having a worse prognosis [104, 105]. A considerable proportion of the tumours are cystic. In a recent paper 46% were predominantly cystic and 36% were mixed solid and cystic. Backlund's use of intracystic Yttrium-90 as part of a multimodality treatment was limited to patients where more than 50% of the tumour was cystic [99].

When considering a patient for GKNS for a craniopharyngioma and when assessing the literature two other factors must be born in mind, both anatomical. The first is tumour volume. In a very recent review on the surgical treatment of these tumours, the mean <u>diameter</u> (volume is not stated) is 4.1 cm. If the tumours were spherical this is equivalent to a <u>mean</u> volume of over 30 cm^3. The reader is asked to bear this size in mind. The second factor is the relationship to the visual pathway. While the relationship between this pathway and pituitary adenomas and/ or meningiomas is mostly visible or predictable, the situation with craniopharyngiomas is different. Firstly, if they have been operated and particularly if cyst fluid has leaked into the subarachnoid space the clear anatomy of the basal cisterns may be blurred by a reaction to the presence of the cyst fluid and clear definition of the anatomy is no longer possible. In addition the craniopharyngioma is THE tumour which has the ability to lie both above and below the visual pathway which places far greater limits on the ability to apply an adequate dose to the tumour margin than is the case with pituitary adenomas or meningiomas where the pathways are usually below or to one side. Moreover, with larger tumours where the visual pathway is obscured the location of the pathway is much less easy to guess because its relationship to craniopharyngiomas is less predictable than in the case of other tumours in this region.

Case Selection

It is clear from this Table 17.1 that the mean volume of these tumours is considerably smaller than the mean volume of the tumours being treated by surgery cited above [106]. It was this author's unpublished experience that while working in Cairo over a 6 year period, 94 patients with craniopharyngiomas were referred. Only 26 could be accepted for treatment mostly because the remainder were too large for treatment. It also be came clear as in the material from Stockholm that when a tumour increased in volume after GKNS it was always as a result of cyst enlargement [105]. This is in keeping with the experience of others quoted above that cystic tumours are more of a problem than solid tumours.

Table 17.1 Volumes of craniopharyngiomas in some of the major GKNS series [101, 103–105, 107–111]

Publication	Number patients	Mean tumour volume cm^3	Range tumour volume cm^3
Amendola et al. [2]	14	3.7	0.1–26.5
Barajas et al. [101]	10	4.5	0.67–14.2
Chung et al. [103]	31	9.0	0.3–28
Chung et al. [108]	21	9.0	0.3–28
Kobayashi et al. [104]	107	3.5	Not specified
Mokry [109]	23	7.0	0.5–32
Niranjan et al. [73]	46	1.0	0.07–8.0
Ulfarsson et al. [105]	21	7.8	0.4–33.0
Yomo et al. [111]	18	1.8	0.12–13.9

Table 17.2 The variation between different series but little clear relationship between dose and control and presumably the variable results reflect the variation in tumours from series to series as indicated above must be unavoidable

Publication	Growth control	Number patients	Mean dose
Yomo et al. [111]	94%	18	11.6
Niranjan et al. [73]	91.6%	46	13.0
Barajas et al. [101]	90%	10	14.0
Chung et al. [103]	87%	31	12.2
Kobayashi et al. [104]	79.6%	107	10.8
Mokry [109]	74%	23	10.8
Chiou et al. [102]	58.3	10	16.4
Amendola et al. [2]	100%	14	14.0

Results of Treatment

In addition in view of the prevalence of multimodality treatment the condition of the tumour and patient presenting in different series for GKNS as one of the modes of treatment will vary perhaps significantly from series to series. One thing is consistent and that is that GKNS is associated with a relative absence of deterioration of vision [100, 103, 104, 108, 110, 112]. Moreover, increased endocrine dysfunction was recorded in only one series which as noted above treated an unusually variable group of tumours [105]. The results in one particular retrospective series did not specify a mean prescription dose as there was such great variation from 3 to 25 Gy. This reflected the great variation in tumour volume as shown in the table above for Ulfarsson et al. However, the series did demonstrate tumour growth control was significantly related to a prescription dose of 6 Gy or more [105]. This series yet again documented that the tumour was more difficult with children. The overall growth control for the 19 patients was 36.4%. Recurrence occurred in 82% of children and 50% of adults. Failure to control growth was always associated with an increase in the volume of the cyst.

The results in terms of tumour control and dose are shown in Table 17.2.

Conclusion

It is hoped that the text above indicates that GKNS will be appropriate only for a minority of craniopharyngiomas and usually as part of a multimodality treatment. However, used sensibly and in particular in tumours with a well visualised optic pathway it has a role to play in the absence of radiotherapy. However, if the tumours are larger or the optic pathways are not well visualised fractionated external beam radiotherapy may well be the more sensible approach.

References

1. Landolt A. History of pituitary surgery. In: 'A History of Neurosurgery: in its Scientific and Professional Contexts', (ed), Greenblatt SD. AANS, Park Ridge, IL: pp 373–400; 1997
2. Takakura K, Hayashi M, Izawa M. Pituitary tumours. In: 'Principles and Practice of Stereotactic Radiosurgery', (eds), Chin LS, Regine WF. Heidelberg: Springer Verlag: pp 299–308; 2008
3. Horsley V. On the techniques of operations on the central nervous system. Br Med J **2**: 411–423; 1906
4. Northfield DWC. The Surgery of the Central Nervous System. Blackwell Scientific Publications, Oxford London: p 308; 1973
5. Northfield DWC. The Surgery of the Central Nervous System. Blackwell Scientific Publications, Oxford London, p 314; 1973
6. Liu JK, Fleseriu M, Delashaw JB Jr, Ciric IS, Couldwell WT. Treatment options for Cushing disease after unsuccessful transsphenoidal surgery. Neurosurg Focus **23(3)**: E8; 2007
7. Degerblad M, Rahn T, Bergstrand G, Thoren M. Long-term results of stereotactic radiosurgery to the pituitary gland in Cushing's disease. Acta Endocrinol (Copenh) **112(3)**: 310–314; 1986
8. Hoybye C, Grenback E, Rahn T, Degerblad M, Thoren M, Hulting AL. Adrenocorticotropic hormone-producing pituitary tumors: 12- to 22-year follow-up after treatment with stereotactic radiosurgery. Neurosurgery **49(2)**: 284–291; 2001
9. Andrews DW. Pituitary adenomas. Curr Opin Oncol **6(1)**: 53–59; 1994
10. Castinetti F, Nagai M, Dufour H, Kuhn JM, Morange I, Jaquet P, Conte-Devolx B, Régis J, Brue T. Gamma knife radiosurgery is a successful adjunctive treatment in Cushing's disease. Eur J Endocrinol **156(1)**: 91–98; 2007
11. Castinetti F, Nagai M, Morange I, Dufour H, Caron P, Chanson P, Cortet-Rudelli C, Kuhn JM, Conte-Devolx B, Régis J, Brue T. Long-term results of stereotactic radiosurgery in secretory pituitary adenomas. J Clin Endocrinol Metab **94(9)**: 3400–3407; 2009
12. Castinetti F, Taieb D, Kuhn JM, Chanson P, Tamura M, Jaquet P, Conte-Devolx B, Régis J, Dufour H, Brue T. Outcome of gamma knife radiosurgery in 82 patients with acromegaly: correlation with initial hypersecretion. J Clin Endocrinol Metab **90(8)**: 4483–4488; 2005
13. Clarke MJ, Erickson D, Castro MR, Atkinson JL. Thyroid-stimulating hormone pituitary adenomas. J Neurosurg **109(1)**: 17–22; 2008
14. Ganz JC. Gamma knife treatment. In: 'Pituitary Adenomas', (eds), Landolt AM, Vance ML, Reilly PL. New York, London: Churchill Livingstone: pp 461–474; 1996
15. Ganz JC. Gamma Knife treatment of pituitary adenomas. Stereotact Funct Neurosurg **64 (Suppl 1)**: 3–10; 1995
16. Ganz JC. Radiosurgery for pituitary adenomas. In: 'Stereotactic and Functional Neurosurgery', (eds), Gildenberg PL, Tasker RR. New York, Elsevier: pp 845–856; 1998
17. Gutt B, Wowra B, Alexandrov R, Uhl E, Schaaf L, Stalla GK, Schopohl J. Gamma-knife surgery is effective in normalising plasma insulin-like growth factor I in patients with acromegaly. Exp Clin Endocrinol Diabetes **113(4)**: 219–224; 2005
18. Iwai Y, Yamanaka K, Yoshioka K, Kanai M. Gamma knife radiosurgery for GH-secreting microadenoma with empty sella. J Clin Neurosci **11(4)**: 418–421; 2004
19. Jane JA Jr, Vance ML, Woodburn CJ, Laws ER Jr. Stereotactic radiosurgery for hypersecreting pituitary tumors: part of a multimodality approach. Neurosurg Focus **14(5)**: e12; 2003
20. Kanter AS, Diallo AO, Jane JA Jr, Sheehan JP, Asthagiri AR, Oskouian RJ, Okonkwo DO, Sansur CA, Vance ML, Rogol AD, Laws ER Jr. Single-center experience with pediatric Cushing's disease. J Neurosurg **103(5 Suppl)**: 413–420; 2005
21. Laws ER, Vance ML, Thapar K. Pituitary surgery for the management of acromegaly. Horm Res **53(Suppl 3)**: 71–75; 2000

22. Locatelli M, Vance ML, Laws ER. Clinical review: the strategy of immediate reoperation for transsphenoidal surgery for Cushing's disease. J Clin Endocrinol Metab **90(9)**: 5478–5482; 2005
23. Mahmoud-Ahmed AS, Suh JH, Mayberg MR. Gamma knife radiosurgery in the management of patients with acromegaly: a review. Pituitary **4(4)**: 223–230; 2001
24. Motti ED, Losa M, Pieralli S, Zecchinelli A, Longobardi B, Giugni E, Ventrella L. Stereotactic radiosurgery of pituitary adenomas. Metabolism **45(8 Suppl 1)**: 111–114; 1996
25. Park YG, Chang JW, Kim EY, Chung SS. Gamma knife surgery in pituitary microadenomas. Yonsei Med J **37(3)**: 165–173; 1996
26. Picozzi P, Losa M, Mortini P, Valle MA, Franzin A, Attuati L, Ferrari da Passano C, Giovanelli M. Radiosurgery and the prevention of regrowth of incompletely removed nonfunctioning pituitary adenomas. J Neurosurg **102(Suppl)**: 71–74; 2005
27. Pollock BE, Cochran J, Natt N, Brown PD, Erickson D, Link MJ, Garces YI, Foote RL, Stafford SL, Schomberg PJ. Gamma knife radiosurgery for patients with nonfunctioning pituitary adenomas: results from a 15-year experience. Int J Radiat Oncol Biol Phys **70(5)**: 1325–1329; 2008
28. Pollock BE, Young WF Jr. Stereotactic radiosurgery for patients with ACTH-producing pituitary adenomas after prior adrenalectomy. Int J Radiat Oncol Biol Phys **54(3)**: 839–841; 2002
29. Sheehan JP, Kondziolka D, Flickinger J, Lunsford LD. Radiosurgery for nonfunctioning pituitary adenoma. Neurosurg Focus **14(5)**: e9; 2003
30. Swords FM, Monson JP, Besser GM, Chew SL, Drake WM, Grossman AB, Plowman PN. Gamma knife radiosurgery: a safe and effective salvage treatment for pituitary tumours not controlled despite conventional radiotherapy. Eur J Endocrinol **161(6)**: 819–828; 2009
31. Tinnel BA, Henderson MA, Witt TC, Fakiris AJ, Worth RM, Des Rosiers PM, Edmondson JW, Timmerman RD, Lo SS. Endocrine response after gamma knife-based stereotactic radiosurgery for secretory pituitary adenoma. Stereotact Funct Neurosurg **86(5)**: 292–296; 2008
32. Vladyka V, Liscak R, Novotny JJr, Marek J, Jezkova J. Radiation tolerance of functioning pituitary tissue in gamma knife surgery for pituitary adenomas. Neurosurgery **52(2)**: 309–316; 2003
33. Attanasio R, Epaminonda P, Motti E, Giugni E, Ventrella L, Cozzi R, Farabola M, Loli P, Beck-Peccoz P, Arosio M. Gamma-knife radiosurgery in acromegaly: a 4-year follow-up study. J Clin Endocrinol Metab **88(7)**: 3105–3112; 2003
34. Jackson IM, Noren G. Role of gamma knife radiosurgery in acromegaly. Pituitary **2(1)**: 71–77; 1999
35. Jackson IM, Noren G. Role of gamma knife therapy in the management of pituitary tumors. Endocrinol Metab Clin North Am **28(1)**: 133–142; 1999
36. Jezkova J, Marek J, Hana V, Krsek M, Weiss V, Vladyka V, Lisak R, Vymazal J, Pecen L. Gamma knife radiosurgery for acromegaly – long-term experience. Clin Endocrinol (Oxf) **64 (5)**: 588–595; 2006
37. Mingione V, Yen CP, Vance ML, Steiner M, Sheehan J, Laws ER, Steiner L. Gamma surgery in the treatment of nonsecretory pituitary macroadenoma. J Neurosurg **104(6)**: 876–883; 2006
38. Sheehan JP, Niranjan A, Sheehan JM, Jane JA Jr, Laws ER, Kondziolka D, Flickinger J, Landolt AM, Loeffler JS, Lunsford LD. Stereotactic radiosurgery for pituitary adenomas: an intermediate review of its safety, efficacy, and role in the neurosurgical treatment armamentarium. J Neurosurg **102(4)**: 678–691; 2005
39. Kobayashi T, Kida Y, Mori Y. Gamma knife radiosurgery in the treatment of Cushing disease: long-term results. J Neurosurg **97(5 Suppl)**: 422–428; 2002
40. Vladyka V, Liscak R, Subrt O, Simonova G, Novotny J. Use of the radiosurgery knife in the treatment of hypophyseal adenomas. Cas Lek Cesk **134(17)**: 539–542; 1995

41. Ma ZM, Qiu B, Hou YH, Liu YS. Gamma knife treatment for pituitary prolactinomas. Zhong Nan Da Xue Xue Bao Yi Xue Ban **31(5)**: 714–716; 2006
42. Pan L, Zhang N, Wang EM, Wang BJ, Dai JZ, Cai PW. Gamma knife radiosurgery as a primary treatment for prolactinomas. J Neurosurg **93(Suppl 3)**: 10–13; 2000
43. Yuan YH, Dong XM, Yu HW, Guan JH, Wang CL. Gamma knife for hypersecreting pituitary adenom: analysis of 120 cases. Zhonghua Wai Ke Za Zhi **44(6)**: 416–419; 2006
44. Zhang N, Pan L, Wang EM, Dai JZ, Wang BJ, Cai PW. Radiosurgery for growth hormone-producing pituitary adenomas. J Neurosurg **93(Suppl 3)**: 6–9; 2000
45. Feigl GC, Bonelli CM, Berghold A, Mokry M. Effects of gamma knife radiosurgery of pituitary adenomas on pituitary function. J Neurosurg **97(5 Suppl)**: 415–421; 2002
46. Jackson IM, Noren G. Gamma knife radiosurgery for pituitary tumours. Baillieres Best Pract Res Clin Endocrinol Metab **13(3)**: 461–469; 1999
47. Kim M, Paeng S, Pyo S, Jeong Y, Lee S, Jung Y. Gamma knife surgery for invasive pituitary macroadenoma. J Neurosurg **105(Suppl)**: 26–30; 2006
48. Losa M, Valle M, Mortini P, Franzin A, da Passano CF, Cenzato M, Bianchi S, Picozzi P, Giovanelli M. Gamma knife surgery for treatment of residual nonfunctioning pituitary adenomas after surgical debulking. J Neurosurg **100(3)**: 438–444; 2004
49. Muacevic A, Uhl E, Wowra B. Gamma knife radiosurgery for nonfunctioning pituitary adenomas. Acta Neurochir Suppl **91**: 51–54; 2004
50. Thoren M, Hoybye C, Grenback E, Degerblad M, Rahn T, Hulting AL. The role of gamma knife radiosurgery in the management of pituitary adenomas. J Neurooncol **54(2)**: 197–203; 2001
51. Wowra B, Stummer W. Efficacy of gamma knife radiosurgery for nonfunctioning pituitary adenomas: a quantitative follow up with magnetic resonance imaging-based volumetric analysis. J Neurosurg **97(5 Suppl)**: 429–432; 2002
52. Sheehan JP, Kondziolka D, Flickinger J, Lunsford LD. Radiosurgery for residual or recurrent nonfunctioning pituitary adenoma. J Neurosurg **97(5 Suppl)**: 408–414; 2002
53. Vladyka V, Liscak R, Simonova G, Chytka T, Novotny J Jr, Vymazal J, Marek J, Hana V, Vavros D. Radiosurgical treatment of hypophyseal adenomas with the gamma knife: results in a group of 163 patients during a 5-year period. Cas Lek Cesk **139(24)**: 757–766; 2000
54. Lim YL, Leem W, Kim TS, Rhee BA, Kim GK. Four years' experiences in the treatment of pituitary adenomas with gamma knife radiosurgery. Stereotact Funct Neurosurg **70(Suppl 1)**: 95–109; 1998
55. Iwai Y, Yamanaka K, Yoshioka K Radiosurgery for nonfunctioning pituitary adenomas. Neurosurgery **56(4)**: 699–705; 2005
56. Mokry M, Ramschak-Schwarzer S, Simbrunner J, Ganz JC, Pendl G. A six year experience with the postoperative radiosurgical management of pituitary adenomas. Stereotact Funct Neurosurg **72(Suppl 1)**: 88–100; 1999
57. Petrovich Z, Yu C, Giannotta SL, Zee CS, Apuzzo ML. Gamma knife radiosurgery for pituitary adenoma: early results. Neurosurgery **53(1)**: 51–59; 2003
58. Ronchi CL, Attanasio R, Verrua E, Cozzi R, Ferrante E, Loli P, Montefusco L, Motti E, Ferrari DI, Giugni E, Beck-Peccoz P, Arosio M. Efficacy and tolerability of gamma knife radiosurgery in acromegaly: a 10-year follow-up study Clin Endocrinol (Oxf); 2009 [epub ahead of print]
59. Seo Y, Fukuoka S, Takanashi M, Sasaki T, Suematsu K, Nakamura J. Gamma knife surgery for Cushing's disease. Surg Neurol **43(2)**: 170–175l; 1995
60. Shin M, Kurita H, Sasaki T, Tago M, Morita A, Ueki K, Kirino T. Stereotactic radiosurgery for pituitary adenoma invading the cavernous sinus. J Neurosurg **93(Suppl 3)**: 2–5; 2000
61. Vik-Mo E, Oksnes M, Pedersen PH, Wentzel-Larsen T, Rodahl E, Thorsen F, Schreiner T, Aanderud S, Lund-Johansen M. Gamma knife sterotactic radiosurgery of Nelson syndrome Eur J Endocrinol **160(2)**: 143–148; 2009

62. Ganz JC, El Shehaby A, Reda WA, Abdelkarim K. Protection of the anterior visual pathways during gamma knife treatment of meningiomas. Br J Neurosurg **24(3)**: 248–258; 2010

63. Pollock BE. Stereotactic radiosurgery for intracranial meningiomas: indications and results. Neurosurg Focus **14(5)**: e4; 2003

64. Rowe JG, Walton L, Vaughan P, Malik I, Radatz M, Kemeny A. Radiosurgical planning of meningiomas: compromises with conformity. Stereotact Funct Neurosurg **82(4)**: 169–174; 2004

65. Jagannathan J, Sheehan JP, Pouratian N, Laws ER, Steiner L, Vance ML. Gamma Knife surgery for Cushing's disease. J Neurosurg **106**: 980–987; 2007

66. Jagannathan J, Sheehan JP, Pouratian N, Laws ER Jr, Steiner L, Vance ML. Gamma knife radiosurgery for acromegaly: outcomes after failed transsphenoidal surgery. Neurosurgery **62(6)**: 1262–1269; 2008

67. Liscak R, Vladyka V, Marek J, Simonova G, Vymazal J. Gamma knife radiosurgery for endocrine-inactive pituitary adenomas. Acta Neurochir **149**: 999–1006; 2007

68. Marek J, Malik J, Fendrych P. Initial experience of an endocrinologist with the treatment of hypophyseal adenomas with the Leksell gamma knife. Cas Lek Cesk **134(17)**: 543–546; 1995

69. Martinez R, Bravo G, Burzaco J, Rey G. Pituitary tumors and gamma knife surgery. Clinical experience with more than two years of follow-up. Stereotact Funct Neurosurg **70(Suppl 1)**: 110–118; 1998

70. Mauermann WJ, Sheehan JP, Chernavvsky DR, Laws ER, Steiner L, Vance ML. Gamma knife surgery for adrenocorticotropic hormone-producing pituitary adenomas after bilateral adrenalectomy. J Neurosurg **106**: 988–993; 2007

71. Pollock BE, Brown PD, Nippoldt TB, Young WF Jr. Pituitary tumor type affects the chance of biochemical remission after radiosurgery of hormone-secreting pituitary adenomas. Neurosurgery **62(6)**: 1271–1276; 2008

72. Pollock BE, Jacob JT, Brown PD, Nippoldt TB. Radiosurgery of growth hormone-producing pituitary adenomas: factors associated with biochemical remission. J Neurosurg **106**: 833–838; 2007

73. Pollock BE, Nippoldt TB, Stafford SL, Foote RL, Abboud CF. Results of stereotactic radiosurgery in patients with hormone-producing pituitary adenomas: factors associated with endocrine normalization. J Neurosurg **97(3)**: 525–530; 2002

74. Pouratian N, Sheehan J, Jagannathan J, Laws ER Jr, Steiner L, Vance ML. Gamma knife radiosurgery for medically and surgically refractory prolactinomas. Neurosurgery **59(2)**: 255–266; 2006

75. Sheehan JM, Vance ML, Sheehan JP, Ellegala DB, Laws ER Jr. Radiosurgery for Cushing's disease after failed transsphenoidal surgery. J Neurosurg **93(5)**: 738–742; 2000

76. Thoren M, Rahn T, Guo WY, Werner S. Stereotactic radiosurgery with the cobalt-60 gamma unit in the treatment of growth hormone-producing pituitary tumors. Neurosurgery **29(5)**: 663–668; 1991

77. Lim YJ, Leem W, Park JT, Kim TS, Rhee BA, Kim GK. Cerebral infarction with ICA occlusion after gamma knife radiosurgery for pituitary adenoma: a case report. Stereotact Funct Neurosurg **72(Suppl 1)**: 132–139; 1999

78. Iwai Y, Yamanaka K, Yoshioka K, Yoshimura M, Honda Y, Matsusaka Y, Komiyama M, Yasui T. The usefulness of adjuvant therapy using gamma knife radiosurgery for the recurrent or residual nonfunctioning pituitary adenomas. No Shinkei Geka **33(8)**: 777–783; 2005

79. Ganz JC, Aanerud S, Mørk S, Smieveoll A-I. Tumour volume reduction following gamma knife radiosurgery: the relationship between X-ray and histological findings. In: 'Advances in Radiosurgery', (eds), Lindquist C, KondziolkaD, Loeffler J. Vienna, New York: Springer Verlag: pp 39–42; 1994

80. Jeffcoate WF. Treating Cushing's disease. Br Med J **296**: 227–228; 1988

81. Choi JY, Chang JH, Chang JW, Ha Y, Park YG, Chung SS. Radiological and hormonal responses of functioning pituitary adenomas after gamma knife radiosurgery. Yonsei Med J **44(4)**: 602–607; 2003

82. Morange-Ramos I, Régis J, Dufour H, Andrieu JM, Grisoli F, Jaquet P, Peragut JC. Short-term endocrinological results after gamma knife surgery of pituitary adenomas. Stereotact Funct Neurosurg **70(Suppl 1)**: 127–138; 1998

83. Pouratian N, Prevedello DM, Jagannathan J, Lopes MB, Vance ML, Laws ER Jr. Outcomes and management of patients with Cushing's disease without pathological confirmation of tumor resection after transsphenoidal surgery. J Clin Endocrinol Metab **92(9)**: 3383–3388; 2007

84. Ayuk J, Sheppard MC. Does Acromegaly enhance mortality? Rev Endocr Metab Disord **9 (1)**: 33–39; 2008

85. Kobayashi T, Mori Y, Uchiyama Y, Kida Y, Fujitani S. Long-term results of gamma knife surgery for growth hormone-producing pituitary adenoma: is the disease difficult to cure? J Neurosurg **102(Suppl)**: 119–123; 2005

86. Wang MH, Liu P, Liu AL, Luo B, Sun SB. Efficacy of gamma knife radiosurgery in treatment of growth hormone-secreting pituitary adenoma. Zhonghua Yi Xue Za Zhi **83 (23)**: 2045–2048; 2003

87. Landolt AM, Haller D, Lomax N, Scheib S, Schubiger O, Siegfried J, Wellis G. Stereotactic radiosurgery for recurrent surgically treated acromegaly: comparison with fractionated radiotherapy. J Neurosurg **88(6)**: 1002–1008; 1998

88. Landolt AM, Haller D, Lomax N, Scheib S, Schubiger O, Siegfried J, Wellis G. Octreotide may act as a radioprotective agent in acromegaly. J Clin Endocrinol Metab **85(3)**: 1287–1289; 2000

89. Killinger D, Gonzales J, Horvath E, Kovacs K, Smyth H. Correlation between pre-operative testing and tumour morphology in acromegaly. In: 'Sandostatin in the Treatment of Acromegaly', (ed), Lamberts SWJ. Berlin, Heidelberg, New York: Springer Verlag: pp 9–16; 1988

90. von Werder K. Prolactinoma: clinical findings and endocrinology. In: 'Pituitary Adenomas', (eds), Landolt AM, Vance ML, Reilly PL. New York, London: Churchill Livingstone: pp 111–126; 1996

91. Jagannathan J, Yen CP, Pouratian N, Laws ER, Sheehan JP. Stereotactic radiosurgery for pituitary adenomas: a comprehensive review of indications, techniques and long-term results using the gamma knife. J Neurooncol **92(3)**: 345–356; 2009

92. Kim MS, Lee SI, Sim JH. Gamma knife radiosurgery for functioning pituitary microadenoma. Stereotact Funct Neurosurg **72(Suppl 1)**: 119–124; 1999

93. Kim SH, Huh R, Chang JW, Park YG, Chung SS. Gamma Knife radiosurgery for functioning pituitary adenomas. Stereotact Funct Neurosurg **72(Suppl 1)**: 101–110; 1999

94. Endocrine-inactive, FSH, LH and α-SU adenomas. In: 'Pituitary Adenomas', (eds), Landolt AM, Vance ML, Reilly PL. New York, London: Churchill Livingstone: pp 127–138; 1996

95. Hayashi M, Izawa M, Hiyama H, Nakamura S, Atsuchi S, Sato H, Nakaya K, Sasaki K, Ochiai T, Kubo O, Hori T, Takakura K. Gamma Knife radiosurgery for pituitary adenomas. Stereotact Funct Neurosurg **72(Suppl 1)**: 111–118; 1999

96. Izawa M, Hayashi M, Nakaya K, Satoh H, Ochiai T, Hori T, Takakura K. Gamma knife radiosurgery for pituitary adenomas. J Neurosurg **93(Suppl 3)**: 19–22; 2000

97. Qiu B, Ma ZM, Liu YS, Hou YH, Tang JB. Gamma knife treatment for pituitary adenomas. Zhong Nan Da Xue Xue Bao Yi Xue Ban **29(4)**: 463–466; 2004

98. Shin M. Gamma knife radiosurgery for pituitary adenoma. Biomed Pharmacother **56(Suppl)**: 1178s–1181s; 2002

99. Backlund EO. Colloidal radioisotopes as part of a multi-modality treatmentof craniopharyngiomas. J Neurosurg Sci **33(1)**: 95–97; 1989

100. Albright AL, Hadjipanayis CG, Lunsford LD, Kondziolka D, Pollack IF, Adelson PD. Individualized treatment of pediatric craniopharyngiomas. Childs Nerv Syst **21(8–9)**: 649–654; 2005

101. Barajas MA, Ramirez-Guzman G, Rodriguez-Vazquez C, Toledo-Buenrostro V, Velasquez-Santana H, del Robles RV, Cuevas-Solorzano A, Rodriguez-Hernandez G. Multimodal management of craniopharyngiomas: neuroendoscopy, microsurgery, and radiosurgery. J Neurosurg **97(5 Suppl)**: 607–609; 2002

102. Chiou SM, Lunsford LD, Niranjan A, Kondziolka D, Flickinger JC. Stereotactic radiosurgery of residual or recurrent craniopharyngioma, after surgery, with or without radiation therapy. Neuro Oncol **3(3)**: 159–166; 2001

103. Chung WY, Pan DH, Shiau CY, Guo WY, Wang LW. Gamma knife radiosurgery for craniopharyngiomas. J Neurosurg **93(Suppl 3)**: 47–56; 2000

104. Kobayashi T, Kida Y, Mori Y, Hasegawa T. Long-term results of gamma knife surgery for the treatment of craniopharyngioma in 98 consecutive cases. J Neurosurg **103(6 Suppl)**: 482–488; 2005

105. Ulfarsson E, Lindquist C, Roberts M, Rahn T, Lindquist M, Thoren M, Lippitz B. Gamma knife radiosurgery for craniopharyngiomas: long-term results in the first Swedish patients. J Neurosurg **97(5 Suppl)**: 613–622; 2002

106. Elliott RE, Hsieh K, Hochman T, Belitskaya-Levy I, Wisoff J, Wisoff JH. Efficacy and safety of radical resection of primary and recurrent craniopharyngiomas in 86 children. J Neurosurg Pediatr **5(1)**: 30–48; 2010

107. Amendola BE, Wolf A, Coy SR, Amendola MA. Role of radiosurgery in craniopharyngiomas: a preliminary report. Med Pediatr Oncol **41(2)**: 123–127; 2003

108. Chung WY, Pan HC, Guo WY, Shiau CY, Wang LW, Wu HM, Lee LS. Protection of visual pathway in gamma knife radiosurgery for craniopharyngiomas. Stereotact Funct Neurosurg **70(Suppl 1)**: 139–151; 1998

109. Mokry M. Craniopharyngiomas: a six year experience with gamma knife radiosurgery. Stereotact Funct Neurosurg **72(Suppl 1)**: 140–149; 1999

110. Niranjan A, Kano H, Mathieu D, Kondziolka D, Flickinger JC, Lunsford LD. Radiosurgery for Craniopharyngioma Int J Radiat Oncol Biol Phys **78(1)**:64–71; 2010

111. Yomo S, Hayashi M, Chernov M, Tamura N, Izawa M, Okada Y, Hori T, Iseki H. Stereotactic radiosurgery of residual or recurrent craniopharyngioma: new treatment concept using Leksell gamma knife model C with automatic positioning system. Stereotact Funct Neurosurg **87(6)**: 360–367; 2009

112. Kobayashi T, Tanaka T, Kida Y. Stereotactic gamma radiosurgery of craniopharyngiomas. Pediatr Neurosurg **21(Suppl 1)**: 69–74; 1994

Chapter 18
Less Common Skull Base Tumours

Introduction

There are a number of different tumour types which are rare and where it has taken time to accumulate information about the results of treatment. There are also tumours sufficiently rare or considered sufficiently inappropriate for GKNS that only case reports exist. A list of diagnoses where information is limited to case reports is given at the end of the chapter.

Benign Skull Base Tumours

Non-vestibular Schwannomas

These are very rare accounting for 0.5% of all intracranial tumours or less.

Trigeminal Schwannoma

This is the non vestibular schwannoma about which most has been written [1–9]. In these papers mean/median follow up varies between 40 and 72 months. There is a total of 276 patients reported with series varying between 15 and 58 with a mean of around 30 patients per series. Thus, today there is a reasonable amount of information on which to base management and patient information. Growth control was between 90 and 100% in all but two papers, both of which are recent. In the one paper the follow up used volumetric analysis which is associated with greater accuracy and tumour volume increase was registered in three patients [8]. In one increasing trigeminal symptoms led to surgery. In the other two the increase in volume was only slight and continued observation has shown stability. Thus, basically only 1 of 26 patients was not adequately controlled, although there was a case of out of field new tumour which required a retreatment and the tumour was

J.C. Ganz, *Gamma Knife Neurosurgery*,
DOI 10.1007/978-3-7091-0343-2_18, © Springer-Verlag/Wien 2011

then controlled. In the other paper where tumour control was less than 90% [1] the authors describe GKNS failure in five patients. In two of these the failure was due to persistent pain associated with radiation induced oedema. They were operated. In the other three failed cases, the tumour volume increased because of inadequate tumour cover with the prescription dose. If the two inadequately covered tumours are excluded then in this series the 10% actuarial control was 91%. Overall the reasons for loss of control were mainly a malignant tumour [3, 5] or inadequate tumour cover [1, 5]. In one patient a tumour cyst developed after treatment [5]. This is a rare but known complication from other schwannomas.

The mean prescription doses used varied between 13 and 16 Gy. In all but two papers the mean tumour volume varied between 3.5 cm^3 and 4.6 cm^3. The two papers [3, 5] where the mean volumes were 10 cm^3 and 8.7 cm^3 were the two papers reporting altogether three patients where tumour cover with the prescription dose was inadequate. Since it is possible with the current editions of the dose-planning software to perform pre-treatment dose plans, it is suggested that this should be done more often in borderline cases.

Clinical improvement is recorded in between 30 and 65% of patients in the various papers. The major symptoms concerned are either ophthalmoplegias or more commonly symptoms related to the trigeminal nerve. By far the commonest complication is increasing trigeminal numbness [1, 3–5, 7, 8]. The frequency of this complication varies between 0 and 17%. There is no clear cut reason for the variation in this finding. The second most common complication is worsening facial pain which may require surgery [1, 8].

GKNS has been used as both a primary treatment and as an adjunct to surgery. Kano et al. [3] found a worse result if the tumour was >8 cm^3 and Hasegawa et al. [1] found a worse result for tumours with a volume more than 15 cm^3. Kano et al. recommend GKNS for tumours of 8 cm^3 or less and Hasegawa et al. recommend surgery first for tumours with a volume greater than 15 cm^3.

It is worth noting that Pollock et al. from the Mayo Clinic pointed out an advantage of GKNS as a primary procedure compared with microsurgery, even though trigeminal numbness increased in 33% of their ten patients [10]. Even though this is a high figure for radiosurgery it is much lower than the complication rate in two papers on microsurgery from two of the worlds most respected neurosurgeons [11, 12]. Pollock noted that 32 of 50 patients treated surgically in the two relevant papers would have been suitable for radiosurgery.

Jugular Foramen Schwannoma

The following remarks are based on a recent review [13]. Due to the rarity of the condition – these tumours account for 3–4% of all intracranial nerve sheath tumours – the only way to review a larger number of these tumours is via a metanalysis of published papers which was done in 2008. One hundred and ninety nine published patients were reviewed. They account for 10–30% of all tumours at the jugular foramen. In this review paper 159 tumours were totally removed, almost total removal was achieved in 6, subtotal removal in 18. In 14 patients the tumour recurred unexpectedly after apparent total removal. The commonest complication was lower cranial nerve morbidity (18.6%) and this was a complication which could be life threatening. There was also a danger to facial nerve function of 13%. In the paper from the Mayo Clinic mentioned earlier Pollock et al. point out the same problem. In one surgical series of 16 patients there was a 19% risk of facial palsy and 6% risk of lower cranial nerve palsy [14]. In another series of 19 patients the risk of facial palsy was 21% and of lower cranial nerve palsies 42% [15]. Pollock assesses that in the first series 63% of the patients could have been treated with GKNS and in the second 84%. In his own series of ten patients treated with GKNS with a mean follow up of 43 months the tumour control rate was 100% and there were no complications of any kind. The dose used was 16 Gy in view of a presumed lower radio-responsiveness.

In three major publications on this topic the results have been as follows. From Pittsburgh in 1999 a series of 17 patients were treated with GKNS [16]. Sixteen of the tumours were controlled. One continued to grow and required microsurgery. Thirteen of these patients had undergone microsurgery and already had substantial cranial nerve defects. Apart from the one failure none of the other 16 GKNS patients suffered any neurological deficit and 35% experienced a clinical improvement. In a second series from Shanghai there were 25 patients of whom 12 had undergone prior surgery [17]. The tumour control rate was 100%. There were no clinical deteriorations. Sixty four per cent of the patients experienced a clinical improvement. The mean dose used was 14.6 Gy and the mean tumour volume was 13.5 cm^3 (range 4.5–35.7 cm^3). The final and most recent series is again from Pittsburgh [18]. This time 35 patients are considered and the mean dose was 14 Gy. This paper focuses on the development of cranial nerve dysfunction after GKNS. Twenty two of these patients had undergone prior microsurgery. There was no definite progressive growth of any tumour. However, there was a temporary increase in volume in four tumours which ultimately regressed. One patient had deterioration of glossopharyngeal and vagus function. There was evidence for increased tumour volume. There was also evidence of central tumour necrosis, so this could have been a radiation induced tumour swelling. There was one out of field recurrence which was treated successfully with a second GKNS. Overall there was improvement in cranial nerve function in 22% of patients and in 47% of patients where GKNS was the sole treatment. The authors suggest that GKNS could be used more as a primary treatment and still remains an excellent second stage treatment for non radical treatment. There seems little question that GKNS is superior to microsurgery in terms of avoiding lower potentially dangerous lower cranial nerve deficits.

Facial Schwannoma

These are also very rare having an incidence of 1.9% of all intracranial schwanno-mas according to one paper from Komaki City in Japan [19]. According to another paper from Pittsburgh they account for 0.15–0.8% of all intracranial tumours [20]. These two papers together report 20 patients while a further 11 are reported from the Marseille group [21]. In all cases the mean prescription dose was 12–13 Gy. The volumes of the tumours varied somewhat between the groups. The mean volume of the Marseille group tumours was 888 mm [22]. On the other hand the mean volume of the Japanese tumours was 5.5 cm^3. The mean volume for the Pittsburgh group was 1.8 cm^3. These tumours may be found in the middle cranial fossa, the cerebellopontine angle, the internal auditory meatus and the geniculate ganglion or combinations of these locations depending on tumour size.

There was one case with deterioration of facial function in the Japanese paper from House-Brackman Grade I to Grade III. It was odd because it occurred one day after radiosurgery. The volume of the tumour is not mentioned but it is tempting to surmise that the larger volume of the tumours in this material may have contributed to the deterioration of facial function. Nonetheless, to explain the deterioration on the basis of radiation damage when it occurred the day after treatment is most unusual.

In the papers from Japan and Pittsburgh 50% of the patients had received prior microsurgery. In the paper from Marseille only 2 of 11 had been operated. The diagnosis in the remainder rested on invasion of the geniculate ganglion or some other portion of the intra-petrous portion of the facial nerve with or without a spontaneous facial paresis. In all the three patients the growth of all the tumours was controlled by GKNS except for one of the French patients whose tumour developed a cyst which required microsurgery.

The results recorded in these papers make a powerful case for using GKNS as the primary treatment of these rare tumours on account of the very low risk for deterioration of facial function after treatment.

Schwannomas of the Nerves Controlling Ocular Movement

There is a single paper on this topic [23]. There were eight tumours. All were controlled by treatment with a mean prescription dose of 12.5 Gy given to tumours with a mean volume of 1.32 cm^3. There were no clinical complications of treatment. There was clinical improvement in the five patients with a trochlear nerve tumor. There was no improvement in the eye movements controlled by three tumours innervated either by the oculomotor or abducent nerves.

Glomus Jugulare Tumor

This tumour particularly if there is an intracranial extension represents a great surgical challenge [24]. The need for resection of lower cranial nerves during surgery is well document in two extensive reviews [25, 26]. Kemeny in a recent editorial covering the current literature makes a convincing argument for the increasing use of GKNS as a primary treatment [24], not least because of the lack of damage to lower cranial nerves that are the inevitable concomitant of microsurgery, even in the most skilled hands. Such damage is unavoidable with a Fisch type D tumour and carries a heavy morbidity and significant mortality. Kemeny specifies that for the time being the treatment should be limited to tumours of up to 3 cm mean diameter; equivalent to 14–15 cm^3.

The majority of reports record tumour control in 100% of patients within a mean follow up of 35 months [27–43]. Tumour shrinkage was registered between 11.1% and 57% of patients [28, 29, 31, 32, 34, 36, 37, 39, 40, 42, 44]. The reports cover 335 patients. In three papers a proportion of tumours increased in volume. The Cleveland Clinic reported on a series of 17 patients with a mean follow up of 4 years. This is the series with the largest number of tumours which increased in volume after treatment [45]. There was a transient increase in volume in seven patients. At the most recent MR there was an increase in volume in four patients. None of the volume increases were great and so far no further measures have been required as there is no correlation between the MR changes and the patients' clinical condition. Two patients experienced deterioration. In both there was persistent hearing loss and in one the development of vertigo. In the first of these patients there was a transient volume increase which then decreased but was still larger than the pre treatment volume (3.7 cm^3 as opposed to 2.0 cm^3). This patient was 85 years old. In the second the tumour shrank by 50%. The hearing loss deteriorated on the 5th day after treatment and the maximum dose to the internal auditory meatus has been 3.5 Gy. It is unusual that this dose should cause hearing loss and it is also unusual that radiation damage, particularly at such a low dose should occur so quickly. The sensitivity to volume increases in this material may well reflect that unlike most series MRI volumetric methods were used to calculate volumes. This is known to be a more sensitive and accurate way of measuring volumes. The second report of post treatment tumour volume increase concerned a 55-year-old male with a left sided tumour with a volume of 98.4 cm^3. The tumour received 15 Gy to the margin and the volume increased to 117.4 cm^3. The patient had undergone four microsurgical procedures prior to the GKNS. This would appear to be an unsuitable tumour for GKNS on grounds of volume and its course suggests an aggressive variant [46]. The third paper reporting growth after treatment was retreated with subsequent control of the tumour [44].

In every GKNS reported series a proportion of the cases have been treated with prior surgery. Usually the percentage of operated cases varies between one and two thirds of all cases. Complications of GKNS were few and certainly not of the order reported in surgical series [24–26]. One case where clinical deterioration was associated with the uncontrolled growth of a large aggressive tumour was mentioned above [46]. However, while complications are uncommon they more usually occur without any relationship to tumour control [34, 36, 37, 39]. Thus in four series including 127 patients deterioration or loss of hearing was reported in 11 patients. Two patients suffered respectively a House-Brackman grade II and grade IV facial palsy respectively [37]. One case of vertigo and ataxia was reported in two papers with a total number of cases of 94 [37, 39]. Finally, in a paper from the Mayo Clinic single cases of dysphonia and facial numbness were reported out of a total number of 42 patients [39]. This same paper also made the point that there was deterioration of hearing in 4 cases and that this could well be the consequence of radiation damage to the cochlea or other intratemporal structures rather than to the intracranial components of the auditory pathway. In another more recent paper one patient with hearing deterioration the loss was from normal to Gardener Robertson 2. The other patient in the same paper who showed a hearing deterioration deteriorated from to Gardner Robertson grade 2 to grade 3. Thus, it may be fairly claimed that the treatment produces few complications.

In one recent report, only 3/14 patients had prior surgery. Moreover 10 of the 14 cases had tumours with a volume from 9.8 to 28.4 cm^3. In consequence the mean prescription dose and median prescription doses were 14.2 and 13.9 respectively which is on the low side for these tumours. Most, users prefer a mean/median dose of around 15 Gy [27–39, 41–46]. However, in the paper under advisement [33] 12 patients had degrees of symptomatic recovery with improvement of dysphagia in five, dysphonia in four, facial numbness in three, ataxia in three and tinnitus in two. Individual patients have experienced improvement in vomiting, vertigo, tongue fasciculation, hearing, headache, facial palsy and accessory paresis. The symptomatic improvement frequently occurred prior to any sign in tumour shrinkage, in keeping with the findings of others [31, 32, 35, 44]. It was proposed that clinical improvement may be a more sensitive indicator of tumour control than changes on the images. The mean follow up period was 28 months (range 6–60 months). This is too short and the final word on tumour control remains to be seen, but it is a promising beginning. If this benefit can be maintained it gains extra value from the fact that all but one of the tumours in this series were Fisch Grade D. These are the tumours with the greatest degree of risk for damage to lower cranial nerves and subtotal removal [25, 26]. In other series a majority of Fisch Grade D tumours have been recorded [33, 34, 43].

Despite this early success, the low dose to relatively large volume tumours could be a source of concern to some colleagues. The majority of papers have controlled the tumours with a somewhat higher dose and to largely smaller tumours. However, a novel approach to this dilemma has been proposed from a group based in Cleveland [38, 43]. They suggest the very sensible solution of removing the middle ear and intramastoid components of the tumour through the canal or a retroauricular approach. This was done as an out-patient same day procedure on five patients. None suffered any facial palsy and no hearing loss. Indeed in some patients a conductive hearing loss improved. No attempt was made to approach the jugular bulb. Then 1 month later the remaining tumour was treated with GKNS. The mean remaining tumour volume was 4.14 cm^3. A dose of 15 Gy was delivered to all the tumours. There was no neurological deficit. At 12 months there has been no tumour growth. This is of course too short a period to determine the final value of this treatment algorithm. Nonetheless, it is in keeping with the guiding principle of this author that the treatment is based on the use of multiple techniques planned harmoniously prior to the treatment of the patient. There is the added advantage that histology of the tumour is made available.

There are two more clinical issues that must be addressed before we leave glomus jugulare tumours. The glomus jugulare tumour may be associated with a mutation of the SDHB gene. If this is the case the chances are that the tumour will be much more likely to be malignant. A genetic analysis prior to treatment is thus advisable. The second issue is the basis of diagnosis in the event that GKNS is used as a primary treatment. Radiological diagnosis is based on computed tomographic and magnetic resonance imaging (MRI; T1-weighted sequence with or without contrast) findings of soft tissue mass in (or arising from) the jugular foramen and causing irregular lytic bony destruction without sclerosis that intensely enhances with contrast. In addition there should be an intense tumor blush and an enlarged ascending pharyngeal artery on carotid and vertebral angiograms.

Finally, there is a speculation. Until the introduction of the Gamma Knife "Perfexion" the portion of glomus jugulare tumours which extended into the neck below the skull were largely inaccessible for GKNS. The new machine should permit the treatment of this extension in many cases, though it will take time to acquire material to support this notion because of the rarity of the tumour. Nonetheless, this is an exciting new possibility in the treatment of these very challenging lesions.

Malignant Skull Base Tumours

Adenoid Cystic Carcinoma

Theodor Billroth, pioneer of abdominal surgery, performing musician and a personal friend of Brahms first coined the term cylindroma for the tumour that is now known as an adenoid cystic carcinoma. It can arise from a variety of locations, including the mouth, the salivary glands and the paranasal sinuses. These locations can be associated with skull base invasion. The tumours also have an unpleasant ability to metastasise and to invade nerves. This makes definitive control difficult and can result in severe pain.

The location and local spread can make radical surgical excision difficult or impossible. The standard therapy is an attempt at radical excision followed by radiotherapy. Various types of radiotherapy have been tried including neutron radiotherapy which is more densely ionising than conventional radiotherapy and produces greater amounts of double strand DNA breaks.

The role of GKNS is clearly limited. To date there is information about its use as an adjunctive treatment when all conventional treatments have failed to control skull base tumour extensions [22, 47, 48]. The prescription doses used varied between 12 Gy up to 20 Gy. The mean volumes treated varied between 12 and 15 cm^3. Obviously the doses were adjusted according to tumour volume and local structure at risk. GKNS is never likely to have a primary role in the treatment of the tumour but has shown itself to be useful in extending the survival of patients who have run out of therapeutic options. It has also been recorded to improve symptoms [22].

Chondrosarcomas and Chordomas

These rare skull base tumours are difficult to manage. The chordoma is histologically benign but behaves aggressively and the chondrosarcoma, despite its name seems to behave less aggressively [49–52]. Their location and diffuse growth makes radical microsurgical removal virtually impossible. Thus, treatment has been multimodal usually with an attempt at radical surgery followed by some form of radiation treatment [1, 6, 49–58]. As the tumours are fairly resistant to conventional fractionated radiotherapy other methods have been used including proton treatment [49, 52, 53, 57, 58]. However, proton treatment is cited as being associated with a relatively high rate of radiation induced toxic complications [52, 53, 57]. It is thus logical to attempt GKNS as a treatment for these lesions following surgery. Figure 18.1 illustrates just such an unpleasant tumour.

For chondrosarcomas satisfactory control of low grade tumours has been recorded [49, 51, 52, 54, 55]. Useful but often less effective control can also be achieved for chordomas [49, 53–55, 58]. Doses have varied between 12 and 20 Gy. Repeat treatment has been necessary in some cases. This was the case with the patient illustrated in Fig. 18.2. It is generally agreed that GKNS represents a useful adjunctive treatment for these unpleasant tumours and that the method is associated with an acceptably low toxicity. However, the rarity of the diseases, and the relatively few reported cases makes more precise assessment of the application

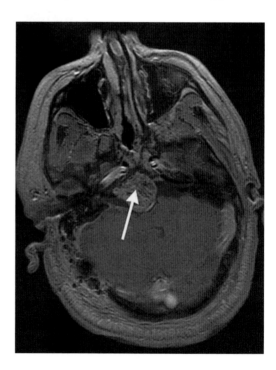

Fig. 18.1 This histologically confirmed chordoma with a volume of 9.4 cm^3 received 18 Gy. The tumour shrank for a year and the patient was better. Thereafter there was rapid uncontrollable growth

Fig. 18.2 This 5.4 cm^3 chondrosarcoma received 12 Gy and was controlled for 4 years. Her presenting headache improved but her ptosis was unchanged. At 4 years she developed a later rectus palsy and the tumour was now 15.3 cm^3. This received 16 Gy. The diplopia resolved and the tumour shrank and was in fine from 6 years after the first treatment

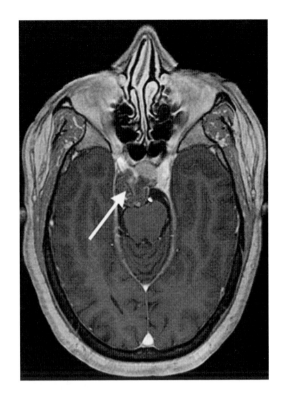

and the optimal technique and timing impossible to determine at the present time. Existing recommendations are few but one paper recommends GKNS for small tumours [57], one suggests up to 20 cm^3 and one up to 30 cm^3.

Neuroblastoma

Esthesioneuroblastomas (olfactory neuroblastomas) despite improvements in neurosurgical technique are rare tumours associated with a high recurrence rate and mortality. There have been only a few papers on the topic and all of them from the department of neurosurgery in Karl Franzens University in Graz, Austria. This short resume is based on their most recent paper. This records the multi-modality treatment of these lesions. The first step is endoscopic sinus surgery. This is followed by GKNS. The prescription doses have varied between 15 and 34 Gy. The tumour volumes have 0.9–22 cm^3. With a mean follow up of 58 months (range 13–128 months), tumour control has been achieved within the treated area in all tumours. It is suggested that this is a promising treatment design for these tumours which merits further assessment.

List of Diagnoses Limited to Case Reports

There are a number of tumours that have been treated using GKNS. However, the reporting is limited to case reports so that it is not possible to comment on principles of treatment. The various conditions concerned are listed below.

Angiofibroma
Carcinoma Hard Palate
Chondroblastoma
Endolymphatic Sac Tumors
Epitheliod Hemangioblastoma
Fibrosarcoma
Hypoglossal Schwannoma
Nasopharyngeal Carcinoma
Spindle Cell Sarcoma
Squamous Cell Carcinoma CPA

References

1. Hasegawa T, Ishii D, Kida Y, Yoshimoto M, Koike J, Iizuka H. Gamma knife surgery for skull base chordomas and chondrosarcomas. J Neurosurg 107: 752–757; 2007
2. Huang CF, Kondziolka D, Flickinger JC, Lunsford LD. Stereotactic radiosurgery for trigeminal schwannomas. Neurosurgery 45(1): 11–16; 1999
3. Kano H, Niranjan A, Kondziolka D, Flickinger JC, Dade LL. Stereotactic radiosurgery for trigeminal schwannoma: tumor control and functional preservation clinical article. J Neurosurg 110(3): 553–558; 2009
4. Nettel B, Niranjan A, Martin JJ, Koebbe CJ, Kondziolka D, Flickinger JC, Lunsford LD. Gamma knife radiosurgery for trigeminal schwannomas. Surg Neurol 62(5): 435–444; 2004
5. Pan L, Wang EM, Zhang N, Zhou LF, Wang BJ, Dong YF, Dai JZ, Cai PW. Long-term results of Leksell gamma knife surgery for trigeminal schwannomas. J Neurosurg 102(Suppl): 220–224; 2005
6. Peker S, Bayrakli F, Kilic T, Pamir MN. Gamma-knife radiosurgery in the treatment of trigeminal schwannomas. Acta Neurochir 149: 1133–1137; 2007
7. Phi JH, Paek SH, Chung HT, Jeong SS, Park CK, Jung HW, Kim DG. Gamma knife surgery and trigeminal schwannoma: is it possible to preserve cranial nerve function? J Neurosurg 107(4): 727–732; 2007
8. Sheehan J, Kondziolka D, Flickinger J, Lunsford LD. Gamma knife surgery for glomus jugulare tumors: an intermediate report on efficacy and safety. J Neurosurg 102(Suppl): 241–246; 2005
9. Sun S, Liu A, Wang C, Luo B, Wang M. Clinical analysis of gamma knife surgery for trigeminal schwannomas. J Neurosurg 105(Suppl): 144–148; 2006
10. Pollock BE. Stereotactic radiosurgery in patients with glomus jugulare tumors. Neurosurg Focus 17(2): E10; 2004
11. Day JD, Fukushima T. The surgical management of trigeminal neuromas. Neurosurgery 42(2): 233–240; 1998
12. Samii M, Babu RP, Tatagiba M, Sepehrnia A. Surgical treatment of jugular foramen schwannomas. J Neurosurg 82: 924–932; 1995

13. Bakar B. The jugular foramen schwannomas: review of the large surgical series. J Korean Neurosurg Soc **44(5)**: 285–294; 2008
14. Samii M, Migliori MM, Tatagiba M, Babu R. Surgical treatment of trigeminal schwannomas. J Neurosurg **82(5)**: 711–718; 1995
15. Mazzoni A, Sanna M, Saleh E, Achilli V. Lower cranial nerve schwannomas involving the jugular foramen. Ann Otol Rhinol Laryngol **106**: 370–379; 1997
16. Muthukumar N, Kondziolka D, Lunsford LD, Flickinger JC. Stereotactic radiosurgery for jugular foramen schwannomas. Surg Neurol **52(2)**: 172–179; 1999
17. Zhang N, Pan L, Dai JZ, Wang BJ, Wang EM, Cai PW. Gamma knife radiosurgery for jugular foramen schwannomas. J Neurosurg **97(5 Suppl)**: 456–458; 2002
18. Martin JJ, Kondziolka D, Flickinger JC, Mathieu D, Niranjan A, Lunsford LD. Cranial nerve preservation and outcomes after stereotactic radiosurgery for jugular foramen schwannomas. Neurosurgery **61**: 76–81; 2007
19. Kida Y, Yoshimoto M, Hasegawa T. Radiosurgery for facial schwannoma. J Neurosurg **106(1)**: 24–29; 2007
20. Madhok R, Kondziolka D, Flickinger JC, Lunsford LD. Gamma knife radiosurgery for facial schwannomas. Neurosurgery **64(6)**: 1102–1105; 2009
21. Litre CF, Gourg GP, Tamura M, Mdarhri D, Touzani A, Roche PH, Régis J. Gamma knife surgery for facial nerve schwannomas. Neurosurgery **60(5)**: 853–859; 2007
22. Miller JP, Semaan M, Einstein D, Megerian CA, Maciunas RJ. Staged gamma knife radiosurgery after tailored surgical resection: a novel treatment paradigm for glomus jugulare tumors. Stereotact Funct Neurosurg **87(1)**: 31–36; 2009
23. Kim IY, Kondziolka D, Niranjan A, Flickinger JC, Lunsford LD. Gamma knife surgery for schwannomas originating from cranial nerves III, IV, and VI. J Neurosurg **109(Suppl)**: 149–153; 2008
24. Kemeny AA. Contemporary management of jugular paragangliomas (glomus tumours): microsurgery and radiosurgery. Acta Neurochir **151(5)**: 419–421; 2009
25. Jackson CG, McGrew BM, Forest JA,Netterville JL, Hampf CF, Glasscock III ME. Lateral skull base surgery for glomus tumors: long-term control. Otol Neurotol **22**: 377–382; 2001
26. Watkins LD, Mendoza N, Cheesman AD, Symon L. Glomus jugulare tumours: a review of 61 cases. Acta Neurochir **130(1–4)**: 66–70; 1994
27. Bari ME, Kemeny AA, Forster DM, Radatz MW. Radiosurgery for the control of glomus jugulare tumours. J Pak Med Assoc **53(4)**: 147–151; 2003
28. Bitaraf MA, Alikhani M, Tahsili-Fahadan P, Motiei-Langroudi R, Zahiri A, Allahverdi M, Salmanian S. Radiosurgery for glomus jugulare tumors: experience treating 16 patients in Iran. J Neurosurg **105(Suppl)**: 168–174; 2006
29. Eustacchio S, Leber K, Trummer M, Unger F, Pendl G. Gamma knife radiosurgery for glomus jugulare tumours. Acta Neurochir **141(8)**: 811–818; 1999
30. Feigl GC, Bundschuh O, Gharabaghi A, Safavi-Abassi SEL, Shawarby A, Samii M, Horstmann GA. Evaluation of a new concept for the management of skull base chordomas and chondrosarcomas. J Neurosurg **102(Suppl)**: 165–170; 2005
31. Foote RL, Coffey RJ, Gorman DA, Earle JD, Schomberg PJ, Kline RW, Schild SE. Stereotactic radiosurgery for glomus jugulare tumors: a preliminary report. Int J Radiat Oncol Biol Phys **38(3)**: 491–495; 1997
32. Foote RL, Pollock BE, Gorman DA, Schomberg PJ, Stafford SL, Link MJ, Kline RW, Strome SE, Kasperbauer JL, Olsen KD. Glomus jugulare tumor: tumor control and complications after stereotactic radiosurgery. Head Neck **24(4)**: 332–338; 2002
33. Ganz JC, Abdelkarim K. Glomus jugulare tumours: certain clinical and radiological aspects observed following gamma knife radiosurgery. Acta Neurochir (Wien) **151(5)**: 423–426; 2009
34. Gerosa M, Visca A, Rizzo P, Foroni R, Nicolato A, Bricolo A. Glomus jugulare tumors: the option of gamma knife radiosurgery. Neurosurgery **59(3)**: 561–569; 2006
35. Leber KA, Eustacchio S, Pendl G. Radiosurgery of glomus tumors: midterm results. Stereotact Funct Neurosurg **72(Suppl 1)**: 53–59; 1999

36. Liscak R, Vladyka V, Simonova G, Vymazal J, Janouskova L. Leksell gamma knife radiosurgery of the tumor glomus jugulare and tympanicum. Stereotact Funct Neurosurg 70(Suppl 1): 152–160; 1998

37. Liscak R, Vladyka V, Wowra B, Kemeny A, Forster D, Burzaco JA, Martinez R, Eustacchio S, Pendl G, Régis J, Pellet W. Gamma knife radiosurgery of the glomus jugulare tumour – early multicentre experience. Acta Neurochir 141(11): 1141–1146; 1999

38. Miller RC, Foote RL, Coffey RJ, Gorman DA, Earle JD, Schomberg PJ, Kline RW. The role of stereotactic radiosurgery in the treatment of malignant skull base tumors. Int J Radiat Oncol Biol Phys 39(5): 977–981; 1997

39. Pollock BE, Foote RL, Stafford SL. Stereotactic radiosurgery: the preferred management for patients with nonvestibular schwannomas? Int J Radiat Oncol Biol Phys 52(4): 1002–1007; 2002

40. Saringer W, Khayal H, Ertl A, Schoeggl A, Kitz K. Efficiency of gamma knife radiosurgery in the treatment of glomus jugulare tumors. Minim Invasive Neurosurg 44(3): 141–146; 2001

41. Sharma MS, Gupta A, Kale SS, Agrawal D, Mahapatra AK, Sharma BS. Gamma knife radiosurgery for glomus jugulare tumors: therapeutic advantages of minimalism in the skull base. Neurol India 56: 57–61; 2008

42. Sheehan J, Yen CP, Arkha Y, Schlesinger D, Steiner L. Gamma knife surgery for trigeminal schwannoma. J Neurosurg 106: 839–845; 2007

43. Willen SN, Einstein DB, Maciunas RJ, Megerian CA. Treatment of glomus jugulare tumors in patients with advanced age: planned limited surgical resection followed by staged gamma knife radiosurgery: a preliminary report. Otol Neurotol 26(6): 1229–1234; 2005

44. Eustacchio S, Trummer M, Unger F, Schrottner O, Sutter B, Pendl G. The role of Gamma Knife radiosurgery in the management of glomus jugular tumours. Acta Neurochir Suppl 84: 91–97; 2002

45. Varma A, Nathoo N, Neyman G, Suh JH, Ros SJ, Par KJ, Barnett GH. Gamma knife radiosurgery for glomus jugulare tumors: volumetric analysis in 17 patients. Neurosurgery 59(5): 1030–1036; 2006

46. Genc A, Bicer A, Abacioglu U, Peker S, Pamir MN, Kilic T. Gamma knife radiosurgery for the treatment of glomus jugulare tumors. J Neurooncol 97(1): 101–108; 2010

47. Douglas JG, Goodkin R, Laramore GE. Gamma knife stereotactic radiosurgery for salivary gland neoplasms with base of skull invasion following neutron radiotherapy. Head Neck 30(4): 492–496; 2008

48. Mori Y, Kobayashi T, Kida Y, Oda K, Shibamoto Y, Yoshida J. Stereotactic radiosurgery as a salvage treatment for recurrent skull base adenoid cystic carcinoma. Stereotact Funct Neurosurg 83(5–6): 202–207; 2005

49. Cho YH, Kim JH, Khang SK, Lee JK, Kim CJ Chordomas and chondrosarcomas of the skull base: comparative analysis of clinical results in 30 patients. Neurosurg Rev 31: 35–43; 2008

50. Feigl GC, Horstmann GA. Intracranial glomus jugulare tumors: volume reduction with Gamma Knife surgery. J Neurosurg 105(Suppl): 161–167; 2006

51. Hasegawa T, Kida Y, Yoshimoto M, Koike J. Trigeminal schwannomas: results of gamma knife surgery in 37 cases. J Neurosurg 106(1): 18–23; 2007

52. Martin JJ, Niranjan A, Kondziolka D, Flickinger JC, Lozanne KA, Lunsford LD. Radiosurgery for chordomas and chondrosarcomas of the skull base. J Neurosurg 107: 758–764; 2007

53. Dassoulas K, Schlesinger D, Yen CP, Sheehan J. The role of gamma knife surgery in the treatment of skull base chordomas. J Neurooncol 94(2): 243–248; 2009

54. Färander P, Rähn T, Kihlström L, Ulfarsson E, Mathiesen T. Combination of microsurgery and Gamma Knife surgery for the treatment of intracranial chondrosarcomas. J Neurosurg 105 (Suppl): 18–25; 2006

55. Kondziolka D, Lunsford LD, Flickinger JC. The role of radiosurgery in the management of chordoma and chondrosarcoma of the cranial base. Neurosurgery 29(1): 38–45; 1991

56. Liu AL, Wang ZC, Sun SB, Wang MH, Luo B, Liu P. Gamma knife radiosurgery for residual skull base chordomas. Neurol Res **30(6)**: 557–561; 2008

57. Muthukumar N, Kondziolka D, Lunsford LD, Flickinger JC. Stereotactic radiosurgery for chordoma and chondrosarcoma: further experiences. Int J Radiat Oncol Biol Phys **41(2)**: 387–392; 1998

58. Pamir MN, Kilic T, Ture U, Ozek MM. Multimodality management of 26 skull-base chordomas with 4-year mean follow-up: experience at a single institution. Acta Neurochir **146(4)**: 343–354; 2004

Part IV
The Gamma Knife and Specific Diseases:
Vascular Diseases

Chapter 19
Gamma Knife for Cerebral Vascular Anomalies

Introduction

This chapter attempts to give a reasonably comprehensive overview of the information currently available to those who wish to treat intracranial vascular malformations with GKNS. This information includes formulae and some scales used in treatment to which frequent mention is made in the literature. Since, these scales and formulae are not always easily available to the reader it is thought that collecting them all in one place will make the text more useful, especially for the beginner. It is again emphasised that the variable nature of the disease means that no single treatment method will be adequate for all cases and a team of combined expertise at specialist centres is required to deliver optimal treatment.

Preamble About Principles

Nature of the Lesion

Cerebral arteriovenous malformations (AVMs) are one kind of blood vessel malformations found in the head. AVMs are considered to be a congenital anomaly, with shunting of blood directly from arteries to veins, without intervening capillaries. They may co-exist with other vascular anomalies including aneurysms, cavernous malformations (CMs) and venous anomalies. Aneurysms may be in the usual location of Berry aneurysm at points of branching along intracerebral arteries. They may however occasionally be found on the feeding arteries and draining veins of the AVM. Nonetheless, the majority of AVMs are solitary lesions. The abnormal arteriovenous shunt is often localised to a nidus or nest; consisting of a network of irregular, pathological blood vessels, with abnormal non-functioning cerebral parenchyma in the interstices. The blood vessel arrangement is shown diagrammatically in Fig. 19.1.

J.C. Ganz, *Gamma Knife Neurosurgery*,
DOI 10.1007/978-3-7091-0343-2_19, © Springer-Verlag/Wien 2011

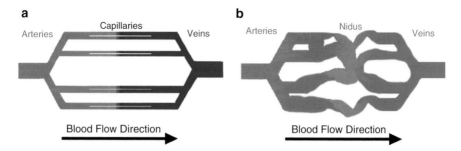

Fig. 19.1 (**a**) Normal anatomy with blood flowing from arteries to veins through capillaries with loss of oxygen and acquisition of waste products. Blood changes from oxygenated to de-oxygenated or in other words from *red* to *blue*. (**b**) Dilated arteries draining blood directly into veins via the abnormal nidus. The veins contain oxygenated red blood under higher pressure than normal. There is no useful exchange of metabolites and waste products

Fig. 19.2 Two dilated arteries (*white arrows*) and one dilated draining vein with arterial red blood is seen (*white arrowhead*). The discoloured vessels (*black arrowhead*) are arteries containing glue following a previous embolisaton

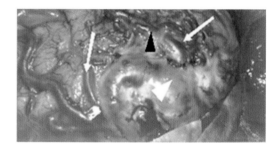

The veins typically contain oxygenated blood which is shown in vivo during an operation in Fig. 19.2.

Their total removal should result in restitution of the surrounding circulation to normal as illustrated in Fig. 19.3. Because there is a localised, apparently space-occupying lesion, these malformations have also been called angiomas in earlier days. However, as stated above, there is a consensus today that they are not neoplastic but congenital in origin.

General Principles of Treatment

The aim of treatment for an AVM is in principle simple. It should be removed. This treatment is not primarily therapeutic but prophylactic for reasons to be outlined below. The practice of AVM management unlike the underlying principle is far from simple. Some of the reasons are as follows.

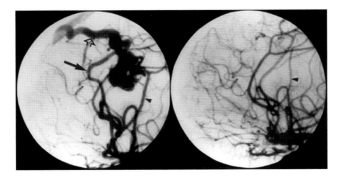

Fig. 19.3 On the left an untreated AVM with hypertrophic feeds (*black arrowhead* and *arrow*) and a large draining vein. Two years after Gamma Knife surgery the abnormal hypertrophic vessel has disappeared. One abnormal vessel has disappeared and one hypertrophic middle cerebral branch is back to normal. The draining vein (*outline arrowhead*) has disappeared. Thus, the images demonstrate the return to normal anatomy after removing an AVM, in this case with Gamma Knife surgery

Sources of Practical Difficulty During Treatment

Anatomical Variation

Size

The anatomy of these lesions is very variable. They vary in size between a few cubic millimetres up to the volume of an entire cerebral lobe or more. The largest of these lesions are almost invariably untreatable.

Vascular Supply

They may be fed by one branch of a cerebral artery or by all the branches of all four carotid arteries and both vertebral arteries. They may drain into any vein or combination of veins both superficial and deep.

Location

An AVM may occur anywhere inside the head and its proximity to or involvement of vital structures complicates its management.

Clinical Picture

AVMs most commonly present with intracranial haemorrhage which is usually subarachnoid and intracerebral or both. It may also be intraventricular. They may also present with epilepsy alone or in addition to the haemorrhage. A third presentation is headache without bleeding. Occasionally, their rapid blood flow steals blood from other parts of the brain and they may present with ischaemic symptoms. Finally, they may be an incidental finding. Apart from emptying haematomas in some cases, there is little the surgeon can do to improve the damage produced by a haemorrhage. Happily, it is quite usual for the clinical damage to be relatively slight in relation to the volume of the haematoma seen on images. Indeed if an intracerebral haematoma is seen on CT or MRI and appears to be larger than the clinical picture would suggest, an AVM should always be considered as an underlying cause. Patients with epilepsy may or may not have their epilepsy controlled with medication. The same applies to the headaches associated with the AVM.

Natural History

The prophylactic nature of treatment requires very strict standards. Removal of an AVM is considered to be the safest method of protecting the patient from future complications in the form of re-bleeding or deteriorating epilepsy. However, the effect of removing an AVM on associated symptoms and signs is uncertain. Since the therapy is essentially preventative, it must be a sine qua non that its consequences are not worse than those of the untreated disease. The re-bleed rate is about 3% per year. For AVMs which have not bled the bleeding rate is about 1% per year. It is characteristic of AVM bleeding that the mortality of an individual bleed is relatively low – about 6%. Thus, the high mortality associated with hypertensive intracerebral haemorrhage and aneurysmal subarachnoid haemorrhage is not a feature of AVMs. On the other hand they occur in a lower age group than the other major causes of intracranial haemorrhage so that there is a longer life expectancy for the accumulation of re-bleed risk. In a recent comprehensive long term follow up study from Finland the mortality rate was 2% per year whether the AVM was ruptured or not. In ruptured AVMs the mortality rate over the series was 35% and in unruptured it was 25%; a significant difference [1, 2]. This finding underlines that failure to rupture does not confer a significant long term benefit. In practice this means that with a ruptured AVM a somewhat higher risk of treatment may be acceptable but even with unruptured AVMs some degree of risk from treatment complications can be accepted in view of the degree of danger represented by the untreated disease. Of course, quantification of these risks for an individual patient is nigh impossible and will need to be assessed on a case by case basis. To this important principle we shall return in the section devoted to Gamma Knife treatment.

The Development of Therapeutic Technology

Given the variety of size, blood supply and location it is natural that no single treatment will suffice in every case. At the present there are three main methods of treatment, microsurgery, radiosurgery and embolisation. Each has its advantages and disadvantages. In many cases it may be necessary to consider using more than one treatment mode. It is also necessary to assess whether treatment is needed at all. From the same Finnish epidemiological study it may be mentioned that patients with obliterated malformations had a mortality rate during the study of 17% compared with 33% in the partially obliterated lesions and 68% in the conservatively treated patients. This is additional evidence to suggest that an active treatment policy where possible, is to be preferred to expectant observation, or as it is sometimes called conservative treatment.

In the 1970s conservative treatment was more popular. Indeed algorithms were developed to indicate when treatment should be implemented and when avoided as propounded by Pellettieri et al. in 1979 [3]. The development of the operating microscope, the development of improved catheterisation techniques and digital subtraction angiography (DSA) has resulted in more and more patients having lesions which may be treated. To these two treatment modalities, radiosurgery was added in the early 1970s in Stockholm following the introduction of the first Gamma Unit in 1968.

Principles of Gamma Knife Treatment

Early Days

The paradigm for the radiosurgical treatment of AVMs is in outline simple. The lesion should be obliterated. The first attempts to achieve this were performed by Ladislau Steiner and his associates in Stockholm. They were entering unchartered terrain under Leksell's guidance. Thus, it was incumbent upon them to move slowly, carefully and to ensure that the documentation was exemplary. Nobody had ever used radiosurgery on AVMs before. It was known that radiotherapy was disappointing [4–7]. The view was taken that treatment should be limited to patients with small AVMs (not more than 2.5 cm in diameter). In addition only AVMs which were at the greatest risk – that is those which had bled – were offered radiosurgery. Over the ensuing years the practice was established that the most effective prescription dose for this subsection of AVMs was 25 Gy and that with this dose a permanent clinical complication rate of 3% could be expected and in addition a 10% temporary complication rate. Taken against the morbidity and mortality noted above these would seem to be acceptable risks. The obliteration rate was around 80%. It was also observed that obliteration occurred in 50% of patients in 1 year and 80% after 2 years.

Thus, within the framework used by the Stockholm group there was apparently enough information to advise a special subgroup of AVM patients about the risks and benefits of GKNS. The risks were less than the risks of the untreated disease. However, seen from the viewpoint of today these results presented an incomplete picture. To begin with the early dose planning was approximate as only angiograms were available for treatment and they project an entire volume into a single plane. Thus precise target definition was impossible and would have to wait upon the development, application and availability of MR images for use in the dose planning. Then, the treatment was mainly limited to AVMs which had bled. Thirdly, the level of complications could be said to be too high and it was reasonable to assess the method with a view to improving the complication rate without at the same time reducing the obliteration rate. The next paragraphs relate how the method has developed in different centres and how new information has affected the way we assess, inform and manage these patients. The various conceptions governing current treatment of AVMs with radiosurgery will now be examined.

Obliteration

It is widely believed that AVMs must be occluded if there is to be no further risk and especially no further bleeding. It is also generally considered that an AVM occluded on angiogram will never bleed again. There have been rare occasions where this has not been true [8–10]. This rare occurrence is considered to be the result of small amounts of overlooked AVM tissue on the control angiogram. It has been suggested that this may be a bit more likely to occur in children [9] with the corollary that follow up must be pursued into adult life even if the paediatric AVM is apparently occluded. How intensive this follow up should be is not clear since these post obliteration re-bleeds are exceptionally rare.

The Obliteration Rate

In the early Steiner material the obliteration rate was given as around 80% after 2 years. More modern work has produced a great variety of results [11–66]. The original Steiner material settled on 25 Gy as a result of slightly misunderstanding the radiobiology of radiation induced haemorrhage in head and neck cancer [32]. However, it turned out to be a happy choice. The lesions treated by Steiner and his group were small (up to 2.5 cm diameter) AVMs which had bled. However, as more experience was gained and more difficult lesions were treated. Obliteration rates under 80% were recorded. The more difficult lesions included larger AVMs and those in a location close to vital structures necessitating a lower dose to reduce the chance of complications. It became clear that a lower dose was associated with a lower obliteration rate [11, 17, 27, 28, 30, 31, 36, 39, 43, 48, 56, 57, 59, 62, 63]. In addition to size and dose it would seem that younger patients have a higher obliteration rate [15, 34, 47, 54, 67–70]. It must be emphasised that it remains the belief of all major centres involved in Gamma Knife surgery, that nothing less than total obliteration will reduce the re-bleed rate. It follows from this that the key parameter for successful obliteration is an adequate **dose**. The correct dose and how to calculate it will be outlined under the section on complications since it is fear of radiation induced cerebral damage which prompts physicians to lower the dose for difficult lesions.

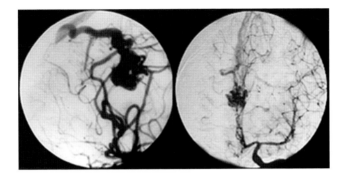

Fig. 19.4 On the left is a fistulous AVM with hypertrophic feeding arteries and a distended draining vein. On the right is a diffuse lesion with no hypertrophic arteries or distended veins. Both AVMs were obliterated. Nonetheless, the best statistical chance was the patient on the right, who was 12 years old at the time of treatment and who also had a diffuse AVM

Another characteristic which has been said to be related to the obliteration rate is the angio-architecture of AVMs. It is suggested that diffuse or Moya-Moya lesions are more easily obliterated than fistulous lesions and that the occlusion rate for a mixture of these two types is intermediate [71], see Fig. 19.4. On the other hand a paper from Zipfel et al. [72] in the respected LINAC centre in Gainsville, found that a diffuse AVMs were less likely to obliterate than more fistulous lesions. This suggests a real conflict of findings until differences in technique are taken into account. Firstly, as with practically all LINAC units the dose planning image mode is primarily CT. This gives a notably less precise definition of an AVM compared with angiogram and MR images used with the Gamma Knife. The term "diffuse" in this paper referred to CT appearance rather than angio-architecture. It reflects a difference between LINAC and GKNS technique.

Attempts to Predict Obliteration Rates

Attempts have been made to calculate the obliteration rate. These have been reviewed by Karlsson et al. [32]. They derived the K-index which remains the best known of these parameters. It was defined as:

Prescription Dose × *Volume* × *1/3*

A value of 27 was considered optimal. Increasing the index over 27 did not improve the obliteration rate. There is little published about index since its introduction. This is perhaps because of a point raised by Friedman in his comments on one of the relevant papers when it was published [73]. He points out that it is not entirely clear

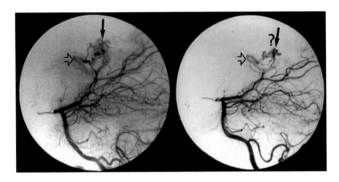

Fig. 19.5   On the left is the pre-treatment AVM indicated by the *solid arrow* and the early draining vein shown by the outline arrowhead. On the right while a hypertophic feeder is seen the AVM itself is not clearly shown. The early draining vein however is still undeniably present. At the time these images were taken this was viewed as grounds for retreatment. Today, we should wait and only consider treatment if the lesion bleeds again, since there is a good change it won't

how it was derived and it is also possible to achieve high K index values with large volumes with moderate doses or small volumes with very high doses.

It is fair to say that the Stockholm margin dose of 25 Gy is still viewed as the most effective and it is also agreed that increasing the dose does not much increase the obliteration rate but will increase the incidence of radiation induced complications. In view of this most attempts to optimize dose have been directed at minimising complications.

In spite of the generally held belief that total obliteration is essential for a safe result there is work indicating that a subtotal obliteration with only an *early filling vein* (Fig. 19.5) is a condition in which new bleeds do not occur. If this is true, then retreatment in this situation would not be necessary [65]. This matter is not decided so further observation is needed and a certain amount of caution when considering retreatment in a given case.

Attempts to Predict and Manage Complication Rates

There are two major complications of GKNS for AVMs. They are a re-bleed and radiation damage to normal brain. There is also a less common complication, namely cyst formation.

Re-bleeding

There is broad agreement that re-bleeding may occur at any time until an AVM is obliterated. The bleeding rate appears to be the same as that of the untreated disease. It is recorded either as an overall bleeding rate [8–11, 17, 18, 20, 25, 26, 28, 30, 31, 33–36, 38, 44, 45, 48, 49, 52, 57, 58, 65, 74–84] for a series or an annual rate [23, 40, 42, 43, 51, 54, 59, 85–87]. The annual rates vary from 1.5% to 4.3%. Overall rates may be that low but are often higher. They represent the total risk to a patient material and vary between 1.3% and 38%. The most important factor which is associated with an increased bleeding risk is AVM volume [23, 48, 75, 85]. This makes sense since larger malformations are either inadequately covered by radiation or compel the use of a lower dose to reduce the risk of complications. This lower dose results in a lower obliteration rate thus leaving tissue which can bleed again. There is also a report that the presence of an uncontrolled proximal aneurysm on an AVM feeding artery can increase the risk of bleeding [80]. Finally, there is Japanese work indicating that the risk of re-bleeding is related to AVM morphology. High flow fistulous AVMs, AVMs with a single draining vein and those with a deep venous drainage have a higher risk of re-bleeding [26].

Adverse Radiation Effects (AREs)

The term adverse radiation effects is a generic term for all damage inflicted by therapeutic radiation on normal tissue. It is not too specific and accurately reflects the state of knowledge of the field. When clinical radiosurgery was started in the late 1960s there were no computerised imaging techniques. Thus, most of the available knowledge on clinically relevant radiation induced brain damage was based on clinical observations. On the other hand, the development of radiosurgery was preceded by intense work on the pathophysiology of radiation induced destruction of tiny volumes of normal brain. This had been done because the original intention was to use radiosurgery to replace open surgery in the performance of such procedures as thalamotomy. This work in days prior to the invention of the Gamma Knife was carried out at the Werner Institute in Uppsala [88, 89]. It was determined amongst other things that a thalamotomy sized lesion could be induced with a maximum dose between 130 and 200 Gy. Within this dose range a limited focal volume of necrosis was produced which did not spread. There was no effect below 130 Gy and 200 Gy was preferred as the lesion developed more quickly. It was also noted that doses above 400 Gy could lead to a spreading necrotic lesion. However, interesting though this is, the lesions are much smaller and the doses much higher than those that are used to treat AVMs. The situations are entirely different. With a thalamotomy the aim is to destroy a tiny volume of anatomically normal brain tissue. With AVMs the aim is to obliterate the AVM without damaging normal brain tissue.

The early work in Stockholm was cautious, since the group was breaking new ground. New cases were initially only treated after the results of treatment on previous patients were known. Moreover, the great majority of the early cases were unresectable AVMs which had bled and which had a diameter preferably not exceeding 2.5 cm. The observation of the patients was the only way to record the frequency of complications. It was known from conventional radiotherapy that increases in dose and irradiated volumes were related to the incidence of radiation induced complications at least in principle [90]. Assessment of the risk of a given

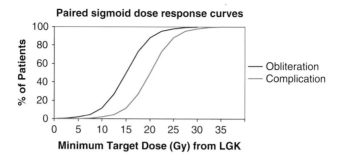

Fig. 19.6 The curves show the obliteration rates of AVMs at different doses and the complication rates at the same doses. The two curves are close together indicating a poor therapeutic ratio. Thus, a consistent 100% obliteration is not feasible because of the high complication rate that would entail

Gamma Knife treatment has since been approached in a number of ways and these will now be outlined. The Stockholm group used a pair of sigmoid dose response curves to indicate the relationship between obliteration and complications (see Fig. 19.6).

Ways of Calculating the Risk of Complications: Post Treatment Assessments

Paired Sigmoid Curves

The paired sigmoid curves were helpful in the early stages. However, they had some weaknesses. They are designed for use in fractionated radiotherapy and not single session radiosurgery. Another major weakness relates to volume. Treatment volume has little effect on complication risk with conventional radiotherapy. With radiosurgery it is far more significant. The dose response curves should take this into account. These weaknesses led the Pittsburgh group, largely in the person of Dr. John Flickinger to provide alternative methods of assessing the risks inherent in any given treatment plan.

The Integrated Logistic Formula [91, 92]

He began with a formulation used in the risk assessment for conventional fractionated radiotherapy to whole brain. It was called the integrated logistic formula. It was then adapted for the specific situation of single fraction treatments of small volumes. The formula exists in two formats. It was meant to calculate the 3% risk for radiation induced damage.

The Linear Form

$$P = 1 - \Pi \left\{ NTD_2(d)/NTD_2(d_{50})^k \right\}^{-v/V}$$

Where

P = The probability of a complication
NTD_2 = The normalized total dose with a prescription of 2 Gy per fraction – this represents the biological effect of the dose
d = The dose delivered
d_{50} = The dose required to give a 50% change of a complication
k = A constant
V = Reference volume usually the whole brain
v = The volume to which the therapeutic radiation is delivered

The Exponential Form

$$P = 1 - \Pi \left[1 + (d/d_{50})^{2k} \right]^{-v/V}$$

Where

P = The probability of a complication
d = The dose delivered
d_{50} = The dose required to give a 50% change of a complication
k = A constant
V = Reference volume usually the whole brain
v = The volume to which the therapeutic radiation is delivered

The latter form seems more useful in the context of radiosurgery risk calculations. It is fair to say that the derivation and significance and the ways of manipulating these formulae are beyond the understanding of those who have not studied fairly advanced mathematics and certainly this understanding is outside the comprehension of many physicians. However, the principle involved is fairly simple. The constants "k" and "d_{50}" can only be derived from observing the effects of treatments on patients. The other parameters relate to elements of dose planning under the control of the physician. Thus, it is these constants which are the key to the risk assessment. Indeed, in the early papers where patient numbers reported were low Flickinger was meticulous about warning that the formula on the basis of the number of patient observations available was not to be considered completely reliable. More data would be added over time.

In the earliest papers on AVMs there were no computerised images on which to observe imaging changes after treatment. However, after Flickinger started his studies MRI was in use for following the patients. It became clear from the use of images that there were post radiation imaging (PRI) changes which were clinically silent. The changes usually consisted of an increase in T2 signal. This is thought to represent at least oedema. This oedema may be local, spreading or expansive. Then there were cases of symptomatic post radiosurgery injury expression (PIE). This distinction represented a problem for the integrated logistic formula which had been worked out for clinical changes. It became clear that the initial formula didn't really work as well as hoped. New updated publications showing improved versions didn't appear. Instead a new, more easily understood parameter was found to be more useful. This was the 12-Gy volume.

The Total 12 Gy Volume [93], PRI PIE and SPIE

During their ongoing analysis of risk factors, the Pittsburgh group came to realise that the only variable which correlated with post radiosurgery imaging (PRI) changes was target volume and the only variable which correlated with PIE was AVM location. A PRI is an image based demonstration of radiation damage or an ARE. Locations were simplified to brainstem and not brainstem [93]. The group analysed a number of questions and found that the best correlation between the development and PRI was the volume of the 12 Gy isodose or the 12 Gy volume as it came to be called. This is presented as a useful parameter since it reflects both dose and volume in a given patient. They demonstrated moreover that PRI without PIE began later and resolved quicker. They could not demonstrate that dose rate was a factor in the development of complications.

They noted that there was a greater chance for PRI with AVMs than with tumours and the authors interpreted this as indicating a difference inherent in AVMs which could contribute to PRI and thus included the AVM volume within the 12 Gy volume as well as the normal brain. No mention was made that the higher doses commonly used in AVMs could account for the higher incidence of PRI. A small number of patients were noted to suffer permanent radionecrosis, defined as imaging or clinical changes persisting beyond two years. It is emphasised in most cases there is no histological evidence available to distinguish between PRI/ARE and necrosis. There was no correlation between the rare development of permanent radiation induced brain damage and any of the parameters examined.

Subsequent papers built on the above work and the 12 Gy volume is still reported in the literature 10 years after its initial description [94]. A year later a new report was made from Pittsburgh dividing up the brain stem locations into subdivision and codifying the locations with numbers [95]. This codification was called the PIE score. The basic findings remained unchanged. It was still not possible to relate the 12 Gy volume and PIE scores to necrosis producing *permanent* loss of function. This matter was in turn addressed by an update paper in 2000 where additional patients were acquired from other centres leading to PIE in 85 cases instead of 30

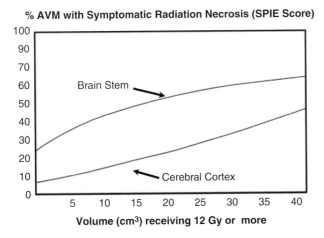

Fig. 19.7 The two lines represent the risk of complications. One for the brainstem and one for the cortex. The risk for symptomatic radiation damage is higher for the brain stem. However, with a volume of 0 there is still a risk of radiation damage according to the curves. That would mean that 12 Gy to 0 cm^3 can give ARE. This is obviously wrong and casts doubt on the validity of this method of calculating the risk of treatment

[96]. This was used to construct a new parameter the Significant Post Radiosurgery Injury Expression or SPIE. These values were derived from a multivariate logistic regression analysis of the effects of location on distinguishing patients who would have *temporary* or *permanent* sequelae. There was enough data to permit this. What was found was that the when the SPIE score was plotted against the 12 Gy volume the different locations gave obviously different curves, indicating that the SPIE score was a good predictor of permanent radiation induced damage. However, there were problems. There was no measure of individual radiosensitivity. Moreover, the curves were in error in one point. The permanent damage percent remained quite high in some locations even when the 12 Gy volume approached zero. Thus, the SPIE score was interesting maybe useful, but still flawed. In this paper as well the whole 12 Gy volume was used. It is of interest that a total 12 Gy volume and 12 Gy volume of normal brain were analysed in this paper. Use of the 12 Gy volume of normal brain did not improve the prediction of the incidence of PIE.

Please note that Fig. 19.7 is a construct for clarification. It looks like the curves in Dr. Flickinger et al.'s paper [96] but is simply a constructed diagram.

Plotting Risk of Symptomatic Radionecrosis for Increasing Total 12 Gy Volume

Then Pollock et al. [97]. from the Mayo clinic published a paper in 2000 on AVM treatment where the 12 Gy volume was divided into total 12 Gy volume and 12

Volume of normal brain = Total 12 Gy volume – Target volume. In this paper, they were testing the dosimetry of treating larger AVMs in a single session or in staged volume treatments. They demonstrated that the staging reduced the dose to the 12 Gy volume as compared to a single session treatment. This effect was more marked for the 12 Gy normal brain volume, underlining that staging protected the normal brain. It did not however assess the relevance of total 12 Gy volume and normal brain 12 Gy volume in respect of complications.

Total 12 Gy Volume and Normal Tissue 12 Gy Volume

More recently, the Pittsburgh group has published a new paper using the 12 Gy volume [94] only this time they specifically use the normal brain 12 Gy volume [94]. The paper records the effects of irradiation on the brain stem. Its findings are not conclusive but serve to underline how difficult it is to apply calculations which reliably inform a physician on what is the appropriate dose. This applies as much to the dose for therapeutic success as the dose for avoiding complications. In this paper about benign brain stem lesions the normal brain 12 Gy volume is recorded as BEV (brainstem exposure volume). Adverse radiation effects on images are renamed Adverse Radiation Imaging Effects (ARIE). There was a linear but not statistically significant relationship between prescription dose and the occurrence of ARIE. There was a relationship between the presence of ARIE and PIE. However, there was no correlation between the presence of ARIE and pathology, margin dose, maximum dose, 12 Gy volume, Brainstem 12 Gy volume and prescription isodose volume. Moreover, there were three patients with minor persisting residual deficits without any ARIE. There was NO clear cut relationship between dose, volume and the development of new neurological deficits. In a group of patients receiving 15–17 Gy prescription dose all the patients with new neurological deficits had cavernomas. The distribution of patients in this material was 23 cavernomas, 8 pilocytic astrocytomas, 7 AVMs and one gangioglioma. This is a disparate group of very different pathological process. This case mix may reasonably explain the lack of useful statistical relationships in such a small material.

The Integral Dose

The author devised a simple "rule of thumb" system for calculating acceptable doses for larger AVMs. The treatment planning software provides a parameter called the 'integral dose' measured in millijoules and reflecting both the dose and the volume being treated [98]. It has been found when reviewing the first hundred AVM patients that doses up to 220 mJ were associated with very few if any significant permanent complications. Subsequently it has seemed reasonable to reduce this acceptable dose to 175 Gy for patients who have not bled.

Ways of Calculating the Risk of Complications: Pre-treatment Assessments

For the surgical management of AVMs a reliable pre-treatment grading system may be used to assess the risk of treatment and on the basis of the grading provide more accurate and useful information to the patient. The traditional grading system to assess the operability of intracranial AVMs is the Spetzler-Martin grade outlined below.

Spetzler-Martin Grade [99]

Parameter	Points
Size of lesion	
Small (<3 cm)	1
Medium (3–6 cm)	2
Large (>6 cm)	3
Location	
Non-eloquent site	0
Eloquent site	1
Pattern of venous drainage	
Superficial only	0
Any deep	1

Grade = Sum of Points. The maximum some of points is Grade 5. However, Spetzler and Martin added a Grade 6 which they characterised as follows. There are certain lesions that should not currently be considered for surgery. Within this group are extremely large diffuse AVM's that are dispersed through critical neurologically eloquent areas, or malformations with a diffuse nidus that encompasses critical structures such as the hypothalamus or brain stem. As surgical resection of such lesions would almost unavoidably be associated with a totally disabling deficit or death, these AVM's fall into a separate category that can be termed "Grade VI" or, more simply, "inoperable."

The Spetzler-Martin grading system is widely used by neurosurgeons as a tool to guide them concerning the risks and benefits of surgery. However, its application to radiosurgery is not completely straightforward. The reasons are as follows. Firstly, the Grade I small is from nothing to 3 cm in diameter. That basically encompasses the range of volumes treated with GKNS and all within one sub-section. The other factor which doesn't work so well for radiosurgery is the eloquent site. This is designed so that the motor cortex, basal ganglia and brain stem all have the same value. The experience of radiosurgery indicates that treatment of superficial lesions is a lot less likely to produce a radiation induced complication than the treatment of deeper lesions. This is presumably related to the dispersal of function in a superficial location.

Radiosurgery Based Grading System [100]

In view of the limited possibilities for applying the Spetzler-Martin grading system for radiosurgery a new system was clearly needed. It is the last and most recent of the risk assessment systems promulgated by the indefatigable Dr. Flickinger, this time in association with Dr. Pollock of the Mayo Clinic. It differs from other systems in that it only records parameters related to the patient and the AVM and does not record treatment parameters. However, its values still assume the dosimetry used by the Mayo Clinic. Thus, it must be applied with caution by those who use different doses than those used by Dr. Pollock's group. While useful, it cannot have the universal applicability that the Spetzler-Martin grading system has for microsurgery. The initial version came out in 2002. The original formula was as follows.

AVM Score $= (0.1)\big(\text{AVM volume in cm}^3\big) + 0.02(\text{patient age in years})$
$\quad\quad + 0.3(\text{Location})$

Locations were scored: Frontal, Temporal $= 0$

Parietal Occipital, Intraventricular, Corpus Callosum,
Cerebellum $= 1$
Basal Ganglia, Thalamus, Brainstem $= 2$

The factors in front of each parameter are derived from regression coefficients obtained during multivariant regression analysis.

The Score would be particularly useful for advising patients and relatives of risk/benefits of treatment if the AVM volume was known beforehand. It is suggested in this paper that the following approximation for determining the AVM volume is as follows.

AVM Volume prior to treatment $= (\pi/6) \times \text{width} \times \text{length} \times \text{height}$ [100]

The scoring system has been found useful so that it was used by the same authors again in 2004 during the reporting of their treatment of deep seated AVMs. Scores of 1.5 or less had noticeably better outcome than higher scores [101].

Finally, it was found reasonable to simplify it since the proposed simplification was found to work just as well as the original.

AVM Score $= (0.1)(\text{AVM volume in cm}^3) + 0.02(\text{patient age in years}) + 0.5$
$\quad\quad (\text{Location})$ [49]

Locations were scored:

Deep $= 1$
Other $= 0$

This Score correlated well with excellent outcomes and deterioration of the Modified Rankin Score [49], a sensitive scoring system for clinical neurological function as shown below.

Modified Rankin Score

0. No symptoms at all
1. No significant disability despite symptoms; able to carry out all usual duties and activities
2. Slight disability; unable to carry out all previous activities, but able to look after own affairs without assistance
3. Moderate disability; requiring some help, but able to walk without assistance
4. Moderately severe disability; unable to walk without assistance and unable to attend to own bodily needs without assistance
5. Severe disability; bedridden, incontinent and requiring constant nursing care and attention
6. Dead

How GKNS Works on AVMs: Changes in Arteries Following Radiation

It is well known that radiation can damage blood vessels [102]. However, most of these effects are considered to affect the small blood vessels particularly small arteries and arterioles. Moreover, most of the tissue examined is pathological so that the exact contribution of the radiation itself can be difficult to determine. While radiation damage to larger vessels is known, with concomitant rupture or occlusion, it is rare.

The treatment of AVMs involves the effects of radiation on what are defined as larger blood vessels in this context. What is common knowledge amongst those who undertake radiosurgery is that radiosurgery occludes pathological AVM vessels while leaving normal adjacent arteries open. It has no known certain direct occlusive effect on draining veins either. One detail that has been known since 1972 is that in experiments with the cat basilar artery, while heavy doses of radiation can damage the vessel wall, arterial occlusion did not occur [103]. This was tried with doses to the basilar artery of this animal varying from 100 to 300 Gy. Marked damage to the adjacent brainstem was achieved and indeed to the blood vessel wall. But as stated, no case of occlusion was seen. This is not definitive information since it applies to a different species, the follow up was short being from 7 to 200 days. However, it does contain a pointer that even high doses or radiation may damage but will most often not occlude a normal blood vessel.

In 1992 Kihlström et al. published their experimental findings based on irradiating the basilar and middle cerebral arteries of rabbits with the Gamma Knife [104]. They demonstrated that doses of 100 Gy produced a marked radionecrosis which had matured within 6 months. The blood vessels in the region of the necrosis were to all intents and purposes normal.

The effect of GKNS on AVMs was a long time in coming. As one might hope there was very little pathological material available to examine. A review in 1997 described the following phenomena [105]. Nine specimens had been obtained 10 months to 5 years after GKNS. The earliest change was endothelial cell damage followed by progressive thickening of the intimal layer caused by proliferation of smooth-muscle cells that make an extracellular matrix including collagen. Over time cellular degeneration and hyaline transformation occurred. The cellular proliferation and elaboration of collagen by smooth-muscle cells contributes to vessel narrowing and eventually occlusion. Workers in Sheffield and Budapest have extended this work with electron microscopy and histochemical studies. They have built on the important concept that AVM interstices are filled with a stroma not found in normal brain tissue. This group also examined tissue taken from 7 GKNS treated patients [106–110]. After irradiation they found spindle cells in this stroma which were identical with the myofibroblasts normally seen in wound healing. In non irradiated AVM tissue these cells were not found. They hypothesised that since these myofibroblasts cells were actively contractile they could contribute to the occlusion of AVM vessels. Whatever the details of the process, the presence of a stroma in AVMs which is not present in normal blood vessels might contribute to the preferential occlusion of AVM arteries compare with normal arteries. Another factor could contribute, though there is to date no evidence to support this notion. The well known principles of Virchow related to intravascular thrombosis could be relevant. The flow in AVMs is known to be turbulent. Add radiation induced irregularities to the endothelium and a situation exists which would be preferential for the generation of a thrombus. However, it is repeated this is a notion. No means of examining this hypothesis has to date been discovered.

Patient Assessment for Gamma Knife Surgery

The Gamma Knife surgeon will require relevant computer imaging studies from the time of the presenting bleed or other symptom. MRI studies are particularly useful for defining the areas of brain, which have been damaged, following bleeding. This can be most useful information when designing a dose-plan. They may be all that is required of images to make a decision on treatment provided they are high quality and include a 3 D T1 series with and without gadolinium and a fine cut T2 series.

However, for smaller, dubious or complex AVMs, high resolution, high-speed digital subtraction angiography remains the examination of choice in this condition. It is the only examination, which gives resolution of the lesion in time. This is very important, because while the draining veins may be the largest structures associated with a malformation, the decision to treat or not is based on the size of the nidus, which is often only clearly defined on the earliest pictures (Fig. 19.4). It is relatively common to find that the actual size of an AVM, at the time of Gamma Knife dose planning is smaller than was assessed on the pre-treatment films. This is because high-speed angiography is consistently used in this context and a complete angiogram series is available and not a selection of pictures. In other words, it is very helpful if the referring physician sends the whole series. In general, any malformation that is not more than 25 mm in all its diameters will be accepted, though the chance of success would appear to decrease with the larger lesions. Nonetheless, larger lesions than this have been managed with success, though it may be necessary to assess the requirement of some other treatment form in addition to the Gamma Knife, in particular a partial resection. As mentioned above, the decisions to treat or not are best made by a team of different relevant specialists.

Informing the Patient (Family)

If a patient meets the criteria outlined in the previous paragraph then that patient may be accepted for treatment. As a Gamma Knife centre becomes known in its area, over time, more and more patients will be referred from places too far away for a face to face discussion with the patient at the time of acceptance. That will have to wait until the patient's admission. Thus, it is very important that the Gamma Knife centre arranges courses symposia and visits to referring physicians and departments to ensure that all involved in the referral and treatment process are properly informed and also kept up to date.

If surgery is a viable alternative, the patients must be made aware of this. Modern AVM grading systems and microsurgery have resulted in a great improvement in the results of open surgery. The fact is, that for surgically accessible malformations of the size appropriate for Gamma Knife treatment, the mortality is today virtually 0%. However, there is the morbidity and cosmetic defect associated with surgery to be considered. In the author's experience the relevance of these considerations varies considerably from patient to patient. Most appear to prefer the Gamma Knife when offered an alternative. However, the choice is more apparent than real, because the majority of patients referred have malformations which are not appropriate for surgery, usually because of their location.

When the patient is admitted, after the various admission routines have been undertaken it will be necessary for an extended discussion about the reasons for treatment, the expectations of treatment and the risks involved. It will also be necessary to inform the patient about the practical aspects of arrival, pre-medication and frame fixation. In the author's experience that is information best left to the nursing staff.

The patient (relatives in case of children) is/are informed that the treatment is, as has been stated, prophylactic. It is not without risk but it is emphasised that the risks of treatment are less than the risk of the untreated disease. The specifics of risk are explained for the particular location, and in respect of any neurological deficit remaining after a haematoma. They are also informed of the delay between treatment and results and the necessary precautions to be taken during that period.

Day of Treatment

Frame

The frame is applied in the normal way. For users with a C model, the placement of the frame will require special care, since an AVM can be anywhere in the head often with a peripheral location. The application is done according to the principles laid out in the Chap. 9 on frame application.

Imaging

The images include three MR series. A T1 3D with and without contrast and a T2 sequence with fine cuts through the affected region have been the most useful. Some users like an MRA in addition but this does not convey a great advantage. This may convey an advantage but it is necessary to ensure that the format of the MRA is consistent with the Gamma Knife dose planning software. This is not always the case and adjustments may need to be made. In addition to the MR examination it will be necessary to perform a DSA. Tiny AVMs or those on the walls of haematomas or those which have been embolised can be difficult to see on MR images no matter how skilful the technique. Thus for tiny lesions MR constitutes just the vaguest of guidelines. The lesion is really only seen on DSA. The details of these procedures are described in Chap. 11.

The treatment of AVMs differs from all other indications. On the one hand it is a histologically benign condition; on the other hand it has, as described above a most aggressive course. The optimal prescription dose would seem to be 25 Gy but this is adjusted in accordance with the concepts laid out in the "principles of treatment"; section above. A knowledge of normal anatomy will help in avoiding important structures. There is an MR diffusion technique under development called diffusion tensor (DT) magnetic resonance imaging. It permits the mapping of anatomical pathways [111–113]. This it is hoped will improve the precision of this method even further. Once the treatment is over and the frame removed the follow up is explained to the patient.

Follow Up

The patients must be followed until the AVM is declared **angiographically obliterated**. However, repeated angiograms are not necessary today. Ideally a 3D MRI examination with contrast every 6 months will suffice with an angiogram either when the AVM is invisible on the MRI or at 2 years, which ever occurs first. If the lesion persists at 2 years one continues with imaging every 6 month until it either disappears or ceases to shrink. When it disappears DSA is appropriate. If it fails to shrink or stops shrinking re treatment must be considered.

On the other hand, some young active patients find the 2-year wait intolerable and request angiographic control at 1 year. Since the chance of obliteration at 1 year is about 50%, this seems reasonable for this restricted patient group. This particular patient category is also extremely appreciative of being shown consideration and declared fit a year earlier. Many are involved in athletics, where taking advantage of their youth is of course of the essence.

Another, issue here is the fate of the tiny AVM. These are in practice essentially impossible to follow on MRI. Thus, the follow up in a very limited number of cases will continue to be DSA. The frequency of this examination should be determined in association with the wishes of the patient.

It also seems to be a characteristic of many patients with AVMs that they remain nervous, even after the AVM is no longer present. This is perhaps understandable, since they will, even in the best situation have suffered the feeling that they have a bomb in their heads that can explode at any minute, for a minimum of over 12 months. Thus, it is incumbent on the physician to show these unfortunate people the greatest possible patience when they ring up or write again and again for reassurance that they really are fit and that the danger is past. In the author's view referral of AVM patients to a psychiatrist at any stage of their treatment is inappropriate, unless they themselves wish it. It cannot be pathological to be anxious about having an AVM in one's head and thus such anxiety is a more sensibly alleviated by reassurance than therapy. However, if the patient wants therapy that too can be an effective form of reassurance. However, if the patient does not want therapy, insisting on it can greatly undermine that patient's relationship with the physician responsible for treating the AVM.

Another often repeated question from AVM patients is to what extent they must restrict their lives and for how long. This seems to be particularly difficult to answer with any degree of confidence, since the relationship of AVM bleeding to short-term energy consuming pursuits is not well defined. However, the restrictions that are to be followed should logically continue until such time as angiographic obliteration of the AVM has been demonstrated.

It seems to the author unreasonable as well as impossible to restrict the every day activities of children, especially pre-school children. However, for school children, avoidance of contact sports where blows to the head are a part of the game seems sensible. These activities carry an unavoidable risk of increasing the load on the circulation, and in many competitive physical games also increase the risk of direct damage to the head. On the other hand walking, jogging, skating, swimming (providing epilepsy is not a contraindication) and in northern regions skiing over familiar terrain all seem reasonable.

Patients are often concerned about how restricted their lovemaking should be. Again there is no simple answer. Advice along the lines of being gentle rather passionate may be helpful. It seems an unreasonable imposition to forbid lovemaking totally. While it is known that a certain number of bleeds occur during sexual activity a far greater number occur at other times. Moreover, a blood pressure rise occurs every time one passes urine, yet this activity cannot be forbidden. To put the problem in perspective, despite the limitations that must pertain to information derived from a single case, the author would like to mention the experience of a particular patient. This lady had been an air stewardess and suffered a cabin decompression at high altitude. She had subsequently changed work and gone to work with horses. During this period of her life she was both kicked on the head and suffered falls on the head. Her malformation finally bled the day after an altercation with a potential mother-in-law. It is really very difficult to assess the dangers of specific activities and while total inactivity is *probably* the safest thing even this is uncertain. In the meanwhile, total compulsory inactivity, if enforced rigorously against the patient's wishes can have serious psychological effects, which can outlast the successful treatment of the malformation, irrespective of the method of treatment involved. However, the inherent delay involved in Gamma Knife treatment makes the careful evaluation of the advice given to patients even more important than is otherwise the case for those suffering from a cerebral arteriovenous malformation.

Epilepsy

This is a slightly special topic in relation to AVMs. Occasionally one or two fits occur immediately after treatment within 24–48 h. One unfortunate taxi driver required two treatments. He had two fits in his entire life and both occurred roughly 4 weeks after each of his LGK treatments. They had little effect on the management of his general health but they were enough to cause him to lose his license as a taxi driver. This post treatment epilepsy normally requires no antiepileptic medication and occurs only once. However, it is alarming and patients need to be gently warned of the possibility even thought it is a rare occurrence.

Results are usually expressed according to the Engels classification of the outcome for patients after surgical treatment for epilepsy. In general epilepsy control can be expected to improve but this cannot be guaranteed.

Engels Classification [114]

Seizure Free
A) Completely seizure free since surgery
B) Aura only since surgery
C) Some seizures since surgery, but seizure free for at least 2 years
D) Atypical generalized convulsion with antiepileptic drug withdrawal only
Rare Seizures ("almost seizure free")
A) Initially seizure-free but has rare seizures now
B) Rare seizures since surgery
C) More than rare seizures since surgery, but rare seizures for at least 2 years
D) Nocturnal seizures only, which cause no disability
Worthwhile improvement
A) Worthwhile seizure reduction
B) Prolonged seizure-free intervals amounting to greater than half the follow-up period, but not less than 2 years

---

(*continued*)

No worthwhile improvement
A) Significant seizure reduction
B) No appreciable change
C) Seizures worse

The more usual situation is that either the patient has never bled and presented with epilepsy or that the patient had a bleed and epilepsy is part of the post-haemorrhagic clinical picture.

The results of the treatment of the GKNS treatment of AVMs with epilepsy have shown the further characteristics. There is a general tendency to improvement [60, 115, 116] with small size and non aggressive pre treatment epilepsy being positive factors [116]. An occasional case has been reported where epilepsy got worse but this is exceptional [117].

Treatment Failure

In addition to complications there is another important unwanted result of treatment and that is treatment failure. Sometimes, the reasons are unavoidable and sometimes not. There is no published series in which all the AVMs have been obliterated. As outlined above, the obliteration rate is determined by a number of AVM characteristics of which the most important are age, volume and location. There is plenty of evidence cited above that the obliteration rate is higher in children. The volume is crucial because it leads to a reduction in dose and as we know a lower dose is associated with a lower obliteration rate. Finally, the AVM location is crucial because again, deep lying AVMs are treated with a lower dose to avoid damage to neighbouring structures. These problems are inherent in the method, unavoidable and while different assessment techniques can to some extent quantify the problems, no solution is currently in sight. Thus, large AVMs and AVMs near crucial structures will receive a lower prescription dose to reduce the risk of complications and the obliteration rate is thus lower.

Nonetheless, there is an avoidable cause of treatment failure. This has been recognised from the earliest days. The Pittsburgh group have written a nice analysis [42]. The problem is that incorrect target definition can lead to part of the AVM receiving an inadequate dose. Six explanations of this error are given. They are classified as "in field" or "out of field" according to the location of the error in relation to the prior delivered prescription dose.

Source of error	In field/out of field
Incomplete cerebral angiography thus missing some nidus	Out of field
Inclusion of unnecessary tissue leading to a larger volume than necessary and thus a lower dose. Large feeding and draining vessels can contribute to this error.	In field
Underestimation of the real nidus because a part of it was hidden by a large draining vein	Out of field
Recanalisation after earlier embolisation	Out of field
Reappearance of compressed nidus vessels after resolution of prior haematoma	In field/out of field
No definitive factors perhaps due to "radiobiological resistance".	In field

It might be expected the out of field tissue may require a slightly higher dose to assure obliteration, since the in field tissue has received on the whole a higher dose at the first treatment and will thus require less a second time round. On the whole the evidence indicated a trend in this direction but nothing that would mean that at present the location of the error should lead to practical changes in the choice or dose given to residual tissue at a retreatment.

A larger problem is the association of an AVM with a haematoma. This can compress the AVM giving a false impression of its size and even its precise location. A latent interval should be allowed of at least three months in which the haematoma can resorb and the AVM regain its normal size and position [37, 82, 118, 119]. This, can be very distressing for anxious patients, but treating too quickly with consequent treatment failure can lead to far more profound delays in the future. However, there is evidence to suggest that the treatment should take place within 6 months of the bleed [118]. There is finally the odd phenomenon of re-bleeding after obliteration has been recorded on DSA as mentioned above.

Repeated Treatment

Repeated treatments are considered here since they are by definition only relevant when primary treatment has failed. Treatments may be repeated in one of two specific situations. The first to be considered in this section is a repeat of a failed treatment. In earlier days it was thought that obliteration would be completed within 2 years. It is now known that it may take considerably longer [18, 32, 33, 55, 62, 120, 121].Thus, so long as an AVM is shrinking on MR or occasionally also on DSA, it is suggested there is no need to treat again. It is in cases where shrinkage stops or where no shrinkage of any kind has been observed within 2 years, that retreatment may be considered.

If treatment fails the first time round a repeat GKNS can often be undertaken. The risks and success rates are quite acceptable [11, 20, 29, 31, 40, 42, 45, 52, 59, 61, 63, 65, 79, 119, 122, 123]. Some authors recorded an increased complication rate [11, 31] but many did not. This is not a situation where other treatments are likely to be relevant since the Gamma Knife is often the last link in the chain of referral for patients whom nobody else wants to treat.

Large AVMs

Although GKNS began as a treatment of AVMs small enough to be included in Spetzler and Martin Grade 1 lesions, there has been a slowly growing body of work concerning the treatment of larger lesions. In principle there are two ways to achieve this aim. One is to treat the whole volume with repeated lower doses, which is a special kind of fractionation The other method is to treat a larger lesion in several sessions with each session treating a specific volume and giving it an effective dose [18, 23, 27, 29, 37, 48, 49, 56–59, 64, 123, 124]. At the next session the same procedure is undertaken for a second volume. This continues at 6 monthly intervals until the entire AVM is treated. The final result of this method is not yet known. However, obliteration rates of vary between 5 and 50–60% for these larger lesions. The information is a little imprecise because there is no cohesion between the dose limits, groupings, prescription doses and locations of the lesions in the various series depicting the treatment of larger AVMs. However, one comes away with the impression that it is possible to offer treatment for lesions in excess of 12 cm^3 with fairly adequate guidelines in the literature. The best results to date have come from a study from the Mayo Clinic where the dose guidelines were as shown in the table below.

Diameter	Volume	Prescription dose
≤2 cm	≤4.2 cm^3	20 Gy
2.1–3 cm	>4.2–14.1 cm^3	18 Gy
>3 cm	>14.1 cm^3	16 Gy

The dose for the lower volumes produced an obliteration rate of about 72% which is low and that dose could well be raised. However, the doses to the middle and higher volumes were associated with an obliteration rate of over 70% with very few complications and these doses are perhaps most appropriate for use as a guideline at present.

Another method of coping with larger volumes is described by another group. This is from Karlsson et al. [30]. The study was designed to treat patients with AVMs with a volume exceeding 9 cm^3 with 15 Gy on the expectation 50% of them would shrink. Then after 3–4 years any residual AVM could be treated again with the same dose, and so on until the AVM had occluded or the accumulated risk of further treatment was considered unacceptable. The treatment achieved an overall occlusion rate of 68% which is high. The complication rate was low and in the context seems acceptable. However, the study design was not tidy and the major disadvantage of this way of treatment is that it necessarily takes a very long time to complete compared with the method of treating different volumes with higher doses as outlined above.

The information about larger AVMs suggests that the Gamma Knife if used cautiously may indeed have a benefit for some larger lesions. At the present the optimal dose and maximum volume that may be treated are not as yet clearly defined. The point to remember is that while GKNS for larger lesions may not be perceived as on optimal treatment, it nonetheless provides hope of clinical improvement for a subgroup of these patients for whom otherwise there is no therapeutic alternative. In other words it can provide a limited benefit.

Combined Treatments

The alternative treatments to GKNS are clearly microsurgery or embolisation. The practice of microsurgery lies outside the scope of this book. However, it is an excellent therapy and its limitations are still largely described within the framework of the Spetzler-Martin grading system. The interested reader is encouraged to search the literature and the library for more detailed information. It is perceived as unavoidable that for a disease as complex and protean as the cerebral arteriovenous malformation that treatment can not be left in the hand of a single individual or even a single speciality. These lesions need to be managed with a team whose members must include a neurosurgeon performing microsurgery on AVMs, a neurosurgeon treating AVMs with the Gamma Knife, a neuroradiologist, a neurologist and a nurse. Other specialities such as ophthalmology can be consulted as required. An oncologist will also be involved in the planning of treatment of those patients who are referred for Gamma Knife treatment.

The role of the neuroradiologist is twofold. This expertise is vital for the treatment of AVMs in the Gamma Knife since DSA pictures are an essential component of the images used during dose planning. Mention in more detail is found in Chap. 11. However, a neuroradiologist may also be an interventionist with the ability to attempt to embolise AVMs. For the surgeon an embolised AVM may be a lot less aggressive during surgery making an operation easier. There is plenty of evidence that respected surgeons find this useful [125, 126]. For the Gamma Knife user the role of embolisation as part of a combined treatment would be to reduce the volume of an AVM thus making it easier to treat. The notion is fine in principle but falls somewhat short in practice.

Endovascular Treatment

The literature on embolisation is extensive and requires special knowledge. The interventionist has a more detailed knowledge of the intracranial vascular anatomy than other specialities. This knowledge is sufficient for the specialist to view the blood vessels from any angle and not from the standard directions to which we others are accustomed. A detailed analysis of this technique is not appropriate for this book. However, there are a number of principles with which the reader should be familiar. The advances in endovascular treatments have depended on improving imaging, improving catheters and improving embolisation materials.

Current imaging is performed using Digital Subtraction Angiography (DSA) which permits digital removal of unwanted parts of an image. This enables the production of images with a much clearer view of the arterial tree than analogue images could achieve. In addition, the images are produced instantly without delay for development. The radiologist can view the images in real time and thus is able to adjust the position of the catheter for delivery of embolic material in just the right place.

Today, the most commonly used catheter is inserted into the femoral artery in the groin. It is made of polyethylene, which is clearly seen on images and it is inserted into position using a flexible guide wire. The catheters are fine enough today to be placed selectively in AVM feeding arteries.

There have been various materials used for embolisation but today there are basically two in common use [127]. The first is *n*-butylcyanoacrylate (NBCA) mixed with the oily dye Lipiodol making it visible on the images. The material is adhesive. The other agent is and ethylene vinyl alcohol copolymer called Onyx which is non adhesive. This property facilitates multiple injections.

There are reports of how embolisation can reduce the volume of AVMs. However, the occlusion rate is reported between 5 and 15% [127, 128]. Moreover, this applies only to a selected population of AVMs with one or at most two feeding arteries. It is accepted that its role is at present adjuvant [127]. The technique is popular prior to surgery since it can reduce the flow through an AVM and make the surgery less exciting. It is also suggested by the proponents of embolisation that it can reduce the volume of AVMs making them easier to treat with radiosurgery [126, 127, 129, 130]. Those who perform GKNS are less certain of this notional benefit and indeed consider that embolisation may have a negative effect on radiosurgery induced obliteration [13, 131]. There is also a LINAC stereotactic radiosurgery centre which voices similar concerns [132]. The present author from his own experience has seen that it is commoner for embolisation to thin out the blood flow through an AVM rather than to reduce its volume. Moreover, the embolisation material can obscure the definition of the remaining nidus. Finally, there is the very real problem of recanalisation of vessels closed by embolisation [37, 119, 133].

There is an additional cause for concern. As indicated embolisation has a limited effect on obliterating an AVM. However, while radiosurgery is minimally invasive, embolisation has a significant morbidity and in unfortunate cases a mortality. In a series of 168 patients there were 11 clinically significant complications, including haemorrhage, aphasia, hemiparesis, visual field defect and changes in mental changes [128]. This is an outstanding paper from the Harvard Medical School with much better results than most. This is illustrated by table of the results at other centres included in the paper. The table includes series published between 2002 and 2004. Here the morbidity ranges between 10 and 22% and mortality is also reported.

Taking all the uncertainties and risks associated with the use of embolisation for the treatment of AVMs it is not possible to state with confidence what the role of this treatment is at present. The current author is convinced of the risks and less convinced of the benefits, though the individual practitioner will have to make his/her own mind up.

Gamma Knife for Cerebral Cavernous Malformations

Cavernous haemangiomas, otherwise known as cavernomas or cavernous malformations (CMs) are one of the diagnoses that are included in the abbreviation AOVM. This stands for Angiographically Occult Vascular Malformation. CMs consist of cavernous, sinusoidal vascular spaces, lined with venous endothelium and without cerebral parenchyma in the interstices. They have been the subject of much discussion and have proven to be complex, variable and unpredictable. In the course of the last few years some degree of clarity has started to emerge. To take a view on whether GKNS is an appropriate treatment for these lesions it is necessary to attempt to clarify the concepts surrounding them. A word about the interstices of the CM may be useful. The AVM has a stroma between its vessels and that stroma maybe important in the process of obliteration after GKNS. It is important to remember that CMs have no brain or stroma in their interstices.

Natural History

Clinical Material

The common clinical presentations are epilepsy, bleeding, headache, neurological deficit and incidental finding. The distribution of these presentations varies between different clinical materials. Thus, in two series obtained by a retrospective review of MR images the commonest presentation was epilepsy [134, 135] In two other materials the patients were referred to a treatment unit. In both these series haemorrhage was the commonest presentation [136, 137]. Thus, the method of acquiring patient material for analysis has a noteworthy effect on the kind of patients being analysed.

What is a Bleed?

This can be one of two things. It can be a bleed within the volume of a CM, which is common [138]. It can also be an overt external or intraparenchymal bleed, which is less common. Not all papers are clear over this distinction in the presentation of the material being analysed. Moreover, while many papers insist on imaging as the basis for a diagnosis of a bleed [134–137, 139, 140] not all papers require this confirmation being content with a clinical ictus at least in some cases [141, 142]. Yet it is known that a clinical ictus can occur in the absence of imaging changes [139, 143, 144].

Location

The brainstem is the most dangerous location for CMs associated with the worst results and the greatest challenges to the physician. It could be said that brainstem CMs should be considered separately from other locations as the natural history and risks of therapy are different [96, 139, 140, 145, 146]. Moreover, there is a tendency for supratentorial lesions to have a greater chance for developing epilepsy.

Bleeding Rate and Re-bleeding Rate

These rates vary greatly between different articles. This is not surprising if one remembers variations in patient acquisition as outlined above. These rates are also expressed in different ways. There is a bleeding rate calculated on the basis that the patient has had the CM all his/her life. There is the re-bleeding rate calculated on the same basis. On the other hand it may be calculated from the first bleed giving a much higher value. Some writers use the first bleed as a starting date but only count the re-bleeding rate for bleeds occurring after the first bleed obtaining a lower result. It is necessary to be clear which measure is being used in a given paper. The table below indicates the recorded bleeding rates before and after radiosurgery, recorded as re-bleeds percent per year. Apart from Aman-Hajani the post radiosurgery rates are quite similar. Kondziolka et al.'s low bleeding rate in the untreated patients is a result of half the patients in that series had never bled. Nonetheless, the table would seem to support the notion that there is an improvement in bleeding rate after radiosurgery. We shall return to this concept a little lower down.

Changes in Size

Changes in size are crucial to an analysis of the effects of radiosurgery. It is generally assumed that shrinkage may be the result of treatment or resorption of a haematoma. However, the observations of Clatterbuck et al. [147] suggest that this may be an over simplification. They recorded changes in CM volume unrelated either treatment or bleeding which they describe as part of the dynamic natural history of the lesions.

Bleeding and Non-bleeding Lesions

This is one area where there seems to be a degree of general agreement. The lesions which bleed are different in terms of natural history and risk compared with those that don't [136, 137, 148–150]. There is ultrastructural evidence that their endothelium has vacuoles and fewer tight junctions between cells promoting the possibility of bleeding. It should be remembered that the pressure inside CMs is not high as in the veins of AVMs so there is less of a pressure for bleeding. Yet they do bleed and now there is the beginning of an understanding about why some bleed and some don't [150]. At all events it is the bleeding lesions which represent the biggest threat to life and function.

Clustering of Bleeding

A recent paper has most interestingly showed that CM bleeds are not evenly distributed over time [151]. They occur in clusters with a tendency to become less and less frequent after a latent period of frequent bleeds lasting about 2 years.

Epilepsy

Epilepsy in some patients can be a major problem and may also be medical therapy resistant. In multiple lesions it can be difficult to know which lesion is responsible for the seizures. CMs with epilepsy seldom bleed. Epilepsy is more commonly present in patients under 40 years of age [152]. It is also been shown that mesial temporal epilepsy is harder to cope with [153, 154] presumably because of the more complex and extensive epileptic focus. Most lesions are thought to have epileptogenesis close to the lesion, maybe related to the deposition of the epileptogenic ferric ions in haemosiderin around a CM.

	Pre-treatment	Re-bleed percent per year after radiosurgery	
	Re-bleed Since first bleed (per cent per year)	≤2 years	>2 years
Aman Hajani et al. [155]	17.4%	22.4%	4.5%
Kondziolka et al. [116]	32.0%	8.8%	1.1%
Hasegawa et al. [148]	33.9%	12.9%	0.76%
Aiba et al. [136]	22.9%	Not Part of these	
Porter et al. [152]	30%	**Reference** studies	
Liu et al. [141]	Not included in this study	10.3%	3.3%
Kondziolka	4.5%[a]	Not included in this study	

[a]This low figure relates to a material were only half the patients had bled. The other papers deal with bleeding patients only

Factors Affecting Outcome

CMs are solitary or multiple. They can be familial or non familial. It would seem bleeding is more aggressive with multiple lesions [156]. However, neurological deficit is associated mainly with either repeat bleeding [135, 137, 150, 152], or an infratentorial location [135, 141, 152, 156, 157]. Other factors such as patient age, sex, and the presence of venous anomalies are reported variously making assessment difficult.

Post Irradiation CMs

It is known that new CMs may arise after radiotherapy [158]. This is almost exclusively a phenomenon limited to fairly young children. While of interest for general understanding of CMs it is not that important a finding in the present context.

Summary of Relevant Natural History

1. CMs are solitary or multiple. They can be familial or non familial.
2. Bleeding CMs are a more dangerous subgroup
3. Location is decisive in terms of risk and decision making

4. Bleeding occurs in clusters with spontaneous improvement
5. CM volume may remain unchanged, increase or decrease spontaneously
6. Some changes in volume may be related to haemorrhages and their resorption but not all
7. An acute clinical ictus my be due to a bleed but it may not
8. The results of published studies in relation to risk and bleeding rates are affected by the inclusion criteria for that study.

Therapy of CMs

Basically there are three therapeutic alternatives; observation, surgery or radio-surgery. The majority of lesions as described in the retrospectively acquired patients from MRI review do not have bleeding and nor do they have progressive neurological deficit. For these patients clinical review will suffice. The groups of patients who require active treatment are those with progressively increasing neurological deficit, usually thought to be associated with repeated bleeds and medically uncontrolled epilepsy. The epilepsy is the lesser problem and will be considered first.

Yoon et al. have proposed a classification of CMs based on MR appearances and suggested how this grading system can help in making decisions about therapy.

Type	MRI findings	Pathology
I	T1: Hyperintense core T2: hyper- or hypointense core with surroundings hypointense	Subacute haemorrhage, surrounded by a rim of haemosiderin-stained macrophages and gliotic brain
II	T1 reticulated mixed signal core T2: reticulated mixed signal core with surrounding hypointense rim	Loculated areas of haemorrhage and thrombosis of varying age, surrounded by gliotic, haemosiderin stained brain; in large lesions, areas of calcification may be seen
III	T1: iso- or hypointense T2: hypointense with a hypointense rim that magnifies the size of the lesion GE: hypointense with greater magnification than T	Chronic resolved haemorrhage, with haemosiderin staining within and around the lesion
IV	T1: poorly seen or not visualized at all T2: poorly seen or not visualized at all – GE: punctate hypointense lesions	May be telangieactasia

Yoon et al.'s study gave the following results.

Type	No. CMs	MR characteristics	Re-bleeds
I	17	Subacute haemorrhage	No Re-bleed
II	23	Mixture of subacute and chronic haemorrhage	6 Re-bleeds
III	10	Area of haemosiderin with small central core	2 Re-bleeds
IV	11	Area of haemosiderin deposition without central core	No Re-bleed

On the basis of these findings Yoon et al. recommended limiting intervention treatments to Types II and III and following types I and IV conservatively.

Treatment of CM Associated Epilepsy

There is one classic paper on this topic and it suggests that GKNS does improve the control of CM related epilepsy [154]. There were two factors that had a negative effect on the success of GKNS treatment of this epilepsy. A mesial temporal location and complex partial seizures did less well. The authors state that a controlled prospective study was required to test the relevance of GKNS vis a vis microsurgery. To date that study has not been done. Apart from the above mentioned multi centre study there are remarks on the control of epilepsy following GKNS for CMs in other studies with improvement registered [159] and also following proton radiosurgery [155]. However, only surgery can remove the epileptogenic ferric ion containing haemosiderin around a CM [150, 153]. Thus, until a randomised trial is completed the role of GKNS remains uncertain, though it could be tempting to try it with multiple CMs where the source of the epilepsy is uncertain. In conclusion, it is perhaps correct to mention that the comments in "Neurosurgery" about the multicentre study [154] were almost all in favour of microsurgery for treatment resistant epilepsy in association with a CM.

Treatment of CM Associated with Haemorrhage

This is of course the key issue. Can GKNS protect a patient from repeated bleeds from a CM. The biggest problem is that CMs are not seen on angiography and the changes on MRI do not disappear. Thus there is no treatment end point similar to the occlusion of AVMs to demonstrate therapeutic success. The only relevant measure is a reduction of the bleeding/re-bleeding rate. To record this takes time and with the variable behaviour of CMs there is room for a variety of interpretations of findings as shown in the table below.

Paper	Mean prescription dose	Number in series	Radiation induced permanent neurological deficit	Re-bleed rate	Assessment
Amin-Hajani et al. [155]	16.5 Gy	98	(3% mortality) 16%	Reduced	Uncertain about GKNS
Kim et al. [159]	14.5 Gy	42	7.1%	Reduced	In favour of GKNS
Liscak et al. [160]	16 Gy	112	4.5%	No change[a]	In favour of GKNS
Hasegawa et al. [148]	16.2 Gy	82	7.3%	Reduced	In favour of GKNS
Kondziolka et al. [149]	16 Gy	47	8.5%	Reduced	In favour of GKNS

(*continued*)

Paper	Mean prescription dose	Number in series	Radiation induced permanent neurological deficit	Re-bleed rate	Assessment
Kim et al. [161]	16.1 Gy	22	9.1%	Reduced	Uncertain about GKNS
Karlsson et al. [143]	18 Gy	23	21.7%	No change	Against GKNS for CM
Pollock et al. [101]	18 Gy	17	41%[a]	Reduced after delay	Doubts GKNS for CM
Seo et al. [162] Stopped using GKNS	15.3 Gy	9	11%	Inadequate	Protection

[a]This series contained 53 patients of 112 who had not bled. Not really comparable with other series where majority had bled

It would seem from this table that a number of workers believe that GKNS reduces the re-bleeding rate from CMs. However, the literature describes a drop in re-bleeding only after 2 years. Another finding illustrated by the table is that it would appear that a prescription dose of 18 Gy is too high and increases the chance of radiation induced permanent neurological deficit. However, the assessments are split more or less evenly concerning the value of GKNS for this condition. The table above deals with radiosurgery only. There is another source of opinion and that is the comments made by surgeons who treat this condition with open surgery. This brings us to the crux of the problem.

A recent study from the experienced group in Taipei specifically attempted to compare the results of GKNS with a craniotomy [163]. This series treated the simpler symptomatic solitary supratentorial lesions. The aim was to see which treatment method was the most effective and under what circumstances. Sixteen were treated with craniotomy and 30 with GKNS. Surgery was significantly better than GKNS at controlling epilepsy ($p < 0.002$). Re-bleeding was slightly better with surgery too though that difference was not significant. The authors concluded that "In the clinical management of solitary supratentorial CM, craniotomy for lesionectomy resulted in better seizure control and re-bleeding avoidance than GKNS."

More Dangerous CMs

It follows from what has been written above that far from all CMs are dangerous. The condition is admittedly protean but the major problem relates to a particular location. The dangerous CMs lie deep in the basal ganglia and the brainstem. The proponents of GKNS for the treatment of these lesions refer to poor surgical results in these locations to justify the use of GKNS in the place of surgery. However, review of the writings of the surgeons shows a slightly different picture.

The Harvard Medical school group admittedly compare microsurgery and radiosurgery using protons with a Bragg Peak technique. Much of the studies were carried out at an earlier time when images and microsurgery were less advanced. Even so, in a centre where physicians were involved in both forms of treatment they came down in favour of microsurgery. They pointed out that patients with more severe pre-operative neurological deficits had worse results [155, 157]. The poorest results were in lesions in the brainstem.

Samii's group in Hannover, also achieved better results with patients who were in a better clinical condition prior to surgery [140]. The results are expressed in relation to the Karnowsky Performance Score. This material deals exclusively with brain stem CMs. Surgery was only indicated if there had been one or more serious bleed. There were 36 patients in this material. All operations were delayed until the acute effects of a haemorrhage had stabilised. There was no mortality. A central point in this paper is that after brain stem haemorrhage only around 14% of patients returned to a normal neurological status prior to surgery. A persisting neurological deficit after treatment was more related to the pre-operative condition than to complications arising from the surgery.

The Barrow Neurological Institute has also published probably the most extensive study on the surgery of CMs and again have concentrated on the most difficult lesions; those in the brain stem [142, 146]. In the earlier paper [146] 24 patients were assessed with CMs in the brainstem. Eight were advised surgery was not appropriate and one of these died. Sixteen were operated without mortality. One patient had permanent surgical morbidity in the form of recurrent symptoms associated with regrowth of her CM. The more recent paper [142] deals with 100 patients with brain stem CMs. Eighty six were operated. The authors state specifically that the latency between radiosurgery and protection from haemorrhage is unacceptable. The authors also point out that the term inoperable is often applied to deep seated CMs by colleagues who are not neurosurgeons. In conclusion they point out that radiosurgery does not remove these lesions.

Conclusions About CMs

- With regard to epilepsy, there is currently not great support for the use of GKNS for CM induced epilepsy with even experienced users like Dr. Kondziolka preferring microsurgery [164].
- Clustering of bleeds has been recorded as a natural phenomenon.
- It is important that those planning treatment for CMs be constantly aware that it is only the significant minority in the basal ganglia and especially the brain stem are the source of problems in treatment. These lesions are capable both of being lethal and of producing the severest morbidity. In this situation an aggressive approach is justified. In this context the danger of modern microsurgery seems to

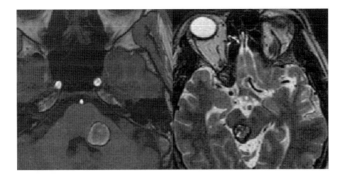

Fig. 19.8 In each image a white arrow indicates the CM. The one of the left is a type I and it did not bleed. The one on the right is a type II and it suffered bleeding

have been exaggerated not least by non-neurosurgeon referring physicians. The results mentioned in these papers are superior to the results achieved with GKNS [140, 142]. These two series relate the management in a decent number of the most severe cases. Also protection from haemorrhage after radical surgery comes immediately.

- If there is a genuine protection from haemorrhage following GKNS the 2-year delay before it comes into effect is worrying.
- Finally, there is the worry about ARE. It would seem that these are less with lower doses but on the other hand, if GKNS is effective for CMs reducing the dose may affect the efficiency of the treatment.

Like every one else the author is swayed by his own personal experience: in this instance in respect of CM patients treated at the Gamma Knife Center, Cairo.

Cairo Patients

The findings were in agreement with those of Yoon et al. [165] cited above, in respect of CM type. There were 16 patients and three were type I of whom none had a re-bleed. There were 12 with type II and of these four re-bled. There was one type III which did not re-bleed. Figure 19.8 shows a type I and type II from our series. The mean and median dose was 14 Gy. Twenty five percent of this little series had clinically significant re-bleeds. Three further patients (18.75%) had symptomatically significant ARE. After the treatment of 16 patients the inadequate protection from haemorrhage together with the clinically expressed complications convinced us to cease treating patients with CMs.

In view of all this uncertainty in the face of such a formidable lesion as a deep sitting, bleeding CM, this author believes that CM treatment with GKNS should be restricted to formally structured scientific studies and should not be on offer on a routine clinical basis.

Gamma Knife for Dural Arteriovenous Fistulae

Over the last 10 years, a small number of experienced departments have treated dural arteriovenous fistulae with the Gamma Knife. Their results can be tabulated as follows.

Paper	Location	Number	Obliteration	
			Total	Partial
Pan et al. [121]	Taipei	20	58%	16%
O'Leary et al. [166]	Sheffield	17	10/17	2/17
Koebbe et al. [167]	Pittsburgh	18	12/18	4/18
Söderman et al. [168]	Stockholm	49	68%	24%

This table would indicate that GKNS is an effective treatment for dural arteriovenous fistulae with a good occlusion rate. Pan et al. make the crucial point that excellent images including MRI, time of flight MRA and stereotactic angiography need to be combined for excellent results. It is suggested this treatment should only be attempted in a centre with top quality neuro-radiological competence. The studies quoted also recall a very useful clinical improvement. However, the current place of GKNS treatment is as an adjunct to surgery and embolisation which are the mainstay. Its final role remains to be determined.

Cerebral Developmental Venous Anomalies

Venous vascular malformations, have also been known as venous angiomas or, more properly, developmental venous anomalies (DVAs). They represent congenital anatomically variant pathways in the normal venous drainage of an area of the brain. Once thought to be rare, they are now considered to be the most common vascular malformation in the CNS occurring [169]. They may occur in as many as 2% of the population. Although for many years DVAs were commonly called venous angiomas, the newer term DVA has been recommended as more appropriate because the involved vessels are not abnormally formed, but apparently merely dilated. (They are still called venous angiomas on the MESH database which is a pity). The majority of DVAs are found incidentally and never cause symptoms, although there are isolated reports of patients with syndromes attributed to DVAs such as haemorrhage or thrombosis. The BNI group specified that in their operative material for CMs all patients had an associated DVA. They also emphasised the importance of not touching them. Thus while there are a few cases of patients with DVAs receiving GKNS, it was never helpful and is now avoided as inappropriate [170–172].

References

1. Hongo K, Koike G, Isobe M, Watabe T, Morota N, Nakagawa H. Surgical resection of cerebral arteriovenous malformation combined with pre-operative embolisation. J Clin Neurosci **7(Suppl 1)**: 88–91; 2000
2. Larsson B. Radiobiological fundamentals in radiosurgery. in Radiosurgery: Baseline and Trends. eds Steiner L et al. Raven Press, New York: pp 3–14; 1992
3. Pellettieri L, Carlsson CA, Grevsten S, Norlén G, Uhlemann C. Surgical versus conservative treatment of intracranial arteriovenous malformations: a study in surgical decision-making. Acta Neurochir Suppl (Wien) **29**: 1–86; 1979
4. Jokura H, Kawagishi J, Sugai K, Akabane A, Boku N, Takahashi K. Gamma knife radiosurgery for arteriovenous malformations: the Furukawa experience. Prog Neurol Surg **22**: 20–30; 2009
5. Kasliwal MK, Kale SS, Gupta A, Kiran NA, Sharma MS, Agrawal D, Sharma BS, Mahapatra AK. Does hemorrhagic presentation in cerebral arteriovenous malformations affect obliteration rate after gamma knife radiosurgery? Clin Neurol Neurosurg **110(8)**: 804–809; 2008
6. Redeskop GJ, Elisevich KV, Gaspar LE, Wiese KP, Drake CG. Conventional radiation therpay of intracranial arteriovenous malformations: long term results. J Neurosurg **78**: 413–422; 1993
7. Tognetti F, Andreoli A, Cuscini A, Testa C. Successful management of an intracranial arteriovenous malformation by conventional irradiation. J Neurosurg **63(2)**: 193–195; 1985
8. Hadjipanayis CG, Levy EI, Niranjan A, Firlik AD, Kondziolka D, Flickinger JC, Lunsford LD. Stereotactic radiosurgery for motor cortex region arteriovenous malformations. Neurosurgery **48(1)**: 70–76; 2001
9. Liscak R, Vladyka V, Simonova G, Urgosik D, Novotny J Jr, Janouskova L, Vymazal J. Arteriovenous malformations after Leksell gamma knife radiosurgery: rate of obliteration and complications. Neurosurgery **60**: 1005–1014; 2007
10. Mizoi K, Jokura H, Yoshimoto T, Takahashi A, Ezura M, Kinouchi H, Nagamine Y, Boku N. Multimodality treatment for large and critically located arteriovenous malformations. Neurol Med Chir (Tokyo) **38(Suppl)**: 186–192; 1998
11. Agid R, Terbrugge K, Rodesch G, Andersson T, Soderman M. Management strategies for anterior cranial fossa (ethmoidal) dural arteriovenous fistulas with an emphasis on endovascular treatment. J Neurosurg **110(1)**: 79–84; 2009
12. Awad I, Jabbour P. Cerebral cavernous malformations and epilepsy. Neurosurg Focus **21(1)**: e7; 2006
13. Barker FG II, Amin-Hanjani S, Butler WE, Lyons S, Ojemann RG, Chapman PH, Ogilvy CS. Temporal clustering of haemorrhages from untreated cavernous malformations of the central nervous system. Neurosurgery **49(1)**: 15–25; 2001
14. Bristol RE, Albuquerque FC, McDoufall CG. The evolution of endovascular treatment for intracranial malformations. Neurosurg Focus **20(6)**: E6; 2006
15. Chang JH, Chang JW, Park YG, Chung SS. Factors related to complete occlusion of arteriovenous malformations after gamma knife radiosurgery. J Neurosurg **93(Suppl 3)**: 96–101; 2000
16. Cheong WY, Tan KP. Cerebral venous angioma – a misnomer? Ann Acad Med Singapore **22** (**5**): 736–741; 1993
17. Chung WY, Shiau CY, Wu HM, Liu KD, Guo WY, Wang LW, Pan DH. Staged radiosurgery for extra-large cerebral arteriovenous malformations: method, implementation, and results. J Neurosurg **109(Suppl)**: 65–72; 2008
18. Cohen-Gadol AA, Pollock BE. Radiosurgery for arteriovenous malformations in children. J Neurosurg **104(6 Suppl)**: 388–391; 2006
19. Del Curling O Jr, Kelly DL Jr, Elster AD, Craven TE. An analysis of the natural history of cavernous angiomas. J Neurosurg **75(5)**: 702–708; 1991

20. Engel J Jr. Outcome with respect to seizures. in Surgical Treatment of the Epilepsies. ed Engel J. Raven Press, New York: pp 553–571; 1987
21. Flickinger JC, Kondziolka D, Pollock BE, Maitz AH, Lunsford LD. Analysis of neurological sequelae from radiosurgery of arteriovenous malformations: how location affects outcome. Int J Radiat Oncol Biol Phys **40(7)**: 274–278; 1998
22. Flickinger JC. The integrated logistic formula and prediction of complications from radiosurgery. Int J Radiat Oncol Biol Phys **17**: 879–885; 1989
23. Hasegawa T, McInerney J, Kondziolka D, Lee JY, Flickinger JC, Lunsford LD. Long-term results after stereotactic radiosurgery for patients with cavernous malformations. Neurosurgery **50(6)**: 1190–1197; 2002
24. Hernesniemi J, Dashti R, Juvela S, Väärt K, Niemelä M, Laakso A. Natural History of Brain Arteriovenous Malformations A Longterm follow up study of risk of haemorrhage in 238 patients. Neurosurgery **63(5)**: 823–831; 2008
25. Husain AM, Mendez M, Friedman AH. Intractable epilepsy following radiosurgery for arteriovenous malformation. J Neurosurg **95(5)**: 888–892; 2001
26. Izawa M, Chernov M, Hayashi M, Iseki H, Hori T, Takakura K. Combined management of intracranial arteriovenous malformations with embolization and gamma knife radiosurgery: comparative evaluation of the long-term results. Surg Neurol **71(1)**: 43–52; 2009
27. Izawa M, Hayashi M, Chernov M, Nakaya K, Ochiai T, Murata N, Takasu Y, Kubo O, Hori T, Takakura K. Long-term complications after gamma knife surgery for arteriovenous malformations. J Neurosurg **102(Suppl)**: 34–37; 2005
28. Johnson RT. Radiotherapy of cerebral angiomas, with a note on some problems in diagnosis. in Cerebral Angiomas. Advances in Diagnosis and Therapy. eds Pia HW, Gleave JRW, Grote E, et al. Springer-Verlag, Berlin, Heidelberg, New York: pp 256–266; 1975
29. Karlsson B, Jokura H, Yamamoto M, Soderman M, Lax I. Is repeated radiosurgery an alternative to staged radiosurgery for very large brain arteriovenous malformations? J Neurosurg **107**: 740–744; 2007
30. Karlsson B, Kihlstrom L, Lindquist C, Ericson K, Steiner L. Radiosurgery for cavernous malformations. J Neurosurg 88(2): 293–297; 1998
31. Karlsson B, Lax I, Soderman M. Risk for haemorrhage during the 2-year latency period following gamma knife radiosurgery for arteriovenous malformations. Int J Radiat Oncol Biol Phys **49(4)**: 1045–1051; 2001
32. Karlsson B, Lindqvist M, Blomgren H, Wan-Yeo G, Soderman M, Lax I, Yamamoto M, Bailes J. Long-term results after fractionated radiation therapy for large brain arteriovenous malformations. Neurosurgery **57(1)**: 42–49; 2005
33. Kemeny AA, Dias PS, Forster DM. Results of stereotactic radiosurgery of arteriovenous malformations: an analysis of 52 cases. J Neurol Neurosurg Psychiatry **52(5)**: 554–558; 1989
34. Kobayashi T, Tanaka T, Kida Y, Oyama H, Niwa M, Maesawa S. Gamma knife treatment of AVM of the basal ganglia and thalamus. No To Shinkei **48(4)**: 351–356; 1996
35. Koebbe CJ, Singhal D, Sheehan J, Flickinger JC, Horowitz M, Kondziolka D, Lunsford LD. Radiosurgery for dural arteriovenous fistulas. Surg Neurol **64(5)**: 392–398; 2005
36. Kurita H, Kawamoto S, Suzuki I, Sasaki T, Tago M, Terahara A, Kirino T. Control of epilepsy associated with cerebral arteriovenous malformations after radiosurgery. J Neurol Neurosurg Psychiatry **65(5)**: 648–655; 1998
37. Laakso A, Seppänen J, Juvela A, Väärt K, Niemelä M, Sankila M, Hernesniemi JA. Long-term excess Mortality in 623 patients with brain arteriovenous malformations. Neurosurgery **63(2)**: 244–255; 2008
38. Lim YJ, Lee CY, Koh JS, Kim TS, Kim GK, Rhee BA. Seizure control of Gamma Knife radiosurgery for non-hemorrhagic arteriovenous malformations. Acta Neurochir Suppl **99**: 97–101; 2006
39. Lindquist C, Guo WY, Karlsson B, Steiner L. Radiosurgery for venous angiomas. J Neurosurg **78(4)**: 531–536; 1993

40. Liscak R, Vladyka V, Simonova G, Vymazal J, Novotny J Jr. Gamma knife surgery of brain cavernous hemangiomas. J Neurosurg **102(Suppl)**: 207–213; 2005

41. Maesawa S, Flickinger JC, Kondziolka D, Lunsford LD. Repeated radiosurgery for incompletely obliterated arteriovenous malformations. J Neurosurg **92(6)**: 961–970; 2000

42. Major O, Szeifert GT, Fazekas I, Vitanovics D, Csonka E, Kocsis B, Bori Z, Kemeny AA, Nagy Z. Effect of a single high-dose gamma irradiation on cultured cells in human cerebral arteriovenous malformation. J Neurosurg **97(5 Suppl)**: 459–463; 2002

43. Maruyama K, Shin M, Tago M, Kishimoto J, Morita A, Kawahara N. Radiosurgery to reduce the risk of first haemorrhage from brain arteriovenous malformations. Neurosurgery **60(3)**: 453–458; 2007

44. Massager N, Régis J, Kondziolka D, Njee T, Levivier M. Gamma knife radiosurgery for brainstem arteriovenous malformations: preliminary results. J Neurosurg **93(Suppl 3)**: 102–103; 2000

45. Mathiesen T, Edner G, Kihlstrom L. Deep and brainstem cavernomas: a consecutive 8-year series. J Neurosurg **99(1)**: 31–37; 2003

46. Nicolato A, Foroni R, Seghedoni A, Martines V, Lupidi F, Zampieri P, Sandri MF, Ricci U, Mazza C, Beltramello A, Gerosa M, Bricolo A. Leksell gamma knife radiosurgery for cerebral arteriovenous malformations in pediatric patients. Childs Nerv Syst **21(4)**: 301–307; 2005

47. Nicolato A, Lupidi F, Sandri MF, Foroni R, Zampieri P, Mazza C, Maluta S, Beltramello A, Gerosa M. Gamma knife radiosurgery for cerebral arteriovenous malformations in children/adolescents and adults. Part I: differences in epidemiologic, morphologic, and clinical characteristics, permanent complications, and bleeding in the latency period. Int J Radiat Oncol Biol Phys **64(3)**: 904–913; 2006

48. Pan DH, Kuo YH, Guo WY, Chung WY, Wu HM, Liu KD, Chang YC, Wang LW, Wong TT. Knife surgery for cerebral arteriovenous malformations in children: a 13-year experience. J Neurosurg Pediatrics **1**: 296–304; 2008

49. Pollock BE, Flickinger JC. Modification of the radiosurgery-based arteriovenous malformation grading system. Neurosurgery **63(2)**: 239–243; 2008

50. Pollock BE, Gorman DA, Coffey RJ. Patient outcomes after arteriovenous malformation radiosurgical management: results based on a 5- to 14-year follow-up study. Neurosurgery **52(6)**: 1291–1296; 2003

51. Pollock BE, Lunsford LD, Kondziolka D, Bissonette DJ, Flickinger JC. Stereotactic radiosurgery for postgeniculate visual pathway arteriovenous malformations. J Neurosurg **84(3)**: 437–441; 1996

52. Régis J, Massager N, Levrier O, Dufour H, Porcheron D, Reyns N, Peragut JC, Farnarier P. Gamma-knife radiosurgery for brainstem arteriovenous malformations. Preliminary results. Neurochirurgie **47(2–3 Pt 2)**: 291–297; 2001

53. Sasaki T, Kurita H, Saito I, Kawamoto S, Nemoto S, Terahara A, Kirino T, Takakura K. Arteriovenous malformations in the basal ganglia and thalamus: management and results in 101 cases. J Neurosurg **88(2)**: 285–292; 1998

54. Shin M, Kawamoto S, Kurita H, Tago M, Sasaki T, Morita A, Ueki K, Kirino T. Retrospective analysis of a 10-year experience of stereotactic radio surgery for arteriovenous malformations in children and adolescents. J Neurosurg **97(4)**: 779–784; 2002

55. Shin M, Maruyama K, Kurita H, Kawamoto S, Tago M, Terahara A, Morita A, Ueki K, Takakura K, Kirino T. Analysis of nidus obliteration rates after gamma knife surgery for arteriovenous malformations based on long-term follow-up data: the University of Tokyo experience. J Neurosurg **101(1)**: 18–24; 2004

56. Sims EC, Plowman PN. Stereotactic radiosurgery XII. Large AVM and the failure of the radiation response modifier gamma linolenic acid to improve the therapeutic ratio. Br J Neurosurg **15(1)**: 28–34; 2001

57. Sirin S, Kondziolka D, Niranjan A, Flickinger JC, Maitz AH, Lunsford LD. Prospective staged volume radiosurgery for large arteriovenous malformations: indications and outcomes in otherwise untreatable patients. Neurosurgery **58(1)**: 17–27; 2006

58. Sirin S, Kondziolka D, Niranjan A, Flickinger JC, Maitz AH, Lunsford LD. Prospective staged volume radiosurgery for large arteriovenous malformations: indications and outcomes in otherwise untreatable patients. Neurosurgery 62(Suppl 2): 744–754; 2008
59. Smyth MD, Sneed PK, Ciricillo SF, Edwards MS, Wara WM, Larson DA, Lawton MT, Gutin PH, McDermott MW. Stereotactic radiosurgery for pediatric intracranial arteriovenous malformations: the University of California at San Francisco experience. J Neurosurg 97(1): 48–55; 2002
60. Sutcliffe JC, Forster DM, Walton L, Dias PS, Kemeny AA. Untoward clinical effects after stereotactic radiosurgery for intracranial arteriovenous malformations. Br J Neurosurg 6(3): 177–185; 1992
61. Valle RD, Zenteno M, Jaramillo J, Lee A, De AS. Definition of the key target volume in radiosurgical management of arteriovenous malformations: a new dynamic concept based on angiographic circulation time. J Neurosurg 109(Suppl): 41–50; 2008
62. Yamamoto M, Hara M, Ide M, Ono Y, Jimbo M, Saito I. Radiation-related adverse effects observed on neuro-imaging several years after radiosurgery for cerebral arteriovenous malformations. Surg Neurol 49(4): 385–397; 1998
63. Yamamoto M, Jimbo M, Hara M, Saito I, Mori K. Gamma knife radiosurgery for arteriovenous malformations: long-term follow-up results focusing on complications occurring more than 5 years after irradiation. Neurosurgery 38(5): 906–914; 1996
64. Yamamoto Y, Coffey RJ, Nichols DA, Shaw EG. Interim report on the radiosurgical treatment of cerebral arteriovenous malformations. The influence of size, dose, time, and technical factors on obliteration rate. J Neurosurg 83(5): 832–837; 1995
65. Yen CP, Varady P, Sheehan J, Steiner M, Steiner L. Subtotal obliteration of cerebral arteriovenous malformations after gamma knife surgery. J Neurosurg 106(3): 361–369; 2007
66. Iwai Y, Yamanaka K, Yoshimura M. Intracerebral cavernous malformation induced by radiosurgery. Case report. Neurol Med Chir (Tokyo) 47(4): 171–173; 2007
67. Crocco A. Arteriovenous malformations in the basal ganglia region: gamma knife radiosurgery as first choice treatment in selected cases. J Neurosurg Sci 46(2): 43–54; 2002
68. Nicolato A, Lupidi F, Sandri MF, Foroni R, Zampieri P, Mazza C, Pasqualin A, Beltramello A, Gerosa M. Gamma Knife radiosurgery for cerebral arteriovenous malformations in children/adolescents and adults. Part II: differences in obliteration rates, treatment-obliteration intervals, and prognostic factors. Int J Radiat Oncol Biol Phys 64(3): 914–921; 2006
69. Ogilvy CS. Radiation therapy for arteriovenous malformations: a review. Neurosurgery 26 (5): 725–735; 1990
70. Tanaka T, Kobayashi T, Kida Y, Oyama H, Niwa M. The comparison between adult and pediatric AVMs treated by gamma knife radiosurgery. No Shinkei Geka 23(9): 773–777; 1995
71. Inoue HK, Ohye C. Haemorrhage risks and obliteration rates of arteriovenous malformations after gamma knife radiosurgery. J Neurosurg 97(5 Suppl): 474–476; 2002
72. Zipfel GJ, Bradshaw P, Bova FJ, Friedman WA. Do the morphological characteristics of arteriovenous malformations affect the results of radiosurgery? J Neurosurg 101(3): 393–401; 2004
73. Ganz JC, Reda WA, Abdelkarim K, Hafez A. A simple method for predicting imaging-based complications following gamma knife surgery for cerebral arteriovenous malformations. J Neurosurg 102(Suppl): 4–7; 2005
74. Aiba T, Tanaka R, Koike T, Kameyama S, Takeda N, Komata T. Natural history of intracranial cavernous malformations. J Neurosurg 83(1): 56–59; 1995
75. Karlsson B, Lindquist C, Steiner L. Prediction of obliteration after gamma knife surgery for cerebral arteriovenous malformations. Neurosurgery 40(3): 425–430; 1997
76. Levy EI, Niranjan A, Thompson TP, Scarrow AM, Kondziolka D, Flickinger JC, Lunsford LD. Radiosurgery for childhood intracranial arteriovenous malformations. Neurosurgery 47 (4): 834–841; 2000

77. Maruyama K, Koga T, Shin M, Igaki H, Tago M, Saito N. Optimal timing for Gamma Knife surgery after haemorrhage from brain arteriovenous malformations. J Neurosurg **109 (Suppl)**: 73–76; 2008

78. Maruyama K, Shin M, Tago M, Kurita H, Kawamoto S, Morita A, Kirino T. Gamma knife surgery for arteriovenous malformations involving the corpus callosum. J Neurosurg **102 (Suppl)**: 49–52; 2005

79. Pedersen PH, Baardsen R, Larsen JL, Thorsen F, Wester K. Stereotactic radiosurgery of cerebral arteriovenous malformations. Tidsskr Nor Laegeforen **122(13)**: 1277–1280; 2002

80. Pollock BE, Flickinger JC, Lunsford LD, Maitz A, Kondziolka D. Factors associated with successful arteriovenous malformation radiosurgery. Neurosurgery **42(6)**: 1239–1244; 1998

81. Pollock BE, Kondziolka D, Flickinger JC, Patel AK, Bissonette DJ, Lunsford LD. Magnetic resonance imaging: an accurate method to evaluate arteriovenous malformations after stereotactic radiosurgery. J Neurosurg **85(6)**: 1044–1049; 1996

82. Pollock BE, Lunsford LD, Kondziolka D, Maitz A, Flickinger JC. Patient outcomes after stereotactic radiosurgery for "operable" arteriovenous malformations. Neurosurgery **35(1)**: 1–7; 1994

83. Shin M, Kawahara N, Maruyama K, Tago M, Ueki K, Kirino T. Risk of haemorrhage from an arteriovenous malformation confirmed to have been obliterated on angiography after stereotactic radiosurgery. J Neurosurg **102(5)**: 842–846; 2005

84. Wara W, Bauman G, Gutin P, Circillo S, Larson D, McDermott M, Sneed P, Verhey L, Smith V, Petti P. Stereotactic radiosurgery in children. Stereotact Funct Neurosurg **64(Suppl 1)**: 118–125; 1995

85. Karlsson B, Lindquist C, Steiner L. Effect of gamma knife surgery on the risk of rupture prior to AVM obliteration. Minim Invasive Neurosurg **39(1)**: 21–27; 1996

86. O'Leary S, Hodgson TJ, Coley SC, Kemeny AA, Radatz MW. Intracranial dural arteriovenous malformations: results of stereotactic radiosurgery in 17 patients. Clin Oncol R Coll Radiol **14(2)**: 97–102; 2002

87. Steiner L, Lindquist C, Adler JR, Torner JC, Alves W, Steiner M. Clinical outcome of radiosurgery for cerebral arteriovenous malformations. J Neurosurg **77(1)**: 1–8; 1992

88. Ledezma CJ, Hoh BL, Carter BS, Pryor JC, Putman CM, Ogilvy CS. Complications of cerebral arteriovenous malformation embolization: multivariate analysis of predictive factors. Neurosurgery **58(4)**: 602–611; 2006

89. Levy DI, Kitz K, Killer M, Richling B. Radiosurgery in the treatment of cerebral AVMs. Acta Neurochir Suppl **63**: 60–67; 1995

90. BhatnagarA, Flickinger JC, Kondziolka D, Niranjan A, Lunsford LD. An analysis of the effects of smoking and other cardiovascular risk factors on obliteration rates after arteriovenous malformation radiosurgery. Int J Radiat Oncol Biol Phys **51(4)**: 969–973; 2001

91. Flickinger JC, Pollock BE, Kondziolka D, Lunsford LD. A dose-response analysis of arteriovenous malformation obliteration after radiosurgery. Int J Radiat Oncol Biol Phys **36(4)**: 873–879; 1996

92. Foron RI, Ricciardi GK, Lupidi F, Sboarina A, De Simone A, Nicolato A, Longhi M, Pizzini F, Ganau M, Beltramello A, Gerosa M. Corticospinal tractography during gamma knife radiosurgery treatment planning for arteriovenous malformations. Acta Neurochir **150**: 989; 2008

93. Flickinger JC, Lunsford LD, Kondziolka D. Assessment of integrated logistic tolerance predictions for radiosurgery with the gamma knife. in Radiosurgery: Baseline and Trends. eds Steiner L et al. Raven Press, New York: pp 15–22; 1992

94. Sharma MS, Kondziolka D, Khan A, Kano H, Niranjan A, Flickinger JC, Lunsford LD. Radiation tolerance limits of the brainstem. Neurosurgery **63(5)**: 728–733; 2008

95. Flickinger JC, Kondziolka D, Pollock BE, Maitz AH, Lunsford LD. Complications from arteriovenous malformation radiosurgery: multivariate analysis and risk modeling. Int J Radiat Oncol Biol Phys **38(3)** 485–490; 1997

96. Flickinger JC, Kondziolka D, Maitz AH, Lunsford LD. An analysis of the dose-response for arteriovenous malformation radiosurgery and other factors affecting obliteration. Radiother Oncol **63(3)**: 347–354; 2002
97. Pollock BE, Kline RW, Stafford SL, Foote RL, Schomberg PJ. The rationale and technique of staged-volume arteriovenous malformation radiosurgery. Int J Radiat Oncol Biol Phys **48** (3): 817–824; 2000
98. Guo WY, Karlsson B, Ericson K, Lindquist M. Even the smallest remnant of an AVM constitutes a risk of further bleeding. Case report. Acta Neurochir **121(3–4)**: 212–215; 1993
99. Spetzler RF, Martin NA. A proposed grading system for arteriovenous malformations. J Neurosurg **65**: 476–483; 1986
100. Pollock BE, Garces YI, Stafford SL, Foote RL, Schomberg PJ, Link MJ. Stereotactic radiosurgery for cavernous malformations. J Neurosurg **93(6)**: 987–991; 2000
101. Pollock BE, Gorman DA, Brown PD. Radiosurgery for arteriovenous malformations of the basal ganglia, thalamus, and brainstem. J Neurosurg **100(2)**: 210–214; 2004
102. Flickinger JC, Kondziolka D, Lunsford DL, Kassam A, Phuong LK, Liscak R, Pollock B. Development of a model to predict premanent symptomatic postradiosurgery injury for arteriovenous malformation patients. Int J Radiat Oncol Biol Phys **46(5)**: 1143–1148; 2000
103. Nilsson A, Wennestrand J, Leksell DG, Backlund EO. Stereotactic gamma irradiation of basilar artery in cat. Preliminary experiences. Acta Radiol Oncol **17**: 150–160; 1978
104. Kim DG, Choe WJ, Paek SH, Chung HT, Kim IH, Han DH. Radiosurgery of intracranial cavernous malformations. Acta Neurochir **144(9)**: 869–878; 2002
105. Schneider GT, Eberhardt DA, Steiner LE. Histopathology of arteriovenous malformatons after gamma knife radiosurgery. J Neurosurg **87(3)**: 352–357; 1997
106. Maruyama K, Kamada K, Shin M, Itoh D, Masutani Y, Ino K, Tago M, Saito N. Optic radiation tractography integrated into simulated treatment planning for gamma knife surgery. J Neurosurg **107**: 721–726; 2007
107. Schneider BF, Eberhard DA, Steiner LE. Histopathology of arteriovenous malformations after gamma knife radiosurgery. J Neurosurg **87(3)**: 352–357; 1997
108. Szeifert GT, Kemeny AA, Timperley WR, Forster DM. The potential role of myofibroblasts in the obliteration of arteriovenous malformations after radiosurgery. Neurosurgery **40(1)**: 61–65; 1997
109. Szeifert GT, Major O, Kemeny AA. Ultrastructural changes in arteriovenous malformations after gamma knife surgery: an electron microscopic study. J Neurosurg **102(Suppl)**: 289–292; 2005
110. Szeifert GT, Timperley WR, Forster DM, Kemeny AA. Histopathological changes in cerebral arteriovenous malformations following gamma knife radiosurgery. Prog Neurol Surg **20**: 212–219; 2007
111. Fournier D, TerBrugge KG, Willinsky R, Lasjaunias P, Montanera W. Endovascular treatment of intracerebral arteriovenous malformations: experience in 49 cases. J Neurosurg **75** (2): 228–233; 1991
112. Kondziolka D, Dempsey PK, Lunsford LD. The case for conservative management of venous angiomas. Can J Neurol Sci **18(3)**: 295–299; 1991
113. Maruyama K, Kawahara N, Shin M, Tago M, Kishimoto J, Kurita H, Kawamoto S, Morita A, Kirino T. The risk of haemorrhage after radiosurgery for cerebral arteriovenous malformations. N Engl J Med **352(2)**: 146–153; 2005
114. Fajardo LF, Morgan Berthrong M, Anderson RE. Cardiovascular system: heart, blood vessels. in Radiation Pathology. Oxford University Press, Oxford England: pp 181–192; 2001
115. Kwon Y, Jeon SR, Kim JH, Lee JK, Ra DS, Lee DJ, Kwun BD. Analysis of the causes of treatment failure in gamma knife radiosurgery for intracranial arteriovenous malformations. J Neurosurg **93(Suppl 3)**: 104–106; 2000
116. Schauble B, Cascino GD, Pollock BE, Gorman DA, Weigand S, Cohen-Gadol AA, McClelland RL. Seizure outcomes after stereotactic radiosurgery for cerebral arteriovenous malformations. Neurology **63(4)**: 683–687; 2004

117. Inoue HK, Kohga H, Kurihara H, Hirato M, Shibazaki T, Andou Y, Ohye C. Classification of arteriovenous malformations for radiosurgery. Neuroimaging, histopathology and radiobiologic effects. Stereotact Funct Neurosurg **64(Suppl 1)**: 110–117; 1995
118. Maruyama K, Kondziolka D, Niranjan A, Flickinger JC, Lunsford LD. Stereotactic radiosurgery for brainstem arteriovenous malformations: factors affecting outcome. J Neurosurg **100(3)**: 407–413; 2004
119. Pollock BE, Kondziolka D, Lunsford LD, Bissonette D, Flickinger JC. Repeat stereotactic radiosurgery of arteriovenous malformations: factors associated with incomplete obliteration. Neurosurgery **38(2)**: 318–324; 1996
120. Kihlström L, Lindquist C, Adler J, Collins P, Karlsson B. Histological studies of gamma knife lesions in normal and hypercholesterolemic rabbits. in Radiosurgery Baseline and Trends. eds Steiner L et al. Raven Press, New York: pp 111–119; 1992
121. Pan DH, Guo WY, Chung WY, Shiau CY, Chang YC, Wang LW. Gamma knife radiosurgery as a single treatment modality for large cerebral arteriovenous malformations. J Neurosurg **93(Suppl 3)**: 113–119; 2000
122. Han JH, Kim DG, Chung HT, Park CK, Paek SH, Kim JE, Jung HW, Han DH. Clinical and neuroimaging outcome of cerebral arteriovenous malformations after Gamma Knife surgery: analysis of the radiation injury rate depending on the arteriovenous malformation volume. J Neurosurg **109(2)**: 191–198; 2008
123. Nicolato A, Foroni R, Crocco A, Zampieri PG, Alessandrini F, Bricolo A, Gerosa MA. Gamma knife radiosurgery in the management of arteriovenous malformations of the Basal Ganglia region of the brain. Minim Invasive Neurosurg **45(4)**: 211–223; 2002
124. Clatterbuck RE, Moriarty JL, Elmaci I, Lee RR, Breiter SN, Rigamonti D. Dynamic nature of cavernous malformations: a prospective magnetic resonance imaging study with volumetric analysis. J Neurosurg **93(6)**: 981–986; 2000
125. Hopkins LN, Ecker RD. Cerebral endovascular neurosurgery. Neurosurgery **62(6 Suppl 3)**: 1483–1502; 2008
126. Richling B, Killer M, Al-Schameri AR, Ritter L, Agic R, Krenn M. Therapy of brain arteriovenous malformations: multimodality treatment from a balanced standpoint. Neurosurgery **59(5 Suppl 3)**: S148–S157; 2006
127. Hou Z, Chen Y, Wu X. The evaluation of MR localization for intracranial arteriovenous malformation treated with gamma knife. Chin Med J Engl **111(11)**: 988–992; 1998
128. Leksell L, Larsson B, Anderson B, Rexed B, Sourander P, Mair W. Lesions in the depth of the brain produced by a beam of high energy protons. Acta Radiol 1960 **54**: 251–264; 1960
129. Bristol RE, Albuquerque FC, Spetzler RF, Rekate HL, McDougall CG, Zabramski JM. Surgical management of arteriovenous malformations in children. J Neurosurg **105(2 Suppl)**: 88–93; 2006
130. Friedman W. Commenting on "Karlsson et al. Prediction of obliteration after gamma knife surgery for cerebral arteriovenous malformations". Neurosurgery **40(3)**: 431; 1997
131. Pollock BE, Flickinger JC. A proposed radiosurgery-based grading system for arteriovenous malformations. J Neurosurg **96(1)**: 79–85; 2002
132. Aoki Y, Nakagawa K, Tago M, Terahara A, Kurita H, Sasaki Y. Clinical evaluation of gamma knife radiosurgery for intracranial arteriovenous malformation. Radiat Med **14(5)**: 265–268; 1996
133. Matsumoto H, Takeda T, Kohno K, Yamaguchi Y, Kohno K, Takechi A, Ishii D, Abiko M, Sasaki U. Delayed haemorrhage from completely obliterated arteriovenous malformation after gamma knife radiosurgery. Neurol Med Chir (Tokyo) **46(4)**: 186–190; 2006
134. Dias PS, Forster DM, Bergvall U. Cerebral medullary venous malformations. Report of four cases and review of the literature. Br J Neurosurg **2(1)**: 7–21; 1988
135. Robinson JR, Awad IA, Little JR. Natural history of the cavernous angioma. J Neurosurg **75(5)**: 709–714; 1991

136. Amin-Hanjani S, Ogilvy CS, Amin Ojemann RG, Crowell RM. Risks of surgical management for cavernous malformations of the nervous system. Neurosurgery **42(6)**: 1220–1227; 1998
137. Kondziolka D. Comment on 'Régis J, Bartolomei F, Kida Y, Kobayashi T, Vladyka V, Liscàk R, Forster D, Kemeny A, Schröttner O, Pendl G. Radiosurgery for epilepsy associated with cavernous malformation: retrospective study in 49 patients. Neurosurgery **47(5)**: 1091–1097; 2000' Neurosurgery **47(5)**: 1097
138. Tung H, GiannottaI SL, Chandrasoma PT, Zee C-S. Recurrent intraparenchymal haemorrhages from angiographically occult vascular malformations. J Neurosurg **73(2)**: 174–180; 1990
139. Kurita H, Kawamoto S, Sasaki T, Shin M, Tago M, Terahara A, Ueki K, Kirino T. Results of radiosurgery for brain stem arteriovenous malformations. J Neurol Neurosurg Psychiatry **68 (5)**: 563–570; 2000
140. Samii M, Eghbal R, Carvalho GA, Matthies C. Surgical management of brainstem cavernomas. J Neurosurg **95(5)**: 825–832; 2001
141. Lunsford LD, Kondziolka D, Flickinger JC, Bissonette DJ, Jungreis CA, Maitz AH, Horton JA, Coffey RJ. Stereotactic radiosurgery for arteriovenous malformations of the brain. J Neurosurg **75(4)**: 512–524; 1991
142. Porter RW, Detwiler PW, Spetzler RF, Lawton MT, Baskin JJ, Derksen PT, Zabramski JM. Cavernous malformations of the brainstem: experience with 100 patients. J Neurosurg **90(1)**: 50–58; 1999
143. Karlsson B, Kihlstrom L, Lindquist C, Steiner L. Gamma knife surgery for previously irradiated arteriovenous malformations. Neurosurgery **42(1)**: 1–5; 1998
144. Porter PJ, Willinsky RA, Harper W, Wallace MC. Cerebral cavernous malformations: natural history and prognosis after clinical deterioration with or without haemorrhage. J Neurosurg **87(2)**: 190–197; 1997
145. Mathis JA, Barr JD, Horton JA, Jungris CA, Lunsford LD, Kondziolka DS, Vincent D, Pentheny S. The efficacy of particulate embolization combined with stereotactic radiosurgery for treatment of large arteriovenous malformations of the brain. Am J Neuroradiol **16 (2)**: 299–306; 1995
146. Zimmerman RS, Spetzler RF, Lee KS, ZabramskiJM, Hargraves RW. Cavernous malformations of the brain. J Neurosurg **75(1)**: 32–39; 1991
147. Coffey RJ, Nichols DA, Shaw EG. Stereotactic radiosurgical treatment of cerebral arteriovenous malformations. Gamma Unit Radiosurgery Study Group. Mayo Clin Proc **70(3)**: 214–222; 1995
148. Heffez DS, Osterdock RJ, Alderete L, Grutsch J. The effect of incomplete patient follow-up on the reported results of AVM radiosurgery. Surg Neurol **49(4)**: 373–381; 1998
149. Kondziolka D, Lunsford LD, Kestle JR. The natural history of cerebral cavernous malformations. J Neurosurg **83(5)**: 820–824; 1995
150. Tu J, Stoodley MA, Morgan MK, Storer KP. Ultrastructural characteristics of hemorrhagic, nonhemorrhagic and recurrent cavernous malformations. J Neurosurg **103(5)**: 903–909; 2005
151. Berge NO, Lindgren M. Relation between field size and tolerance of rabbit's brain to roentgen irradiation (200 kv) via a split-shaped field. Acta Radiol **1**: 147; 1963
152. Robinson JR Jr, Awad IA, Magdinec M, Paranandi L. Factors predisposing to clinical disability in patients with cavernous malformations of the brain. Neurosurgery **32(5)**: 730–736; 1993
153. Back AG, Vollmer D, Zeck O, Shkedy C, Shedden PM. Retrospective analysis of unstaged and staged Gamma Knife surgery with and without preceding embolization for the treatment of arteriovenous malformations. J Neurosurg **109(Suppl)**: 57–64; 2008
154. Régis J, Bartolomei F, Kida Y, Kobayashi T, Vladyka V, Liscàk R, Forster D, Kemeny A, Schröttner O, Pendl G. Radiosurgery for epilepsy associated with cavernous malformation: retrospective study in 49 patients. Neurosurgery **47(5)**: 1091–1097; 2000

155. Andrade-Souza YM, Ramani M, Scora D, Tsao MN, terBrugge K, Schwartz ML. Emboliza-tion before radiosurgery reduces the obliteration rate of arteriovenous malformations. Neurosurgery **60(3)**: 443–451; 2007

156. Pozzati E, Acciarri N, Tognetti F, Marliani F, Giangaspero F. Growth, subsequent bleeding, and de novo appearance of cerebral cavernous angiomas. Neurosurgery **38(4)**: 662–670; 1996

157. Amin-Hanjani S, Ogilvy CS, Candia GJ, Lyons S, Chapman PH. Stereotactic radiosurgery for cavernous malformations: kjellberg's experience with proton beam therapy in 98 cases at the Harvard cyclotron. Neurosurgery **42(6)**: 1229–1236; 1998

158. Pozzati E, Giangaspero F, Marliani F, Acciarri N. Occult cerebrovascular malformations after irradiation. Neurosurgery **39(4)**: 677–682; discussion 682–684; 1996

159. Kiran NA, Kale SS, Vaishya S, Kasliwal MK, Gupta A, Sharma MS, Sharma BS, Mahapatra AK. Gamma Knife surgery for intracranial arteriovenous malformations in children: a retrospective study in 103 patients. J Neurosurg **107**: 479–484; 2007

160. Liu KD, Chung WY, Wu HM, Shiau CY, Wang LW, Guo WY, Pan DH. Gamma knife surgery for cavernous hemangiomas: an analysis of 125 patients. J Neurosurg **102(Suppl)**: 81–86; 2005

161. Kim MS, Pyo SY, Jeong YG, Lee SI, Jung YT, Sim JH. Gamma knife surgery for intracranial cavernous hemangioma. J Neurosurg **102(Suppl)**: 102–106; 2005

162. Seo Y, Fukuoka S, Takanashi M, Nakagawara J, Suematsu K, Nakamura J, Nagashima K. Gamma knife surgery for angiographically occult vascular malformations. Stereotact Funct Neurosurg **64(Suppl 1)**: 98–109; 1995

163. Shih YH, Pan DH. Management of supratentorial cavernous malformations: craniotomy versus gammaknife radiosurgery. Clin Neurol Neurosurg **107(2)**: 108–112; 2005

164. Kupersmith MJ, Kalish H, Epstein F, Yu G, Berenstein A, Woo H, Jafar J, Mandel G, De Lara F. Natural history of brainstem cavernous malformations. Neurosurgery **48(1)**: 47–54; 2001

165. Yoon PH, Kim DI, Jeon P, Ryu YH, Hwang GJ, Park SJ. Cerebral cavernous malformations: serial magnetic resonance imaging findings in patients with and without gamma knife surgery. Neurol Med Chir (Tokyo) **38(Suppl)**: 255–261; 1998

166. Pan DH, Chung WY, Guo WY, Wu HM, Liu KD, Shiau CY, Wang LW. Stereotactic radiosurgery for the treatment of dural arteriovenous fistulas involving the transverse-sigmoid sinus. J Neurosurg **96(5)**: 823–829; 2002

167. Koga T, Maruyama K, Igaki H, Tago M, Saito N. The value of image co-registration during stereotactic radiosurgery. Acta Neurochir **151(5)**: 465–471; 2009

168. Soderman M, Edner G, Ericson K, Karlsson B, Rahn T, Ulfarsson E, Andersson T. Gamma knife surgery for dural arteriovenous shunts: 25 years of experience. J Neurosurg **104(6)**: 867–875; 2006

169. Choe JG, Im YS, Kim JS, Hong SC, Shin HJ, Lee JI. Retrospective analysis on 76 cases of cerebral arteriovenous malformations treated by gamma knife radiosurgery. J Korean Neu-rosurg Soc **43(6)**: 265–269; 2008

170. Douglas JG, Goodkin R. Treatment of arteriovenous malformations using Gamma Knife surgery: the experience at the University of Washington from 2000 to 2005. J Neurosurg **109 (Suppl)**: 51–56; 2008

171. Kondziolka D, Lunsford LD, Flickinger JC, Kestle JR. Reduction of haemorrhage risk after stereotactic radiosurgery for cavernous malformations. J Neurosurg **83(5)**: 825–831; 1995

172. Lindquist M, Karlsson B, Guo WY, Kihlstrom L, Lippitz B, Yamamoto M. Angiographic long-term follow-up data for arteriovenous malformations previously proven to be obliter-ated after gamma knife radiosurgery. Neurosurgery **46(4)**: 803–808; 2000

Part V
The Gamma Knife and Specific Diseases: Functional Indications

Chapter 20
Trigeminal Neuralgia

Introduction

Writing a chapter on one particular treatment for the condition known as trigeminal neuralgia is one of the more daunting tasks for the author of a book such as this. There are few conditions for which there are so many different treatment options and so much disagreement amongst experts as to the optimal treatment and treatment sequence in a given case. As is usual in such situations, this disagreement reflects the complexity of the condition and its frequent resistance to treatment. Thus, because of this complexity more detail than usual of the various areas of knowledge and ignorance, of theory and practice need to be outlined if the reader is to be able to find his/her way through the labyrinth of available information. Let us begin with a consideration of the definition of this clinical condition, where the diagnosis is almost wholly dependent on what the patient says. The definitions below are quoted from the "Headache Classification Subcommittee of the International Headache Society: The International classification and diagnostic criteria for headache disorders, cranial neuralgia and facial pain. Ed 2" [1]. The first unquestionable description of the disease is attributed to Nicolaus André in 1756 [2]. He coined the phrase "tic douloureux" to describe the muscular twitches associated with the lightning like attacks of pain.

Classical Trigeminal Neuralgia [1]

Description

Trigeminal neuralgia is a unilateral disorder characterised by brief electric shock-like pains, abrupt in onset and termination, limited to the distribution of one or more divisions of the trigeminal nerve. Pain is commonly evoked by trivial stimuli including washing, shaving, smoking, talking and/or brushing the teeth (trigger

J.C. Ganz, *Gamma Knife Neurosurgery*,
DOI 10.1007/978-3-7091-0343-2_20, © Springer-Verlag/Wien 2011

factors) and frequently occurs spontaneously. Small areas in the nasolabial fold and/or chin may be particularly susceptible to the precipitation of pain (trigger areas). The pains usually remit for variable periods.

Diagnostic Criteria

(a) Paroxysmal attacks of pain lasting from a fraction of a second to 2 min, affecting one or more divisions of the trigeminal nerve and fulfilling criteria b and c
(b) Pain has at least one of the following characteristics:
　　1. Intense, sharp, superficial or stabbing
　　2. Precipitated from trigger areas or by trigger factors
(c) Attacks are stereotyped in the individual patient
(d) There is no clinically evident neurological deficit[1]
(e) Not attributed to another disorder

Symptomatic Trigeminal Neuralgia

Description

Pain indistinguishable from *Classical trigeminal neuralgia* but caused by a demonstrable structural lesion other than vascular compression. There may be sensory impairment in the distribution of the appropriate trigeminal division. *Symptomatic trigeminal neuralgia* demonstrates no refractory period after a paroxysm, unlike *Classical trigeminal neuralgia*.

　　We shall now move on to the concepts and beliefs relating to the underlying pathology and pathogenesis of the condition.

Pathology and Pathophysiology

Histopathology

There has been much debate about the nature of the pathological and pathophysiological processes which underlie this clinical condition. Over the years agreement has developed on a number of points. Firstly, demyelination is a component in the process.

---

[1]There is evidence from Pittsburgh that ultra thorough clinical examination and neurophysiological examinations can demonstrate consistent abnormalities in these patients, despite the above definition [3].

While not exclusive to trigeminal nerves or root entry zones corresponding to neural-gia, demyelination is found far more extensively and commonly in nerves which give rise to neuralgia [4, 5]. A great number of other changes were described in the early papers cited but subsequent work dismisses these as artefactual [6]. This later study confirms the finding of demyelination moreover a consistent observation has been apposition of demyelinated fibres with very few surrounding glial or inflammatory cells. This apposition would provide the basis for ephaptic transmission between the fibres. This is transmission crossing over from a touch nerve fibre to a pain nerve fibre. This is proposed as the pathophysiological basis of the clinical picture.

Secondary Factors

However, since trigeminal demyelination is found without trigeminal neuralgia and since treatment manoeuvres which do not affect demyelination directly result in symptom relief, demyelination is considered to be only a part of the pathological basis of the symptoms [4, 5]. From an early stage, at operation findings of structures compressing the trigeminal root were described, including vascular loops, veins, aneurysms, arteriovenous malformations, various tumours and thickened dura [4–7]. Through the work of Janetta in the 1960s and onwards it became increasingly accepted that compression of the nerve by neighbouring blood vessels, often the superior cerebellar artery was the cause of trigeminal neuralgia [6, 8–10]. This was called microvascular compression (MVC) and the notion was it could be relieved by separating the compressing arterial loop from the relevant part of the nerve by an operation called microvascular decompression (MVD). However, there are those who think this may be an oversimplification. Another view expressed at the same time was that the causes of trigeminal neuralgia might include pathological changes within the adjacent CNS [11].

Trigeminal Nerve Compression

In April 1951, using a posterior fossa approach, a Danish neurosurgeon called Palle Taarnhøj operated on a 31-year-old man with classical trigeminal neuralgia. The reason for the surgery in those days before computer imaging was the conviction that the disease was probably due to an epidermoid; an impressive feat of clinical acumen. The diagnosis was correct and the trigeminal root was noted to be under some pressure. The next day the man was cured of his neuralgia [12]. This experience led Taarnhøj to believe that pressure on the trigeminal nerve might cause neuralgia in other patients. He reasoned that the only location for such pressure was the dural channel through which the root runs into the Cave of Meckel. He devised an operation to decompress the root in this location. However, the operation never really caught on. It was widely believed that the important thera-peutic factor was not the decompression but the manipulation of the nerve root as quoted with evidence in a review [13].

Contribution of Microvascular Compression (MVC) as an Aetiological Factor: Arguments for and Against

The first surgeon to notice the presence of lesions compressing the trigeminal nerve in association with trigeminal neuralgia was the great Walter Dandy. He performed 250 sections of the trigeminal root with 96% pain relief and a mean follow up of 4.5 years [14]. He observed compression of the nerve by arterial loops, tumours and veins etc. in around a third of the patients; thus suggesting arterial loops were a common but not a majority finding. However, truth to tell he was operating without a microscope. Adams on the other hand performing the same operation with modern equipment in 55 patients found an arterial loop compressing the nerve during only five operations [15]. Both these surgeons were performing rhizotomies not MVDs. At present we are not concerned with results but with pathophysiology, so that arguments about the preferred treatment come later. Jannetta claims to find a compressing blood vessel in 96% of patients [16]. Linskey et al. finds pathological vessels in 100% of cases [17]. Adams as stated finds it in only 11%. Moreover, Taarnhøj found compressing arteries in 14% and veins in 6.6% of his operations, a finding more consistent with Adams than with Janetta. Clearly there is a discrepancy. It could be argued that the failure to find more is because Adams' paper was written prior to the availability of modern computerised imaging methods and this might mitigate the significance of the results. However, that argument is in a sense contradicted by Casey, Janetta's colleague at the Allegheny General Hospital who states "The sensitivity of MR imaging alone for determining the vessel(s) or site of cross-compression is poor" (PJ Jannetta, personal communication 2003) [18]. This view is shared by Brisman et al. [19].

On this basis Adams observations appear to be worthy to stand with those of his colleagues whose observations differ from his. Another factor explaining varying findings could be the experience of the surgeon. In one of the most recent reviews of Jannetta's enormous experience of over 7,000 MVD operations it is stated that negative explorations are related to experience [20]. Klun mentions this and underlines the fact that his experience is the reverse of Adams' who did not find more compressing vessels as his experience increased [21]. Nonetheless, Adams restated his arguments that the microvascular compression MVC was not necessarily the cause of trigeminal neuralgia in a lucid review [13] which provoked an acrimonious correspondence [22]. He makes the suggestion, refuted in the correspondence, that trauma to the nerve or its neighbourhood may be responsible for post operative clinical improvement. Please note that he specifically states that "MVD produce(s) good results in two thirds of patients". There is no suggestion that he is trying to decry the efficacy of the treatment. His remarks are only about the pathophysiological basis of the operation's success. It is a debate about theory. One is reminded of Bernard Shaw's the Doctor's Dilemma where two competing panaceas are forcefully proposed by their protagonists. "Stimulate the phagocytes" or "Excise the Nuciform Sac". Adams review is not basically asking the reader to make a choice about optimal treatment. Rather he asking of those who would stimulate the phagocytes "how would that work?" and of those who would excise the Nuciform Sac "where is it?". This is the way science advances.

Interestingly, in 2001 the Pittsburgh Gamma Knife group demonstrated small pontine infarcts or perineural scarring in nearly 60% of patients coming for GKNS after failed MVD, lending weight to Adams notions [23]. Further discussion of this debate lies outside the scope of this book but the interested reader will find the references make unusually emotional reading for scientific publications. However, the significance of the disagreements between Adams and his opponents is ironically enough reflected in recent words of Jannetta himself [9]. He was describing the difficulties of getting MVD accepted in the early days and he wrote "I learned . . . . . that I was not going to convince 'the Big Professor at Wherever U' that he was wrong and I was right, but that all I did was drive him crazy as he drove me crazy". Adams finds himself somewhat in the same position in respect of the MVD supporters.

Finally, the wisest words in the debate were written by the late Dr. William F Collins, the then editor of the Journal of Neurosurgery. In the introduction to the correspondence he wrote concerning Adams review article which was as stated sceptical to whole notion of MVC. "The paper was accepted not to propose the invalidation of the hypothesis of vascular compression for trigeminal neuralgia, but to allow a member of the profession to express a contrary opinion. I believe there is no proof for any hypothesis concerning the etiology of trigeminal neuralgia, but the hypothesis that compression of the sensory input area of the pons is a cause which receives strong support, as evidenced by the letters received." This statement is reminiscent of the definition of scientific truth which this author's mentor Professor Nicolas Zwetnow liked to teach. "Scientific truth is what you can convince your peers is true today". These matters are discussed in some detail because understanding the pathophysiology of any disease is a prerequisite for rational treatment. The above text would suggest this understanding is currently at best partial and that passions can run high.

The Part of the Trigeminal Root Related to a Blood Vessel

However, there are even more areas where the data is not entirely clear. It is not just enough that there should be a relationship between an artery and the nerve. It must be with the right part of the nerve if the concept of arterial root compression as an aetiological factor is to hold up. The portion which produces trigeminal neuralgia when under compression should be the proximal part of the root at the dorsal root entry zone or DREZ. The nerve fibres here are covered by oligodendroglia and are thought to be more at risk than the part of the nerve covered with Schwann cells. The border between these two regions is called the Obersteiner-Redlich zone. Jannetta suggests that this border may extend more distally than is commonly believed [10]. Evidence for its importance is underlined in the case of facial hemispasm, where an compressing artery was also involved. This artery was responsible for symptoms in 97% of cases which were proximal to the oligodendroglial/Schwann cell margin. In principle this finding should hold good for the trigeminal nerve which is known to have a longer segment of oligodendroglial myelin than the facial nerve [24]. Thus, if a vessel is thought to be the cause of trigeminal neuralgia it must be situated posteriorly along the nerve behind the Obstersteiner-Redlich zone.

The Nature of the Relationship Between the Blood Vessel and the Nerve

This is a book about GKNS, where the operation findings are only mentioned above as part of a discussion concerning pathophysiology. As with other closed procedures the findings upon which GKNS must rely are those shown on images. Yet here again there is disagreement. Opinions are divided about the requirements of a blood vessel which is to be considered significant as a potential contributor to trigeminal neuralgia. Linskey et al. considers for example that grooving of the nerve demonstrated at operation is not necessary. Contact by small arteries or veins will suffice [17]. Often the nature of operative findings is not specified as clearly as in the Linskey paper. Thus, the work of Klun et al. merely mentions proximity/compression of vessels without specifying the precise relationship [18]. The reason for mentioning this point in this section is that the MR will necessarily only show larger vessel. Is contact enough or must a nerve be grooved? At present nobody seems to know. The Mayo Clinic is clear in considering MVD only if there is MR evidence of nerve root compression [25].

In respect of the significance of the relationship between blood vessels and the trigeminal nerve, the evidence is divided. Brisman et al. found that contact between nerve and a blood vessel was associated with a better result of GKNS on trigeminal pain. However, the study classifies the relationship between the nerve and vessel as none, close but not touching, touching without deformation, contact with deformation and contact with deformation of the nerve and brainstem. However, the paper specifies that this relationship refers to the cisternal portion of the nerve and no indication is given as to the proximity of contact to the vital DREZ [19]. In another examination from Pittsburgh, compression and/or distortion of the nerve was found in 67% of a series of patients located in the correct region posteriorly adjacent to the DREZ [23]. Masur et al., using high quality MR images and a double blind assessment procedure to ensure the radiologist had no knowledge of the side of the neuralgia found that compression or distortion on the MR was associated with neuralgia but that contact was not [26]. This paper does not specify the precise location of the compression in the text but the single illustration showing this change illustrates compression at the DREZ as is appropriate. Sheehan et al. have made an attempt to semi-quantify the degree of trigeminal compression observed on the MR examinations used during GKNS for neuralgia [27]. There was compression in 59.4% of patients. However, the study did not mention where along the trigeminal nerve the compression occurred and in figure one of this paper, the demonstrated relationship between blood vessel and nerve appears to be distal. Another study again uses different methodology. Lorenzoni et al. studied 89 patients treated with GKNS of whom only seven had no neurovascular compression

[28]. It is not possible in this study to register a difference between the effect of the presence or absence of compression. However, regrettably this group consider contact equivalent to compression and make no comparison of patients with mere contact compared with those with both compression and or distortion.

It does not seem unfair to comment that the variation in methodologies used in different groups makes it quite difficult for the reader to understand the significance of results from once centre in respect of those from another.

The Question of Veins

Then there is the question of the veins. Dandy himself recorded intimate relationships between the veins and the trigeminal nerve during his operations [14]. The current author has a difficulty in understanding how veins can compress the nerve they drain. The pressure of the blood in a draining vein must necessarily be lower than the pressure of the blood in the vessels of the tissue being drained or else the blood could not flow. It is undeniable that veins are associated with grooves in structures. The author has a large parasagittal frontal bone groove which houses a large subcutaneous vein. It has been there since he was a small boy. It seems doubtful that this groove was produced by pressure on the bone but rather by the interaction between venous and osseous tissue during the processes of development. The author is also fairly sure the vein does not give rise to the headaches from which he does not suffer. Thus, it is suggested that veins cannot compress the trigeminal nerve and contribute to neuralgia. This is not an eccentric personal opinion. Jannetta's own group mentions worse results in patients where the responsible vessel at operation was a vein [20]. Inferior results are also reported by other groups where a vein is the vessel associated with the nerve [21, 29, 30].

Treatment Principles

A Vital Principle

It cannot be stated too strongly that a consistent characteristic of the treatment of trigeminal neuralgia is that no matter what method is used, over time it will cease to work in a proportion of patients and some other treatment will be required.

Aim of Treatment

The aim of treatment is to abolish pain without inducing neurological deficit or other unwanted complications. The most undesired complications are damage to other cranial nerves, altered painful trigeminal sensations and corneal anaesthesia and analgesia with suppression of the corneal reflex. This is perhaps the commonest unwanted effect and carries with it the risk of keratitis, the need for tarsorrhaphy and in occasional cases scarring and blindness. All serious workers have been at pains to ensure their technique spares the ophthalmic division of the nerve in all cases where the neuralgia is not located within the area of its distribution. It is universally agreed that the first line of treatment should be medical and interventions shall be restricted to those patients in whom medical treatment has failed. It has not always been so as outlined in the history section below.

Medical Treatment

Anti-epileptic drugs (AEDs) have formed the backbone of treatment for years and carbamazapine (tegretol) remains the first drug of choice. The first use of tegretol for the treatment of trigeminal neuralgia was published from Uppsala in 1962 [31]. Thus, prior to that time there was no effective medical treatment. As with most drugs affecting the CNS it can have side effects which make its use intolerable. It may then be replaced with alternatives. Details about drugs, their indications and applications can be found in standard texts and will not be set out in more detail here. An excellent review is found in the new text book on stereotactic radiosurgery [32]. In terms of failure or intolerance of treatment, between 25 and 50% of cases the medical treatment will cease to have an effect which satisfies the patient [33]. This is the time for referral for interventional treatment.

The Development of Interventional Treatments

Classification

Interventional treatments can be divided up in one of two ways. There are those which require open surgery and there are closed procedures. All the closed procedures rely on destruction of trigeminal nerve fibres as the basis of treatment. Open operations today consist of destruction of trigeminal root or parts of it (rhizotomy), as with closed procedures or with MVD aimed at relieving the pressure on the nerve without damaging it.

Failure of Medical Treatment

What is failed medical treatment? Interventional treatments are restricted to this subgroup of patients. The definition of failed medical treatment is not universal. Some authors relate the degree of pain to a pain scale. On the whole, however, reports state the indication for intervention as failed medical treatment which implies a subjective assessment of the treating physician to which the suffering patient gives consent. This situation does rather lend itself to variability of reporting. Thus, while the results of a single clinic or physician may be consistent, comparison of results between clinics is less so. A simple clinical detail illustrates this. A patient with uncontrolled trigeminal neuralgia with triggers which are activated during eating and drinking could be expected to lose weight and many do; many but not all. Some patients claiming severe grades of intolerable pain look remarkably well. How does the physician choose in this group of patients whom shall be referred for intervention and who shall not. It is reasonable to believe that different people will find an indication for intervention that varies from that of other colleagues. On the other hand all of us would be inclined to treat the cachectic patient in obvious pain. So from the very start there is an unavoidable built in difficulty in interpreting the work of colleagues even before the sections on technique, results and discussion have been read.

Effects of Open Surgery

Before we can proceed to the role of the Gamma Knife in the treatment of trigeminal neuralgia it is necessary and indeed unavoidable to describe in outline the alternative treatments of this condition. It remains a leading principle that Gamma Knife neurosurgery should only be preferred if it is a superior treatment and this applies also for trigeminal neuralgia. For the reader to gain understanding of the use of GKNS the strengths and weaknesses of alternative techniques need to be described. With trigeminal neuralgia there are rather a lot of them. To understand the state of current knowledge a short description of the development of interventional treatments follows with a short historical introduction outlining how the treatments developed.

Early Attempts

Surgery was in fact the earliest form of effective treatment. There were of course analgesics used but the most common were Morphine which is addictive and Aconite which whether used topically or systemically is poisonous. Horsley was amongst the first to describe a series of patients treated surgically. Most of the cases he reported involved the surgical removal of peripheral branches or divisions of the nerve. These procedures achieved pain relief for limited periods of some months in most patients [34].

Rhizotomy

Horsley did perform one subtemporal trigeminal root avulsion through an *intradural* approach but the patient died [34]. Better procedures were necessary. The surgical techniques continued to develop until Frazier of Philadelphia devised what became one of the standard procedures. The operation which bears his name is an *extradural* rhizotomy [35]. He found that bleeding from 3 sources was the major problem. The middle meningeal artery lying directly lateral to the mandibular branch of the trigeminal nerve would be routinely cut between two ligatures in these pre-diathermy days. This provided access to the most adherent dura lying adjacent to the foramen ovale and foramen rotundum. Haemostasis was achieved with hot saline on cotton pledgets. The original paper by Spiller and Frazier was published in 1901 and bone wax was not used, although Horsley had described its use in 1892, 9 years earlier, in the British Medical Journal. The final potential source of bleeding was the cavernous sinus. Frazier quotes Cushing who advised that this haemorrhage was most likely as the internal aspect of the ganglion was approached. Frazier followed Cushing's advice to "conduct these manipulations as near as possible to the sensory root, since this is the safest point". Frazier also found that he could preserve the motor root. Conclusion 3 at the end of his pioneer paper describing his assessment of the operation reads "Its execution is, comparatively speaking simple". Others would disagree. The author's mentor Richard Johnson of the Manchester Royal Infirmary used to quote another neurosurgical pioneer from the generation after Frazier. What Sir Geoffrey Jefferson is reported to have said was if you could perform Frazier's operation in any patient you had mastered neurosurgery (personal communication).

Cushing himself had developed an *extradural* ganglionectomy [36], the secret of which was to operate low and be able to retract the middle meningeal artery which was elevated but not transected. He experimented on fresh cadavers to develop the right feel for the operation. He split the ganglionic sheath of dura and exposed it and lifted the dura away from the top of the ganglion. The ganglion having been "liberated" was resected. A debate developed between Cushing and Frazier reflecting the merits of their two operations but in the end Cushing adopted the simpler safer operation of Frazier. Frazier attempted in the majority of cases where the ophthalmic division of the nerve was not involved to avoid cutting the fibres of this division, reducing the chance of loss of sensation to the cornea and the concomitant risk of keratitis.

In 1932 Dandy published a series of 250 cases where he approached the trigeminal root through an *intradural* cerebellar approach. Like Frazier he too attempted to spare ophthalmic and motor fibres. He claimed the operation was simpler and more effective than the Frazier operation [14]. The discussion published after this paper's presentation gave Frazier the chance to express his forcefully formulated disagreement [14]. Here the argument was every bit as passionate as that concerning MVD quoted above. The author of this book has only seen the Frazier operation performed in Manchester during his time as a resident. Adams at Oxford as quoted above preferred the Dandy method [13, 15]. Dandy stated a 96% success rate but duration of follow up and complications are not mentioned. Adams stated that in his 55 patient followed for a mean of 4.5 years after the Dandy type rhizotomy, 52 had no significant pain. Two patients with partial root section required subsequent total root section. One patient had an MVD after developing post-rhizotomy painful dysaesthesia. One patient developed anaesthesia dolorosa. In 46 patients followed up personally by the author there was sensory deficit in the fields of the divided fibres. This is a smaller material than Dandy's but the results are better recorded and the success rate is similar.

Taarnhøj's Operation

The rationale for this procedure is described above. It involved opening the roof of the Cave of Meckel and incising the dura over the root all the way back through the greater superficial petrosal sinus. Taarnhøj specifies that the ganglion was not touched [37]. On the other hand it was apparently important to run a hook along the root to ensure that it was adequately decompressed. He reported his findings after 30 years in 1982 [38]. There was a 1.1% mortality. There was an overall long term relief of pain in 64.3% of patients. In 2.3% there was no relief and in 32.3% neuralgia recurred. There were very infrequent complications of which by far the commonest was some degree of reduced facial sensation. This was slight in 8.3% of patients and marked in 2.7%. No dysaesthesias or anaesthesia dolorosa was reported. There were no ophthalmic complications

Recording of Results

No matter what the method of treatment, some easily reproducible, comprehensible and applicable means of registering the result needs to be applied if varying publications are to be compared. This weakness in reporting has been noted previously and remains yet another source of uncertainty in the understanding of the significance of published results [39]. Inevitably there are a number of such systems in use. In the GKNS reporting the systems from BNI and Marseille predominate. They are in fact very similar and throughout this chapter the BNI system will be used where possible as the basis for comparison of results.

BNI Pain Intensity Scale [40]

1. No trigeminal pain, no medication
2. Occasional pain, not requiring medication
3. Some pain, adequately controlled with medication
4. Some pain, not adequately controlled with medication
5. Severe pain/no pain relief

MVD

Introduction

Today the great majority of open operations performed for medically resistant trigeminal neuralgia are MVDs while a minority of surgeons continue to perform rhizotomies [13, 15] and sometimes rhizotomies are performed when no compressing vessel was found at surgery or when MVD failed to relieve the pain [21, 29, 41]. An vital point concerning the results is that the patient should actually be suffering from classical trigeminal neuralgia [21]. There is broad agreement that MVD is the most effective treatment for immediate relief of pain even amongst Gamma Knife users [17, 42–45].

Success Rate

The difficulty of reporting as quoted above is relevant. The Pittsburgh pioneers of MVD have used a system where excellent is essentially the same as BNI grades 1 and 2. The group still refers to a paper published in 1996 as their largest published series [46]. In a study of 1,165 patients they recorded excellent results immediately after operation in 82% of patients and 1 year excellent results in 75% and 10 year excellent results in 64%. These results show the pattern that most failures occur in the first year after treatment. It also, in keeping with all treatments demonstrates that recurrences occur. Thus, it is important when comparing techniques, and different centres that the results be recorded in relation to the time after treatment.

Complications

There were some operative complications but of recent times the most frequent was hearing loss in 1% of patients without coincident facial palsy. No explanation is given for this. There a 2 cases of permanent trochlear nerve dysfunction. Severe facial numbness occurred in only 22 patients. Four patients had dysaesthesias. These are impressive results especially with regard to lack of serious trigeminal dysfunction. It is the excellence of the results and the paucity of side effects which has gained the operation its reputation. However, as stated there are recurrences. Moreover, as argued above, while the operation undoubtedly works, how it works remains a matter of doubt and thus an area for further research with an aim, in this functional disease of obtaining the same result without opening the head.

In conclusion it may be mentioned that the post operative disappearance of pain after an MVD may sometimes be delayed for up to a week or two instead of being immediate. The mechanism for this latent interval is debated but currently unknown, however it is considered to be associated with an increased chance of recurrence.

Alcohol or Phenol Injections into a Peripheral Trigeminal Branch or the Gasserian Ganglion

This topic needs to be mentioned if one is to understand the attitudes of colleagues treating this disease today. There are problems with certain interventions which are consequently no longer in use. The treatments that have fallen out of use are the injection of alcohol into the Gasserian ganglion or into peripheral branches of the trigeminal nerve. It is documented in a paper from Swansea in 1994 that relief is quick but temporary and that the process is painful [47]. This paper is published in Acta Neurochirugica and the chief editor Dr. Loew commented on it that it was included to remind neurosurgeons that colleagues in other specialities were still using this outmoded technique and that the results they reported documented the inefficiency of their method [48]. The current author has performed these procedures himself as a resident in training and can confirm that while technically simple they were painful and the results were disappointing. Anyone interested in deepening their knowledge on peripheral nerve injections is referred to the above paper.

Radiofrequency Lesions

This technique was introduced by the legendary Dr. WH Sweet with his colleague Dr. Wepsic in 1974 [49]. In the introduction to the paper it is explained that at the time the percutaneous treatment of choice was alcohol injection into the trigeminal ganglion. A consistent finding of this method was loss of corneal sensitivity, irrespective of which division was involved in the pain and in a substantial number of the patients with corneal anaesthesia, keratitis requiring tarsorrhaphy was necessary. Moreover, it was pointed out that most complications of the method were not due to mechanical damage by a misplaced needle but by the spread of toxic chemicals in unwanted directions. Thus, it was considered necessary to find a technique which avoided this complication. The thought was raised that heat might produce lesions in a more controllable fashion. Others had tried thermocoagulation of the trigeminal ganglion using relatively crude techniques. The paper under advisement insists that a precisely controllable radiofrequency generator be used to make the lesion. There is much detail about the correct way in which to insert the cannula which will guide the radiofrequency electrode to its correct location. The authors also mention that the hypothesis behind the method is that less myelinated fibers are responsible for pain transmission and that the heat damage can selectively damage these fibres.

The method was designed to produce trigeminal sensory loss, but only to pin prick not to light touch. It became clear that this could be achieved. The retention of touch sensation made the patient's experience after the procedure more comfortable. If loss of pin prick sensation was not achieved the chance of recurrence was greater. Reporting on 154 patients 91% showed initial relief from neuralgia. Only two patients developed unpleasant paraesthesiae. Twenty two per cent had recurrence in a follow up of 2.5–6 years. It was noted that there was a tendency to progressive recurrence as time passed. This is in contrast with MVD where most recurrences appear within the first year. Keratitis leading to blindness following corneal anaesthesia occurred in only one patient. Some degree of masseter weakness was present in over half the patients but this was considered acceptable since the deficit usually normalises.

Broggi et al. reviewing 1,000 patients with a mean follow up of more than 8 years found a similar rate of pain relief and recurrence [50]. However, there were a considerable number of permanent complications with nearly 10% with permanent masseter weakness, corneal anaesthesia in 20%. Six patients required surgery for keratitis and 15 had a painful anaesthesia and a further 52 required heavy medication for dysaesthesias. It is worth noting that in the discussion of the paper Apfelbaum congratulated the authors on the low numbers of complications.

In a highly selected metanalysis paper Lopez et al. [39] recorded a 3 year success rate of around 60% in three reported series. Troublesome dysesthesias were reported in almost 4% of cases with anaesthesia dolorosa in 1.6%. Keratitis occurred in 1.3%.

Glycerol Injection

In the early days of radiosurgery Leksell was interested in using the Gamma Knife for trigeminal neuralgia. His junior colleague Dr. Håkonsson was instructed to inject tantalum powder suspended in glycerol into the subarachnoid space around the Gasserian ganglion to permit visualisation of the ganglion as a "lion's paw" for use in the Gamma Knife procedure. However, it was not possible to continue the treatment on the day of instillation of the tantalum in glycerol mixture. The following morning the patients were pain free. This started an investigation which concluded with Dr. Håkonsson's doctoral thesis concerning the use of glycerol in the subarachnoid space around the Gasserian ganglion as a superior method to the injection of alcohol into the ganglion. The method remains in use to the present day [51]. It may be mentioned in passing that Leksell did publish an anecdotal report of GKNS treatment of some patients in 1971 [52] but the systematic use of the Gamma Knife for trigeminal neuralgia would not begin until later.

In Håkonsson's original paper the glycerol technique made 86% of patients pain free after 1–2 injections. The recurrence rate was 18% after 17 months [51]. Dr WH Sweet visited Stockholm and was so impressed with the method that he stated in an article directly following Håkonsson's paper in "Neurosurgery" "We conclude that the method is probably going to be an improvement over radiofrequency heating for the treatment of trigeminal neuralgia in many situations" [12]. Thereby, Sweet showed a generosity of spirit and a scientific objectivity unusual in debates about the nature and management of this disease. He was particularly impressed at the relatively slight trigeminal neurological deficit following the treatment. Subsequent analyses have however been disappointing. The glycerol technique undoubtedly works quickly and in the majority of patients. However, in the metanalysis of Lopez et al. only half the patients retained pain relief at 3 years [39]. Moreover, persisting troublesome sensory disturbances were present in 10.5% of patients. In addition there is evidence that its success is related to persistent sensory loss, as with other destructive lesions [50]. One study found a 72% recurrence rate and 29% unpleasant dysaesthesias [53]. Yet another showed treatment failure at 18 months in 50% [54]. While another reported 38% troublesome dysaesthesia [55]. The discrepancies in the results may relate to variations in technique. Lunsford et al. using exactly the same technique as Håkonsson achieved excellent pain relief in 67% and good in 23% and no loss of facial sensation in 73% [56]. Moreover, it has been observed that the quality of the results depends on previous treatments. Prior interventions were associated with worse results [57].

Balloon Compression

Balloon compression was pioneered by Mullan and Lichtor in 1983 [58]. Ignoring glycerol and other toxic substances their article begins with a brief review of various operative procedures. Part of this material is devoted to pointing out the unwanted complications or recurrence rates of rhizotomies, Taarnhøj's operation or MVD. The other major part of the introduction is related to discussing the mechanisms of the various procedures and arguing that of the two mechanical alternatives of decompression of the trigeminal ganglion and compression, the latter gives better results. Their starting point is the early work of Shelden who proposed that compression of the nerve could produce adequate relief of pain with minimal trigeminal deficit [59]. This early paper had only a short follow up. Nonetheless Mullan believed that the concepts behind this earlier work were correct and proposed that compression could be obtained by introducing a Fogarty catheter into Meckel's cave percutaneously. The paper describes the technique in detail. Initial relief of pain was obtained in all but one patient. There was a recurrence of pain requiring treatment in 6 of the 50 patients (12%). In three of these a repeat compression produced lasting pain relief. The other three patients sought other means of pain relief. The reported sustained pain relief in subsequent papers has been 74% [60]. In another paper with many patients and a long follow up initial pain relief was 99% [61]. However, recurrence was 19.2% at 5 years and 31.9% over a study period of from 2 to 22 years (mean 10.7 years). There were symptomatic dysaesthesias in 3.8% of patients. However, there was no anaesthesia dolorosa and no corneal anaesthesia. It is the preservation of corneal sensation which is the one of the strongest arguments in favour of this technique. Experimental work has shown that this is probably because compression selectively damages medium and large myelinated fibres and that the corneal reflex is mediated by small fibres [60]. Comparatively speaking these are really excellent results and it is not altogether clear why balloon compression has not been used more widely.

Gamma Knife Treatment

Introduction

The above text which is not about GKNS must seem very lengthy in a book devoted to that subject. It is considered necessary because of the variety of opinion and argument around the topic of the management of trigeminal neuralgia. There are competing therapies. If a physician is to advise about a given treatment it is necessary to know what else is available and the pros and cons of the alternative treatment methods.

Maybe the reader is now expecting to enter the calmer waters around a single methodology. One of the strengths of the Gamma Knife has always been that its use is consistent from centre to centre. For most indications this is true. For trigeminal neuralgia it is not. There is indeed a fair amount of discussion amongst GKNS users as to the optimal method for using the technique.

The Mechanism by Which GKNS Can Affect Trigeminal Neuralgia

There is to date just one structured paper on the experimental histological findings following doses of 80 or 100 Gy given to the trigeminal nerve of baboons [62]. This produced MR changes in the nerve without changes in the nearby pons. 80 Gy produce non specific axonal degeneration in nerve fibres of all sizes and degrees of myelinisation. 100 Gy could lead to partial necrosis. A second piece of histological evidence comes from a rhizotomy performed on a lady whose GKNS had succeeded for 16 months and then been repeated with a more anteriorly placed dose and without effect. The tissue showed no signs of necrosis [63]. There is currently no other histological information on this topic. It is currently believed the basis of this limited data that anatomical neuronal damage is required to produce the therapeutic effect.

In the discussion section of the Kondziolka paper mentioned above [62], Donlin Long makes the point that if trigeminal neuralgia is due to MVC at the DREZ region, the GKNS treatments reported in the literature are usually located anteriorly to that region and he speculates as to why lesions anterior to the pathology should result in pain relief. Presumably, it works in the same way as previous outmoded peripheral treatments by reducing the amount of impulse traffic passing through the pathological region. However, this is an interesting question requiring elucidation considering the debate around MVC as the major aetiological factor in trigeminal neuralgia.

In addition to this excellent paper there are two other case reports reporting histological findings on patients who had received GKNS for trigeminal neuralgia. In one paper [63] the patient received a more anterior dose of 85 Gy with pain relief for 16 months (BNI III). On recurrence a more distal location was treated with 70 Gy. The pain continued unabated and she was subjected to a posterior fossa rhizotomy. A small portion of the proximal to "mid cisternal" nerve was sent for biopsy. No pathological changes were shown. The authors draw the conclusion that anatomical nerve damage is necessary to produce pain relief. In the other paper [64], the treatment sequence was the reverse. The patient first received 90 Gy to the distal end of the nerve. The quality of the improvement is not stated but the patient received 70 Gy to the proximal part of the nerve 10 months later. Again the quality of pain relief is not mentioned. Since the patient died of a stroke shortly after the second treatment it was possible to obtain histological material from the treated nerve. Acute and chronic radiation damage were found in the appropriate locations. This paper concludes that 90 Gy produces an adequate lesion. These two papers provide information obviously but their significance is hard to place. In the first treatment reported [63] 16 months of pain relief was produced followed by no relief and yet there was no visible radiation damage in the biopsy tissue. On the other hand in the second paper there was clear cut radiation damage of different ages relating to the treatments given and yet the clinical improvement though not stated, must from the timing and sequence of treatments have been less effective than in the first paper [63]. Thus, currently there remains much to learn about the mechanism of GKNS on trigeminal neuralgia and certain of the clinical findings suggest that the mechanism may be more complex than just simple axonal destruction.

Development of Radiosurgery for Use with Trigeminal Neuralgia

Leksell wrote only one English language and much misquoted paper specifically related to this topic [52]. In this paper he describes the effect of the radiosurgical treatment of the neuralgia using a Müller MG 300 kV industrial X-ray unit working at 280 kV, 10 mA attached to the arc of the stereotactic instrument. Two patients were treated in the above mentioned paper and both did well [52]. The paper mentions in the discussion section that trigeminal neuralgia would be treated by the Gamma Knife in future. In the same year, in a Swedish paper reviewing the neurophysiology and management of trigeminal neuralgia and headed with a very dashing picture of the author ten patients are mentioned who has been treated with the first Gamma Unit [65]. There was immediate pain relief in eight of the ten patients but Leksell commented that the follow up was too short to draw any definite conclusions. In a review of radiosurgery based on a lecture to the Sir Hugh Cairns Memorial Lecture of 1981 delivered to the Society of British Neurological Surgeons, Leksell listed up the 762 patients who had been treated with the Gamma Knife. Of these 63 had trigeminal neuralgia. No mention is made of either technique or result. There is additional information of this material from a later review where 46 patients are mentioned [66]. In 24 localisation was made from bony landmarks and in 22 from cisternography. The results were unsurprisingly not that good with pain control in four patients after two and a half years. It may be believed that the serendipitous discovery of the effects of retro-Gasserian glycerol injection may have distracted Leksell's main interest in the disappointing effects of the Gamma Knife for this particular indication [51].

  Real interest in treating trigeminal neuralgia was awakened by Rand in an article describing the somewhat varied treatment of patients with very differing histories and therapeutic backgrounds [3]. A multi-institutional study from respected centres provided a basis for increasing interest [67]. Since then GKNS has become an increasingly popular method for treating drug resistant trigeminal neuralgia.

GKNS Technique in the Treatment of Trigeminal Neuralgia

Frame Application

Sagittal MR images taken prior to treatment can show the direction of the trigeminal nerve and the frame can be applied so that the base is parallel with the nerve. This usually means the frame is tilted slightly in the sagittal plane with the anterior border being slightly higher than the posterior border. This will ensure that a maximal length of the nerve is visualised.

Imaging

Technique

The author has found the both a T1 3D acquisition with and without contrast together with a CISS series are helpful. The use of gradient echo 3D axial images is in keeping with the experience of other workers [23, 67–69]. The use of CISS images which may improve the visualisation of relevant vascular structures is advocated by yet other groups [27, 70, 71].

Findings

It is of course necessary to reveal the trigeminal nerve. It is preferable to visualise any structures impinging upon it. Further matter of interest are anatomically visible changes in the nerve or root entry zone. These can include atrophy [71–73], distortion or dislocation of the nerve by a vessel [28, 41, 73] infarcts [23, 46] and scarring [23]. Many of the above mentioned changes may be related to previous interventional treatments.

Treatment Technique

Target Location

The location of the radiation shot varies in different series. An anterior location [67, 73–85] is preferred by some workers. Others prefer a proximal location as close to the DREZ as possible usually specifying 2–4 mm from the DREZ [17, 19, 40, 43, 62, 63, 68, 86–113]. A few refer to placement in the middle of the nerve, but nearly always when the initial treatment was posterior and a retreatment is being undertaken [63, 99, 108, 109]. There is a single paper which compares the effects of posterior against anterior placement. The conclusion was that a posterior placement gave a better pain control [114].

There is a slight problem interpreting what is actually meant by a described location. To begin with the actual length of trigeminal nerves varies. Moreover, the apparent length of the nerve on axial MR images also varies depending on the angulation of the stereotactic frame in respect of the nerve in the sagittal plane. Even supposing the imaging of the nerve is ideal, many of the quoted papers with a proximal localisation specify that they aim at placing the shot at 2–4 mm from the root entry zone. However, this information is then qualified by the extra information that only the 20 or 30% isodose is allowed to touch the pons. If this is the case the shot will have to be moved distally and one suspects, though cannot prove that many shots are closer to the middle of the nerve than the root entry zone, irrespective of the originally intended location. It seems likely that the BNI group in Phoenix, who place the 50% isodose in contact with the pons probably have the most proximally placed lesion and that which is most likely to be in the root entry zone affecting nerves covered with oligodendroglia. As mentioned above one paper reported that a posterior location gave better results in terms of pain relief [114]. However, this advantage was only shortly after treatment. The complication rate in terms of trigeminal nerve dysfunction was higher in the anterior group but there was a tendency for a higher dose to be used in this location. It is not easy to interpret these results.

It can be stated that the location along the nerve cannot be crucial because all the methods produce fairly similar results in respect of pain relief and recurrence, as outlined below. The significance of position will be mentioned further under the effects of method on results.

Dose

This varies between 70 and 90 Gy for a single session [17, 40, 42–44, 62, 63, 67, 68, 74, 75, 81–92, 94, 95, 98–107, 110–127]. Lower doses were used once in a trial of larger treatment volume [120] and three times as part of dose escalation studies. Since that time 70–90 Gy has remained the standard [67, 68, 104]. Other occasions where lower doses are used generally refer to re-treatments [77, 78, 96, 128]. The variation in dose is seldom clarified explicitly though the reason is obvious to any GKNS user who treats this condition. It is however specified at least once and relates to material outlined above about minimising the dose to the brain stem. No matter what dose is desired it is modified in relation to the length of the nerve to be treated and the desire to spare the brain stem excessive radiation dose. It would seem that the desirable dose is between 70 and 90 Gy but there is no clear cut evidence to support either dose in view of variations in other parameters such as shot location, previous treatment and the use of plugs.

There are a number of methods used as measures of sparing the brain stem. Some workers ensure that only the 20% isodose touches the brain stem [39, 67, 68, 75, 82, 85, 90, 91, 94, 99, 107, 110, 129]. Some prefer the 30% isodose [27, 67, 99, 100, 104, 125, 130]. A few prefer the 40% isodose [82, 110]. A few specify brain stem protection in terms of ensuring that the isodose touching the pons is less than 50%

[92, 131]. Some workers take a different approach and shape the dose, so that the maximum dose to the brain stem is only 12 Gy. Another group makes sure that no more than 20 mm^3 receive 15 Gy. Finally, the group in Brussels works to ensure that only 10 mm^3 receive 12 Gy and only 1 mm^3 receives 15 Gy.

Thus it may be seen that there is no consensus about either dose or the best way to protect the brain stem. However, the greater the emphasis on brain stem protection is considered the greater the tendency will be for a final shot placement to drift anteriorly or for the dose rate to be affected by the use of plugging to shape the dose.

There is one paper which mentions 100 Gy but that is purely experimental and 100 Gy was found to be the necrotising dose [62].

The Number of Shots and the Use of Plugs

The great majority of papers report the use of a single 4 mm shot [17, 40, 43, 63, 67–69, 74–76, 78–82, 85–89, 91, 93, 94, 96–103, 106–108, 110–114, 120, 122, 125, 126]. A few use a mixture of one or two 4 mm shots [92, 104, 109, 116, 130]. A couple use two shots consistently [105, 132]. So it may be seen that a single shot is by far the most favoured technique even if there is as indicated above, variation in the location of that shot. Occasional use of an 8 mm shot in association with a 4 mm shot or alone has been used without any benefit being demonstrated.

In a relatively small number of papers plugs have been used to shape the dose and keep it away from the brainstem [80, 81, 91, 96, 122, 130]. Most workers have avoided this practice. Those who use it have compared its use with the initial success rate after treatment claiming an advantage in terms of pain relief but the significance of this reporting is not clear.

Success Rates and Recurrence

Success rates in major series give good initial results in between 69 and 94% of series. The success rates depend on the nature of the reporting [40, 67, 88, 104, 107, 110, 113, 131]. The median latency to a good result in these papers varies between 2 and 8 weeks though mostly it is achieved within 4 weeks. However, the latency period can be as much as 120 days and in very rare cases even longer. In general, it may be stated that shorter latencies are associated with better results.

Reported recurrence rates vary between 6 and 56% [40, 42, 43, 45, 67, 74, 76, 82, 86, 88, 91, 92, 94, 95, 98, 100, 102, 104, 105, 107, 110, 114, 126, 129, 133]. In general, the longer follow up is associated with higher recurrence rates. Retreatment is possible again with variations in management. Some workers like to use either a lower dose or a different location for the shot. Initial the BNI results from 1 to 3 achieved in most repeat treatment series were similar to those in primary treatments [75, 78, 96, 97, 112, 128]. There was however an increased chance of trigeminal deficit after a second treatment.

Trigeminal Deficit

While GKNS may take a bit longer to work than other interventional treatments, there is plenty of evidence that it is associated with a lower rate of sensory dysfunction of the trigeminal nerve. Sensory disturbance, mostly numbness is reported at rates between 2.7% and 73% [42, 43, 45, 67, 75, 82, 93, 100–102, 106–108, 110, 111, 113, 125, 130]. Bothersome sensory disturbance, again mostly numbness but also paraesthesia is a lot less common being reported in between 4 and 19% of cases [79, 82, 90, 91, 93, 101, 102, 108, 117, 134]. A better clinical response is reported in the presence of sensory deficit [75, 82, 109, 111, 125, 135]. There is also broad agreement that previous interventions decrease the chance of a good result [82, 87, 99, 101–104, 107, 117, 130, 134].

MVC and GKNS

There is no convincing evidence that MVC compression of the trigeminal nerve on the side with neuralgia has an effect on the results of treatment [98, 121]. There is one complex paper which found contact between nerve and blood vessel was associated with improved results [87]. However, the registration of improvement does not conform to the BNI, Marseille or McGill methods of result registration and the report includes proximity and not just compression or distortion of the nerve in the group of patients with where the blood vessel could be a contributory factor. This makes the paper difficult to interpret in respect of other work.

MVD After Failed GKNS

While GKNS after any previous intervention including MVD gives worse results the reverse is not true. MVD seems to work just as well after GKNS as without it [124].

Secondary Trigeminal Neuralgia and Atypical Facial Pain

Trigeminal pain either typical neuralgia or atypical facial pain can occur in the presence of visible pathology of which the commoner examples are space occupying lesions [84, 132, 136, 137] and MS [87, 121, 138]. GKNS can produce useful results thought they are less consistent than with primary trigeminal neuralgia. Régis et al. introduced the notion that the treatment with tumours should be dictated by the anatomy. The dose and location of the dose would depend on the visibility of the trigeminal nerve. In the first instance the tumour would be treated with a normal tumour dose. Only if this did not relieve the neuralgia would a specific treatment with a higher dose be directed at visible trigeminal nerve when that was possible. This advice was not followed in a recent paper reporting two patients with trigeminal neuralgia and an adjacent tumour [139]. The tumour was treated but the neuralgia did not improve. The patients were not then treated with a high dose to the clearly visible trigeminal nerve but were operated with MVD. This is a respectable treatment strategy but the possibility exists that retreatment along the lines advocated by Régis could have avoided the need for open surgery.

It has also been shown that GKNS may relieve atypical facial pain although the results are less certain than with classical trigeminal neuralgia [88, 90, 121].

Conclusions

The Nature of GKNS Treatment

It would appear that GKNS is an ablative technique like all the other techniques quoted above. It has the advantage that it is associated with a low rate of complications in particular keratitis is not reported although one paper describes how to avoid a tiny minority of patients suffering from a dry eye [122]. Anaesthesia dolorosa does not occur though occasional troublesome dysaesthesias do occur though usually in patients subject to prior intervention. However, it is fair to state that while trigeminal dysfunction is attractively infrequent its presence is associated with a high rate of pain relief.

It is suggested that the location of the shot is not crucial as similar results are obtained with varying shot locations. The user may choose from among the various options described above.

It is suggested that the individual user make a selection from the various brainstem protecting techniques as none has been shown to be better than others.

Pain recurrence increases over the passage of time as it does with all treatments for this condition. A second treatment has been shown to be effective and worthwhile with satisfactory pain relief in nearly as many patients as with a primary treatment but a higher risk of trigeminal dysfunction. It is probably wise to use a similar dose at both treatments.

The disadvantage of the treatment is the latent interval between treatment and result. If the patient is in a desperate condition from the data accumulated above it would seem a balloon compression would be a suitable alternative treatment.

MVC and MVD

From a reading of the literature and the debates the reaction of those who support MVD for MVC to those who express doubt is similar to that of devout Christians to an unmannered apostate who spits in church. The current author believes there is an overwhelming literature demonstrating the benefits of MVD on trigeminal neuralgia. However, the case for the mechanism of the success of the operation is believed to be in doubt and the following reasons are given. Firstly, the quotation of the editor of the Journal of Neurosurgery prior to a vitriolic correspondence seems absolutely fair and balanced. Secondly the finding that nearly 60% of patients undertaking MR for failed MVD showed post-operative scarring of the nerve or pontine infarcts. This opens the door at least to the notion that mechanisms other than decompression could result in pain relief.

This author does NOT know the answer but believe the debate should be ongoing and above all calm and courteous.

Considerations About the Sequence of Interventional Treatments for Trigeminal Neuralgia

The following are no more than suggestions, but they are suggestions which follow logically from what has been written above. The author does not expect anything close to total agreement with the following simple algorithm but hopes that it will be accepted as a carefully assessed view and worthy at least of consideration.

1. The starting point for this final set or recommendations is that all treatments of trigeminal neuralgia fail in a proportion of cases. There can be no doubt that previous intervention reduces the effectiveness of GKNS.
2. Even in the best hands MVD is open surgery and carries a greater risk than a closed procedure. Moreover it is not universally successful as the significant number of patients coming to GKNS after failed MVD indicates.
3. A patient whose situation is extreme should not be exposed to a treatment which only works after a latent interval. Balloon compression seems particularly well suited in this situation because of rapid effect and low complication rate.
4. For the patient who might be considered for MVD it is at least worth considering using GKNS first. It is non-invasive and amongst the safest of the treatments. Like all others it will inevitably fail in a number of cases. These cases could then be considered for MVD since previous GKNS does not seem to affect the difficulty or nor reduce the effectiveness of MVD.

References

1. Headache Classification Subcommittee of the International Headache Society: The International classification and diagnostic criteria for headache disorders, cranial neuralgia and facial pain. Ed 2 Cephalalgia **24 Suppl 1**: 9–160; 2004
2. Eboli P, Stone JL, Aydin S, Slavin KV. Historical characterization of trigeminal neuralgia. Neurosurgery **64(6)**: 1183–1187; 2009
3. Rand RW, Jacques DB, Melbye RW, Copcutt BG, Levenick MN, Fisher MR. Leksell gamma knife treatment of tic douloureux. Stereotact Funct Neurosurg **61(Suppl 1)**: 93–102; 1992

4. Kerr FW. Evidence for a peripheral etiology of trigeminal neuralgia. J Neurosurg **26(1 Suppl)**: 168–174; 1967
5. Kerr FW. Pathology of trigeminal neuralgia: light and electron microscopic observations. J Neurosurg **26(1 Suppl)**: 151–156; 1967
6. Love S, Coakham HB. Trigeminal neuralgia. Pathology and pathogenesis. Brain **124(12)**: 2347–2360; 2001
7. Malis LI. Petrous ridge compression and its surgical correction. J Neurosurg **26(1 Suppl)**: 163–167; 1967
8. Jannetta PJ. Arterial compression of the trigeminal nerve at the pons in patients with trigeminal neuralgia. J Neurosurg **26(1 Suppl)**: 159–162; 1967
9. Jannetta PJ. Trigeminal neuralgia. Neurosurg Focus **18(5)**: Intro; 2005
10. Jannetta PJ, McLaughlin MR, Casey KF. Technique of microvascular decompression. Technical note. Neurosurg Focus **18(5)**: E5; 2005
11. King RB. Evidence for a central etiology of tic douloureux. J Neurosurg **26(1 Suppl)**: 175–180; 1967
12. Sweet WH, Poletti CE, Macon JB. Treatment of trigeminal neuralgia and other facial pains by retrogasserian injection of glycerol. Neurosurgery **9(6)**: 647–653; 1981
13. Adams CB. Microvascular compression: an alternative view and hypothesis. J Neurosurg **70(1)**: 1–12; 1989
14. Dandy WE. The treatment of trigeminal neuralgia by the cerebellar route. Ann Surg **96**: 787–795; 1932
15. Adams CB, Kaye AH, Teddy PJ. The treatment of trigeminal neuralgia by posterior fossa microsurgery. J Neurol Neurosurg Psychiatry **45(11)**: 1020–1026; 1982
16. Janetta PJ. Treatment of Trigeminal Neuralgia by Micro-operative decompression ed 3. Saunders, Philadelphia; 1990
17. Linskey ME, Ratanatharathorn V, Penagaricano J. A prospective cohort study of microvascular decompression and Gamma Knife surgery in patients with trigeminal neuralgia. J Neurosurg **109(Suppl)**: 160–172; 2008
18. Casey KF. Role of patient history and physical examination in the diagnosis of trigeminal neuralgia. Neurosurg Focus **18(5)**: E1; 2005
19. Brisman R, Khandji AG, Mooij RB. Trigeminal nerve-blood vessel relationship as revealed by high-resolution magnetic resonance imaging and its effect on pain relief after gamma knife radiosurgery for trigeminal neuralgia. Neurosurgery **50(6)**: 1261–1266; 2002
20. Cohen DB, Oh MY, Jannetta PJ. Trigeminal neuralgia: surgical perspective. in (eds) Chin LS, Regine WF. Principles and Practice of Stereotactic Radiosurgery. Springer Science+Business Media LLC, New York: pp 527–534; 2008
21. Klun B. Microvascular decompression and partial sensory rhizotomy in the treatment of trigeminal neuralgia: personal experience with 220 patients. Neurosurgery **30(1)**: 49–52; 1992
22. Møller AR, Heros RC, Apfelbaum RI, Aoki N, Ambrosetto P, Silbergeld D. Views on microvascular compression: to the editor. J Neurosurg **71(3)**: 459–464; 1989
23. Jawahar A, Kondziolka D, Kanal E, Bissonette DJ, Lunsford LD. Imaging the trigeminal nerve and pons before and after surgical intervention for trigeminal neuralgia. Neurosurgery **48(1)**: 101–106; 2001
24. Campos-Benitez M, Kaufmann AM. Neurovascular compression findings in hemifacial spasm. J Neurosurg **109(3)**: 416–420; 2008
25. Pollock BE, Ecker RD. A prospective cost-effectiveness study of trigeminal neuralgia surgery. Clin J Pain **21(4)**: 317–322; 2005
26. Masur H, Papke K, Bongartz G, Vollbrecht K. The significance of three-dimensional MR-defined neurovascular compression for the pathogenesis of trigeminal neuralgia. J Neurol **242(2)**: 93–98; 1995

27. Sheehan JP, Ray DK, Monteith S, Yen CP, Lesnick J, Kersh R, Schlesinger D. Gamma knife radiosurgery for trigeminal neuralgia: the impact of magnetic resonance imaging-detected vascular impingement of the affected nerve. J Neurosurg 113: 53–58; 2010

28. Lorenzoni J, David P, Devriendt D, Desmedt F, De WO, Massager N. Patterns of neurovascular compression in patients with classic trigeminal neuralgia: a high-resolution MRI-based study Eur J Radiol: 2010 [Epub ahead of print]

29. Burchiel KJ, Clarke H, Haglund M, Loeser JD. Long-term efficacy of microvascular decompression in trigeminal neuralgia. J Neurosurg 69(1): 35–38; 1988

30. Kolluri S, Heros RC. Microvascular decompression for trigeminal neuralgia. A five-year follow-up study. Surg Neurol 22(3): 235–240; 1984

31. Blom S. Trigeminal neuralgia: its treatment with a new anticonvulsant drug (G-32883). Lancet 1(7234): 839–840; 1962

32. Parker NC. Trigeminal neuralgia: medical management perspective. in (eds) Chin LS, Regine WF. Principles and Practice of Stereotactic Radiosurgery. Springer Science+Business Media LLC, New York: pp 535–540; 2008

33. Dalessio DJ. Trigeminal neuralgia. A practical approach to treatment. Drugs 24(3): 248–255; 1982

34. Horsley V, Taylor J, Colman WS. Remarks on the various surgical procedures devised for the relief of trigeminal neuralgia (tic douloureux). Br Med J 2: 1249–1252; 1891

35. Speller WG, Frazier WG. The division of the sensory root of the trigeminus for the relief of tic douloureux; an experimental, pathological and clinical study with a preliminary report of one surgically successful case. The Philadelphia Medical Journal 8: 1039–1049; 1901

36. Cushing H. A method of total extirpation of the Gasserian ganglion for trigeminal neuralgia. By a route through the temporal fossa and beneath the middle meningeal artery. J. Am Med Ass 34: 1035–1041: 1900

37. Taarnhøj P. Decompression of the trigeminal root and the posterior part of the ganglion as treatment in trigeminal neuralgia. Preliminary communication. J Neurosurg 9(3): 288–290; 1952

38. Taarnhøj P. Decompression of the posterior trigeminal root in trigeminal neuralgia. A 30-year follow-up review. J Neurosurg 57(1): 14–17; 1982

39. Lopez BC, Hamlyn PJ, Zakrzewska JM. Systematic review of ablative neurosurgical techniques for the treatment of trigeminal neuralgia. Neurosurgery 54(4): 973–982; 2004

40. Rogers CL, Shetter AG, Fiedler JA, Smith KA, Han PP, Speiser BL. Gamma knife radiosurgery for trigeminal neuralgia: the initial experience of The Barrow Neurological Institute. Int J Radiat Oncol Biol Phys 47(4): 1013–1019; 2000

41. Theodosopoulos PV, Marco E, Applebury C, Lamborn KR, Wilson CB. Predictive model for pain recurrence after posterior fossa surgery for trigeminal neuralgia. Arch Neurol 59(8): 1297–1302; 2002

42. Kondziolka D, Zorro O, Lobato-Polo J, Kano H, Flannery TJ, Flickinger JC, Lunsford LD. Gamma Knife stereotactic radiosurgery for idiopathic trigeminal neuralgia. J Neurosurg 112 (4): 758–765; 2010

43. McNatt SA, Yu C, Giannotta SL, Zee CS, Apuzzo ML, Petrovich Z. Gamma knife radiosurgery for trigeminal neuralgia. Neurosurgery 56(6): 1295–1301; 2005

44. Pollock BE Comparison of posterior fossa exploration and stereotactic radiosurgery in patients with previously nonsurgically treated idiopathic trigeminal neuralgia. Neurosurg Focus 18(5): E6; 2005

45. Régis J, Metellus P, Hayashi M, Roussel P, Donnet A, Bille-Turc F. Prospective controlled trial of gamma knife surgery for essential trigeminal neuralgia. J Neurosurg 104(6): 913–924; 2006

46. Barker FG 2nd, Jannetta PJ, Bissonette DJ, Larkins MV, Jho HD. The long-term outcome of microvascular decompression for trigeminal neuralgia. N Engl J Med 334(17): 1077–1083; 1996

47. Fardy MJ, Zakrzewska JM, Patton DW. Peripheral surgical techniques for the management of trigeminal neuralgia – alcohol and glycerol injections. Acta Neurochir 129(3–4): 181–184; 1994

48. Loew F. Peripheral surgical techniques for the management of trigeminal neuralgia–alcohol and glycerol injections – editorial comments. Acta Neurochir **129(3–4)**: 185; 1994
49. Sweet WH, Wepsic JG. Controlled thermocoagulation of trigeminal ganglion and rootlets for differential destruction of pain fibers. 1. Trigeminal neuralgia. J Neurosurg **40(2)**: 143–156; 1974
50. Broggi G, Franzini A, Lasio G, Giorgi C, Servello D. Long-term results of percutaneous retrogasserian thermorhizotomy for "essential" trigeminal neuralgia: considerations in 1000 consecutive patients. Neurosurgery **26(5)**: 783–786; 1990
51. Håkanson S. Trigeminal neuralgia treated by the injection of glycerol into the trigeminal cistern. Neurosurgery **9(6)**: 638–646; 1981
52. Leksell L. Sterotaxic radiosurgery in trigeminal neuralgia. Acta Chir Scand **137(4)**: 311–314; 1971
53. Fujimaki T, Fukushima T, Miyazaki S. Percutaneous retrogasserian glycerol injection in the management of trigeminal neuralgia: long-term follow-up results. J Neurosurg **73(2)**: 212–216; 1990
54. Burchiel KJ. Percutaneous retrogasserian glycerol rhizolysis in the management of trigeminal neuralgia. J Neurosurg **69(3)**: 361–366; 1988
55. Slettebø H, Hirschberg H, Lindegaard KF. Long-term results after percutaneous retrogasserian glycerol rhizotomy in patients with trigeminal neuralgia. Acta Neurochir **122(3–4)**: 231–235; 1993
56. Lunsford LD, Bennett MH. Percutaneous retrogasserian glycerol rhizotomy for tic douloureux: part 1. Technique and results in 112 patients. Neurosurgery **14(4)**: 424–430; 1984
57. Saini SS. Reterogasserian anhydrous glycerol injection therapy in trigeminal neuralgia: observations in 552 patients. J Neurol Neurosurg Psychiatry **50(11)**: 1536–1538; 1987
58. Mullan S, Lichtor T. Percutaneous microcompression of the trigeminal ganglion for trigeminal neuralgia. J Neurosurg **59(6)**: 1007–1012; 1983
59. Shelden CH, Pudenz RH, Freshwater DB, Crue BL. Compression rather than decompression for trigeminal neuralgia. J Neurosurg **12(2)**: 123–126; 1955
60. Brown JA, McDaniel MD, Weaver MT. Percutaneous trigeminal nerve compression for treatment of trigeminal neuralgia: results in 50 patients. Neurosurgery **32(4)**: 570–573; 1993
61. Skirving DJ, Dan NG. A 20-year review of percutaneous balloon compression of the trigeminal ganglion. J Neurosurg **94(6)**: 913–917; 2001
62. Kondziolka D, Lacomis D, Niranjan A, Mori Y, Maesawa S, Fellows W, Lunsford LD. Histological effects of trigeminal nerve radiosurgery in a primate model: implications for trigeminal neuralgia radiosurgery. Neurosurgery **46(4)**: 971–976; 2000
63. Foy AB, Parisi JE, Pollock BE. Histologic analysis of a human trigeminal nerve after failed stereotactic radiosurgery: case report. Surg Neurol **68**: 655–658; 2007
64. Szeifert G, Salmon I, Lorenzoni J, Massager N, Levivier M. Pathological findings following trigeminal neuralgia radiosurgery. in (eds) Szeifert GT, Kondziolka D, Levivier M, Lunsford LD. Basel, Karger. Prog Neurol Surg 20: pp 244–248; 2007
65. Leksell L. Trigeminus neuralgi – Några neurofysiologiska aspekter och en ny behandlings metod. Läkartidningen **68(45)**: 5145–5148; 1971
66. Lindquist C, Kihlström L, Hellstrand E. Functional neurosurgery – a future for the gamma knife? Stereotact Funct Neurosurg **57**: 72–81; 1991
67. Kondziolka D, Lunsford LD, Flickinger JC, Young RF, Vermeulen S, Duma CM, Jacques DB, Rand RW, Régis J, Peragut JC, Manera L, Epstein MH, Lindquist C. Stereotactic radiosurgery for trigeminal neuralgia: a multiinstitutional study using the gamma unit. J Neurosurg **84(6)**: 940–945; 1996
68. Cheuk AV, Chin LS, Petit JH, Herman JM, Fang HB, Regine WF. Gamma knife surgery for trigeminal neuralgia: outcome, imaging, and brainstem correlates. Int J Radiat Oncol Biol Phys **60(2)**: 537–541; 2004
69. Massager N, Abeloos L, Devriendt D, Op de Beeck M, Levivier M. Clinical evaluation of targeting accuracy of gamma knife radiosurgery in trigeminal neuralgia. Int J Radiat Oncol Biol Phys **69(5)**: 1514–1520; 2007

70. Erbay SH, Bhadelia RA, Riesenburger R, Gupta P, O'Callaghan M, Yun E, Oljeski S. Association between neurovascular contact on MRI and response to gamma knife radiosurgery in trigeminal neuralgia. Neuroradiology **48(1)**: 26–30; 2006

71. Zerris VA, Noren GC, Shucart WA, Rogg J, Friehs GM. Targeting the cranial nerve: microradiosurgery for trigeminal neuralgia with CISS and 3D-flash MR imaging sequences. J Neurosurg **102(Suppl)**: 107–110; 2005

72. Erbay SH, Bhadela RA, O'Callaghan M, Gupta P, Riesenburger R, Krackov W, Polak JF. Nerve atrophy in severe trigeminal neuralgia: noninvasive confirmation at MR imaging – initial experience. Radiology **238(2)**: 689–692; 2006

73. Lorenzoni JG, Massager N, David P, Devriendt D, Desmedt F, Brotchi J, Levivier M. Neurovascular compression anatomy and pain outcome in patients with classic trigeminal neuralgia treated by radiosurgery. Neurosurgery **62(2)**: 368–375; 2008

74. Dellaretti M, Reyns N, Touzet G, Sarrazin T, Dubois F, Lartigau E, Blond S. Clinical outcomes after gamma knife surgery for idiopathic trigeminal neuralgia: review of 76 consecutive cases. J Neurosurg **109(Suppl)**: 173–178; 2008

75. Dvorak T, Finn A, Price LL, Mignano JE, Fitzek MM, Wu JK, Yao KC. Retreatment of trigeminal neuralgia with gamma knife radiosurgery: is there an appropriate cumulative dose? Clinical article. J Neurosurg **111(2)**: 359–364; 2009

76. Hasegawa T, Kondziolka D, Spiro R, Flickinger JC, Lunsford LD. Repeat radiosurgery for refractory trigeminal neuralgia. Neurosurgery **50(3)**: 494–500; 2002

77. Huang CF, Chuang JC, Tu HT, Chou MC. Microsurgical outcomes after failed repeated gamma knife surgery for refractory trigeminal neuralgia. J Neurosurg **105(Suppl)**: 117–119; 2006

78. Huang CF, Chuang JC, Tu HT, Lin LY. Repeated gamma knife surgery for refractory trigeminal neuralgia. J Neurosurg **105(Suppl)**: 99–102; 2006

79. Massager N, Lorenzoni J, Devriendt D, Desmedt F, Brotchi J, Levivier M. Gamma knife surgery for idiopathic trigeminal neuralgia performed using a far-anterior cisternal target and a high dose of radiation. J Neurosurg **100(4)**: 597–605; 2004

80. Massager N, Murata N, Tamura M, Devriendt D, Levivier M, Régis J. Influence of nerve radiation dose in the incidence of trigeminal dysfunction after trigeminal neuralgia radiosurgery. Neurosurgery **60(4)**: 681–687; 2007

81. Massager N, Nissim O, Murata N, Devriendt D, Desmedt F, Vanderlinden B, Régis J, Levivier M. Effect of beam channel plugging on the outcome of gamma knife radiosurgery for trigeminal neuralgia. Int J Radiat Oncol Biol Phys **65(4)**: 1200–1205; 2006

82. Pollock BE, Phuong LK, Gorman DA, Foote RL, Stafford SL. Stereotactic radiosurgery for idiopathic trigeminal neuralgia. J Neurosurg **97(2)**: 347–353; 2002

83. Régis J, Arkha Y, Yomo S, Murata N, Roussel P, Donnet A, Peragut JC. Radiosurgery in trigeminal neuralgia: Long-term results and influence of operative nuances. Neurochirurgie **55(2)**: 213–222; 2009

84. Régis J, Metellus P, Dufour H, Roche PH, Muracciole X, Pellet W, Grisoli F, Peragut JC. Long-term outcome after gamma knife surgery for secondary trigeminal neuralgia. J Neurosurg **95(2)**: 199–205; 2001

85. Zheng LG, Xu DS, Kang CS, Zhang ZY, Li YH, Zhang YP, Liu D, Jia Q. Stereotactic radiosurgery for primary trigeminal neuralgia using the Leksell Gamma unit. Stereotact Funct Neurosurg **76(1)**: 29–35; 2001

86. Balamucki CJ, Stieber VW, Ellis TL, Tatter SB, Deguzman AF, McMullen KP, Lovat OJ, Shaw EG, Ekstrand KE, Bourland JD, Munley MT, Robbins M, Branch C. Does dose rate affect efficacy? The outcomes of 256 gamma knife surgery procedures for trigeminal neuralgia and other types of facial pain as they relate to the half-life of cobalt. J Neurosurg **105(5)**: 730–735; 2006

87. Brisman R. Gamma knife radiosurgery for primary management for trigeminal neuralgia. J Neurosurg **93(Suppl 3)**: 159–161; 2000

88. Brisman R. Gamma knife surgery with a dose of 75 to 76.8 Gray for trigeminal neuralgia. J Neurosurg **100(5)**: 848–854; 2004

89. Brisman R, Mooij R. Gamma knife radiosurgery for trigeminal neuralgia: dose-volume histograms of the brainstem and trigeminal nerve. J Neurosurg **93(Suppl 3)**: 155–158; 2000
90. Dhople A, Kwok Y, Chin L, Shepard D, Slawson R, Amin P, Regine W. Efficacy and quality of life outcomes in patients with atypical trigeminal neuralgia treated with gamma-knife radiosurgery. Int J Radiat Oncol Biol Phys **69(2)**: 397–403; 2007
91. Dhople AA, Adams JR, Maggio WW, Naqvi SA, Regine WF, Kwok Y. Long-term outcomes of gamma knife radiosurgery for classic trigeminal neuralgia: implications of treatment and critical review of the literature. Clinical article. J Neurosurg **111(2)**: 351–358; 2009
92. Flickinger JC, Pollock BE, Kondziolka D, Phuong LK, Foote RL, Stafford SL, Lunsford LD. Does increased nerve length within the treatment volume improve trigeminal neuralgia radiosurgery? A prospective double-blind, randomized study. Int J Radiat Oncol Biol Phys **51(2)**: 449–454; 2001
93. Gellner V, Kurschel S, Kreil W, Holl E, Ofner-Kopeinig P, Unger F. Recurrent trigeminal neuralgia: long-term outcome of repeat gamma knife radiosurgery. J Neurol Neurosurg Psychiatry **79(12)**: 1405–1407; 2008
94. Han JH, Kim DG, Chung HT, Paek SH, Kim YH, Kim CY, Kim JW, Kim YH, Jeong SS. Long-term outcome of gamma knife radiosurgery for treatment of typical trigeminal neuralgia. Int J Radiat Oncol Biol Phys **75(3)**: 822–827; 2009
95. Henson CF, Goldman HW, Rosenwasser RH, Downes MB, Bednarz G, Pequignot EC, Werner-Wasik M, Curran WJ, Andrews DW. Glycerol rhizotomy versus gamma knife radiosurgery for the treatment of trigeminal neuralgia: an analysis of patients treated at one institution. Int J Radiat Oncol Biol Phys **63(1)**: 82–90; 2005
96. Herman JM, Petit JH, Amin P, Kwok Y, Dutta PR, Chin LS. Repeat gamma knife radiosurgery for refractory or recurrent trigeminal neuralgia: treatment outcomes and quality-of-life assessment. Int J Radiat Oncol Biol Phys **59(1)**: 112–116; 2004
97. Huang CF, Tu HT, Liu WS, Chiou SY, Lin LY. Gamma knife surgery used as primary and repeated treatment for idiopathic trigeminal neuralgia. J Neurosurg **109(Suppl)**: 179–184; 2008
98. Jawahar A, Wadhwa R, Berk C, Caldito G, DeLaune A, Ampil F, Willis B, Smith D, Nanda A. Assessment of pain control, quality of life, and predictors of success after gamma knife surgery for the treatment of trigeminal neuralgia. Neurosurg Focus **18(5)**: E8; 2005
99. Kondziolka D, Lunsford LD, Flickinger JC. Stereotactic radiosurgery for the treatment of trigeminal neuralgia. Clin J Pain **18(1)**: 42–47; 2002
100. Kondziolka D, Perez B, Flickinger JC, Habeck M, Lunsford LD. Gamma knife radiosurgery for trigeminal neuralgia: results and expectations. Arch Neurol **55(12)**: 1524–1529; 1998
101. Little AS, Shetter AG, Shetter ME, Bay C, Rogers CL. Long-term pain response and quality of life in patients with typical trigeminal neuralgia treated with gamma knife stereotactic radiosurgery. Neurosurgery **63(5)**: 915–923; 2008
102. Little AS, Shetter AG, Shetter ME, Kakarla UK, Rogers CL. Salvage gamma knife stereotactic radiosurgery for surgically refractory trigeminal neuralgia. Int J Radiat Oncol Biol Phys **74(2)**: 522–527; 2009
103. Longhi M, Rizzo P, Nicolato A, Foroni R, Reggio M, Gerosa M. Gamma knife radiosurgery for trigeminal neuralgia: results and potentially predictive parameters – part I: idiopathic trigeminal neuralgia. Neurosurgery **61(6)**: 1254–1260; 2007
104. Maesawa S, Salame C, Flickinger JC, Pirris S, Kondziolka D, Lunsford LD. Clinical outcomes after stereotactic radiosurgery for idiopathic trigeminal neuralgia. J Neurosurg **94(1)**: 14–20; 2001
105. Morbidini-Gaffney S, Chung CT, Alpert TE, Newman N, Hahn SS, Shah H, Mitchell L, Bassano D, Darbar A, Bajwa SA, Hodge C. Doses greater than 85 Gy and two isocenters in Gamma Knife surgery for trigeminal neuralgia: updated results. J Neurosurg **105(Suppl)**: 107–111; 2006

106. Nicol B, Regine WF, Courtney C, Meigooni A, Sanders M, Young B. Gamma knife radiosurgery using 90 Gy for trigeminal neuralgia. J Neurosurg **93(Suppl 3)**: 152–154; 2000
107. Petit JH, Herman JM, Nagda S, DiBiase SJ, Chin LS. Radiosurgical treatment of trigeminal neuralgia: evaluating quality of life and treatment outcomes. Int J Radiat Oncol Biol Phys **56 (4)**: 1147–1153; 2003
108. Pollock BE, Foote RL, Link MJ, Stafford SL, Brown PD, Schomberg PJ. Repeat radiosurgery for idiopathic trigeminal neuralgia. Int J Radiat Oncol Biol Phys **61(1)**: 192–195; 2005
109. Pollock BE, Foote RL, Stafford SL, Link MJ, Gorman DA, Schomberg PJ. Results of repeated gamma knife radiosurgery for medically unresponsive trigeminal neuralgia. J Neurosurg **93(Suppl 3)**: 162–164; 2000
110. Pollock BE, Phuong LK, Foote RL, Stafford SL, Gorman DA. High-dose trigeminal neuralgia radiosurgery associated with increased risk of trigeminal nerve dysfunction. Neurosurgery **49(1)**: 58–62
111. Rogers CL, Shetter AG, Ponce FA, Fiedler JA, Smith KA, Speiser BL. Gamma knife radiosurgery for trigeminal neuralgia associated with multiple sclerosis. J Neurosurg **97(5 Suppl)**: 529–532; 2002
112. Urgosik D, Liscak R, Novotny J Jr, Vymazal J, Vladyka V. Treatment of essential trigeminal neuralgia with gamma knife surgery. J Neurosurg **102(Suppl)**: 29–33; 2005
113. Young RF, Vermulen S, Posewitz A. Gamma knife radiosurgery for the treatment of trigeminal neuralgia. Stereotact Funct Neurosurg **70(Suppl 1)**: 192–199; 1998
114. Matsuda S, Serizawa T, Nagano O, Ono J. Comparison of the results of 2 targeting methods in Gamma Knife surgery for trigeminal neuralgia. J Neurosurg **109(Suppl)**: 185–189; 2008
115. Alberico RA, Fenstermaker RA, Lobel J. Focal enhancement of cranial nerve V after radiosurgery with the Leksell gamma knife: experience in 15 patients with medically refractory trigeminal neuralgia. AJNR Am J Neuroradiol **22(10)**: 1944–1948; 2001
116. Alpert TE, Chung CT, Mitchell LT, Hodge CJ, Montgomery CT, Bogart JA, Kim DY, Bassano DA, Hahn SS. Gamma knife surgery for trigeminal neuralgia: improved initial response with two isocenters and increasing dose. J Neurosurg **102(Suppl)**: 185–188; 2005
117. Drzymala RE, Malyapa RS, Dowling JL, Rich KM, Simpson JR, Mansur DB. Gamma knife radiosurgery for trigeminal neuralgia: the Washington University initial experience. Stereotact Funct Neurosurg **83(4)**: 148–152; 2005
118. Fountas KN, Lee GP, Smith JR. Outcome of patients undergoing gamma knife stereotactic radiosurgery for medically refractory idiopathic trigeminal neuralgia: Medical College of Georgia's experience. Stereotact Funct Neurosurg **84(2–3)**: 88–96; 2006
119. Friedman DP, Morales RE, Goldman HW. Role of enhanced MRI in the follow-up of patients with medically refractory trigeminal neuralgia undergoing stereotactic radiosurgery using the gamma knife: initial experience. J Comput Assist Tomogr **25(5)**: 727–732; 2001
120. Kanner AA, Neyman G, Suh JH, Weinhous MS, Lee SY, Barnett GH. Gamma knife radiosurgery for trigeminal neuralgia: comparing the use of a 4-mm versus concentric 4- and 8-mm collimators. Stereotact Funct Neurosurg **82(1)**: 49–57; 2004
121. Martinez-Moreno NE, Martinez-Alvarez R, Rey-Portoles G, Gutierrez-Sarraga J, Burzaco-Santurtun J, Bravo G. Gamma knife radiosurgery treatment of trigeminal neuralgia and atypical facial pain. Rev Neurol **42(4)**: 195–201; 2006
122. Matsuda S, Serizawa T, Sato M, Ono J. Gamma knife radiosurgery for trigeminal neuralgia: the dry-eye complication. J Neurosurg **97(5 Suppl)**: 525–528; 2002
123. Shaya M, Jawahar A, Caldito G, Sin A, Willis BK, Nanda A. Gamma knife radiosurgery for trigeminal neuralgia: a study of predictors of success, efficacy, safety, and outcome at LSUHSC. Surg Neurol **61(6)**: 529–534; 2004
124. Shetter AG. Trigeminal neuralgia: the impact of magnetic resonance imaging-detected vascular impingement of the affected ner, Zabramski JM, Speiser BL Microvascular decompression after gamma knife surgery for trigeminal neuralgia: intraoperative findings and treatment outcomes. J Neurosurg **102(Suppl)**: 259–261; 2005

125. Tawk RG, Duffy-Fronckowiak M, Scott BE, Alberico RA, Diaz AZ, Podgorsak MB, Plunkett RJ, Fenstermaker RA. Stereotactic gamma knife surgery for trigeminal neuralgia: detailed analysis of treatment response. J Neurosurg 102(3): 442–449; 2005
126. Young RF, Vermeulen SS, Grimm P, Blasko J, Posewitz A. Gamma knife radiosurgery for treatment of trigeminal neuralgia: idiopathic and tumor related. Neurology 48(3): 608–614; 1997
127. Zorro O, Lobato-Polo J, Kano H, Flickinger JC, Lunsford LD, Kondziolka D. Gamma knife radiosurgery for multiple sclerosis-related trigeminal neuralgia. Neurology 73(14): 1149–1154; 2009
128. Wang L, Zhao ZW, Qin HZ, Li WT, Zhang H, Zong JH, Deng JP, Gao GD. Repeat gamma knife radiosurgery for recurrent or refractory trigeminal neuralgia. Neurol India 56: 36–41; 2008
129. Brisman R. Microvascular decompression vs. gamma knife radiosurgery for typical trigeminal neuralgia: preliminary findings. Stereotact Funct Neurosurg 85(2–3): 94–98; 2006
130. Fountas KN, Smith JR, Lee GP, Jenkins PD, Cantrell RR, Sheils WC. Gamma knife stereotactic radiosurgical treatment of idiopathic trigeminal neuralgia: long-term outcome and complications. Neurosurg Focus 23: E8; 2007
131. Sheehan J, Pan HC, Stroila M, Steiner L. Gamma knife surgery for trigeminal neuralgia: outcomesand prognostic factors. J Neurosurg 102(3): 431–444; 2005
132. Huang CF, Tu HT, Liu WS, Lin LY. Gamma knife surgery for trigeminal pain caused by benign brain tumors. J Neurosurg 109(Suppl): 154–159; 2008
133. Kang JH, Yoon YS, Kang DW, Chung SS, Chang JW. Gamma knife radiosurgery for medically refractory idiopathic trigeminal neuralgia. Acta Neurochir Suppl 101: 35–38; 2008
134. Brisman R. Repeat gamma knife radiosurgery for trigeminal neuralgia. Stereotact Funct Neurosurg 81(1–4): 43–49; 2003
135. Pollock BE. Radiosurgery for trigeminal neuralgia: is sensory disturbance required for pain relief? J Neurosurg 105(Suppl): 103–106; 2006
136. Chang JW, Chang JH, Park YG, Chung SS. Gamma knife radiosurgery for idiopathic and secondary trigeminal neuralgia. J Neurosurg 93(Suppl 3): 147–151; 2000
137. Régis J, Metellus P, Lazorthes Y, Porcheron D, Peragut JC. Effect of gamma knife on secondary trigeminal neuralgia. Stereotact Funct Neurosurg 70(Suppl 1): 210–217; 1998
138. Cheng JS, Sanchez-Mejia RO, Limbo, M, Ward MM, Barbaro NM. Management of medically refractory trigeminal neuralgia in patients with multiple sclerosis. Neurosurg Focus 18 (5): E13; 2005
139. Miller JP, Acar F, Burchiel KJ. Trigeminal neuralgia and vascular compression in patients with trigeminal schwannomas: case report. Neurosurgery 62(4): E974–E975; 2008

Chapter 21
Diverse Functional Indications

Introduction

This chapter concerns functional indications other than trigeminal neuralgia. Tic douloureux has established itself as a major indication whilst the contribution of GKNS to other functional indications is a lot less clear. This is mildly ironic since the original Gamma Unit was specifically designed to treat Parkinson's disease and attempts were also made to treat cancer related pain.

Parkinson's Disease and Essential Tremor

As stated in an earlier part of the book the idea of gamma radiosurgery was to create small punched out volumes of brain in the locations normally used for the performance of thalamotomies or pallidotomies. The development of new pharmacological agents rendered all types of surgical intervention in the treatment of Parkinson's disease as less interesting than they had been. It took a while before the side effects of dopamine agonists made the use of thalamotomy more interesting again as a means of treating the tremor of Parkinson's disease.

In this context the Gamma Knife has been used for the treatment of Parkinson's disease in a number of centres. The treatment suffers from the same difficulties which concern all surgeons who attempt to produce lesions to obtain a given functional result. One of these is agreement about the appropriate target. This was well illustrated in 1985 by Laitenen who made contact with 16 of the world's leading functional neurosurgeons for information about the point they targeted [1]. He received nearly 16 different answers concerning location and a fair amount of variation in concerning the route to the target and the technique of lesion making. This is reflected in the Gamma Knife literature. Some workers have favoured thalamotomy [2–12]: using the VIM. One study has preferred the VOA or VOP [13]. Some use has been made of pallidotomy [9, 11, 12, 14–16] for the treatment of rigidity and bradykinesia. Gamma Knife pallidotomy has also been used for L-dopa

J.C. Ganz, *Gamma Knife Neurosurgery*,
DOI 10.1007/978-3-7091-0343-2_21, © Springer-Verlag/Wien 2011

induced dyskinesias [11, 12, 16]. There have also been reports of caudatotomy for the treatment of bradykinesia and rigidity [3, 13]. All of these papers report few if any complications. All of them record a latency of months to a year between treatment and effect. These reports claim success with thalamotomy for tremor in between 66% and over 84% of patients [2, 4–6, 8–13, 15]. The reports on pallidotomy for rigidity and bradykinesia are from one centre optimistic [11, 12, 16]. In all of the above reports the complications are listed as minor. GKNS has also been used against essential tremor with a similar pattern of good results and few significant complications [17–20].

Despite the enthusiasm from a few centres there seems to be a need for caution. The possession of a piece of technical equipment, in this case the Gamma Knife, does not automatically qualify its user to treat any condition that is technically possible to treat. It has been a theme of this book that modern treatment of many of the indications where GKNS may be used should be in the hands of a multi modality team who can bring their varying expertise to bear on the management. Nowhere, is this more true than in the surgical treatment (open or radiosurgical) than in the case of Parkinson's disease and Essential Tremor and other dyskinesias. To begin with, interventional methods are only appropriate in the face of failed medical treatment. The primary medical treatment is in the hands of the neurologist so that it is he/she who decides if intervention is possible. The surgeon's role is directed at deciding which method is most appropriate for the given patient in discussion with the neurologist and the neuroradiologist. In addition, the assistance of the neurophysiologist will be vital in assessing the investigation of the patient before and after any form of treatment. In the absence of an entire team experience in the management of these complex lesions, it would be inappropriate for a surgeon who has acquired a Gamma Knife to start using it for movement disorders without the necessary clinical and scientific backup team.

There is more. Over recent years new technology has been developed. There has always been a feeling that destroying a piece of anatomically normal brain tissue to repair a functional disorder is in a sense a mutilation. Today, there are ways of treating the malfunctioning brain by stimulation, so called deep brain stimulation (DBS) which is adjustable and replaceable. This method does require maintenance and is costly but is increasingly regarded as the surgical treatment of choice for movement disorders, when intervention is required. The Gamma Knife at best is an alternative to a destructive lesion.

Then there is the matter of complications. In a paper from the Cleveland Clinic, eight patients were reported with serious complications [15]. The paper concerned has one weakness in terms of its importance in that the dose used is not discussed. In four of the patients a dose of 200 Gy was used which is very high compared to the more usual 120–160 Gy reported in other series. However, in four of the patients lower doses were used. The seriousness of the complications recorded from such a distinguished centre is somewhat disquieting.

This paper also quotes a reference where there can be a difference of 1.5 mm between the desired target on a CT image and the actual stereotactic location within the frame. The paper refers to another paper which quotes the same inaccuracy [21].

This paper in term is quoting from the actual source paper, which should be obligatory reading for anyone using a stereotactic frame [22]. This study of accuracy demonstrates that realistically taking all the factors into account, using 1 mm CT slices. The paper includes a number of factors the measurement of which lies outside the competence of the physician and emphasises at least implicitly the importance of having a physicist on the team to make sure that the frame is used as accurately as humanly possible. This seminal paper on stereotactic accuracy which is still quoted was written 15 years ago. It is necessary for the physicist in each centre to check the accuracy of the technique being used in his/her particular centre and to put in place routines to ensure the maintenance of optimal levels of accuracy. It is perhaps relevant to quote from the above mentioned paper [22] that the maximum unavoidable error due to uncertainty of the precise location of a point within a 1 mm thick CT voxel was 1.36 mm. All of this is relevant to the current argument because it suggests that in terms of lesion making within the tolerances concerned, anatomical localisation without physiological confirmation of the correct location cannot ever be as reliable as a localisation technique. Yet anatomical localisation is the basis for lesion making using GKNS for thalamotomies or other lesions.

There is yet another factor. Patients' individual radiosensitivity is variable. Thus, even if the dose is delivered to the right location there is no certainty as to how the lesion will develop nor in which direction from around its centre. In a balanced review from the Pittsburgh Gamma Knife Centre and the University of Maryland in Baltimore it is suggested that the current level of information is too sparse and the long term follow up too short for definitive guidelines to be laid down for the use of GKNS for these functional indications [23]. They sensibly advise that GKNS ablative surgery should be restricted to those patients where intervention is strongly indicated and where the patient's medical condition precludes other treatments. They also consider that GKNS should only be used for Parkinson's disease and Essential Tremor and that its use in other cases remains an open question.

Finally, the current author would like to repeat that such treatment should definitely be restricted to centres which have a well established thalamotomy program in place before the Gamma Knife is installed, ensuring that all the necessary management expertise is already in place.

Epilepsy

Epilepsy number is not a disease but a pathological reaction of the brain to a wide variety of abnormal situations. Epilepsy is defined as the occurrence of two or more unprovoked seizures. There are a great variety of seizure syndromes. Some forms of epilepsy may be focal. The first treatment of all forms of epilepsy is medical using antiepileptic drugs (AEDs). It is only when AEDs fail that surgical intervention may be considered. There have been many attempts to perform the removal of epileptic foci mapped at corticography, a painstaking and frustrating technique. It is interesting to note that in the chapter "Epilepsy: Surgery Perspective" in the recent text book on radiosurgery, this treatment alternative is barely mentioned [24]. It has long been realised that the most useful form of surgical intervention for epilepsy concerned epilepsy based on anatomical definition, rather than physiological location of the epileptic focus. Thus, epilepsy associated with space occupying lesions may well improve following removal of the lesion, such lesions include hypothalamic hamartomas. Again, the most commonly performed surgical procedures are for mesial temporal epilepsy and there has been some success with corpus callosotomy.

Epilepsy Associated with Treatment Aimed Primarily at a Visible Lesion

It has been known for a while that epilepsy in association with AVMs could improve after GKNS [25–30]. This was first recorded in 1992 more or less from the Stockholm group and from the group in Sheffield [30, 31]. Further work on the topic was done from the ASAN Medical Center in Seoul, where Dr. Jin Whang presented two reports on the effectiveness of GKNS for epilepsy associated with non-growing space occupying lesions, for which surgery was not desired [32, 33]. There was gradual improvement with time so that the number of Engels class 1 results improved from 6 to 24 months after treatment. There were no clinical neurological deficits. Two patients developed asymptomatic post treatment oedema. The cautious Dr. Whang did not mention the prescription dose in his publications but he indicated in lectures that maybe 20 Gy was necessary for consistent results.

There is another series of tumours reported where the aim was to control the tumour and epilepsy. This came from Graz and had a particular notion that has not been subsequently repeated [34]. The great majority of the tumours were low grade gliomas and for the mean follow up of 2.25 years all were controlled by the GKNS. However, the major purpose was the control of epilepsy. The tumour volume and 10 Gy volume and the 10 Gy/tumour volume ratio were all recorded. When the 10 Gy volume/tumour volume was more than 3 the control of epilepsy and quality of epilepsy result was better. There were also better results in the temporal lobe tumours and for tumours with epilepsy lasting less than 2.5 years. The notion was in keeping with the teaching of Barcia Solario in aiming to treat a large volume with a low dose rather than a small volume with a large dose [35, 36].

Epilepsy Where the Epilepsy is the Reason for Treatment

Mesial Temporal Lobe Epilepsy is the Reason for Treatment

The first GKNS paper published on epilepsy based on physiological localisation came from the Stockholm group [37]. These early results were not encouraging but the notion had been created. The first consistently successful results were published from Marseille. The first paper came out in 1995 [38]. This concerned an elegant case report emphasising the advantage of applying the frame parallel with the temporal horn. The target was indicated graphically and the delayed result of treatment with necrosis of the irradiated area at 10 months is illustrated. The patient had been seizure free during the for 16 months of follow up but was still taking AEDs. A similar effect is shown at 9 months in a patient treated in Cairo who achieved an Engels I result (Fig. 21.1).

In 2000 the group then designed a very precise protocol and published the results on 16 patients followed for more than 24 months [39]. They required perfect agreement of all electro-physiological, radiological and medical data. The patients had to be suffering from medically refractory mesial temporal lobe epilepsy MTLE. The definition of medically refractory is not given, but then that is the decision of the responsible neurologist. The region to be irradiated including the amygadaloid complex (sparing the upper and mesial part) the head and anterior half of the body of the hippocampus, and the anterior part of the para-hippocampal gyrus. In addition the anterior part of the entorhinal area was included. The target should be covered by two 18 mm collimators and the margin dose should be 20–25 Gy delivered to the 50% isodose. The volume of the isodose should be between 6.5 and 7.5 mm [2]. The visual pathway should not receive more than 8 Gy and the brain stem should not receive more than 12 Gy. Thirteen (81%) of the patients were seizure free within 2 years. The median latency to cessation of seizures was 10 months. When the expansive necrosis appeared on MR the patients were routinely treated with corticosteroids till the changes improved. The paper lays weight on the fact that the epilepsy control was as good or better than with surgery

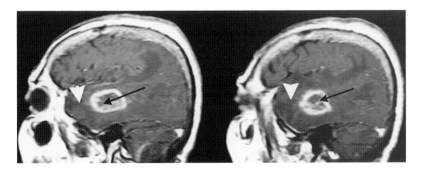

Fig. 21.1 These images were taken 9 months after treatment. The appropriate region had received 25 Gy to the 50% isodose created from two 18 mm shots. The maximum dose to the visual pathway was 6.5 Gy. The black arrow indicates the region of necrosis as shown by Gadolinium leakage on a T1 image with contrast. The white arrowhead indicates the region of oedema around the necrosis. Three months after this MR the patient deteriorated quite seriously and required dexamethasone for severe headache, which finally resolved leaving her with an Engels I result

and that there were negligible complications. Several other publications have come from this group on this topic [40–44]. In 1996 the team demonstrated in the laboratory that between 56 and 90 days after a delivering a dose of 100 Gy through the 4 mm collimator to the striatum of the rat, there developed an increase in neuroinhibitory transmitters and a decrease in neuroexcitatory transmitters [45]. This is thought to provide a potential basis for the decreased electric activity associated with control of epilepsy. However, how the radiation achieves this effect was not clear. The latest results from Marseille were published in 2008. Both papers show a seizure free rate of 60% at 5 years or more. The only neurological complication was asymptomatic quadrantinopsia in one patient and a hemianopsia in one patient [25]. A number of patients suffered a period of headache, treated with steroids [40]. One patient developed an asymptomatic post treatment temporal lobe cyst [25]. However, one patient died during an epileptic attack 6 months after treatment; a victim of the latent interval between treatment and effect.

The question then arises as to what extent other centres have been able to achieve similar results. A recent multicenter paper from the USA involved 30 patients followed for 3 years [46]. They were divided into two groups, one receiving 20 Gy and the other receiving 24 Gy. There was no significant difference between the two groups in terms of results but the overall freedom from seizures was 67%. There was a tendency for improvement to begin a bit quicker with the higher dose. There was no difference in complication rates between the two groups. Some patients in both groups required steroids for headache associated with brain swelling in association with necrosis. There was one patient who had a serious visual deficit and steroid resistant papilloedema and blind spot increase. This patient underwent a temporal lobectomy and the visual symptoms resolved. When seizures recurred after 18 months a second lobectomy rendered him seizure free. These results are closest to those from Marseille with the one difference that there was a serious loss of vision in one patient.

A series from Lille in France, whose patients were treated in Marseille had a slightly different experience. However, this was because the epileptogenic zone extended outside the typical MTLE region in some of their cases. In the 10 with the zone restricted to the MTLE region 60% were seizure free.

However, not every worker has a similar positive experience. Susan Spencer from Yale comments that the latent interval with possibility for increased mortality and slightly lower response rate plus the need for a longer period on medication could be considered to outweigh the advantages of a non-invasive method [47].

The group in Prague reported 15 patients with a mean follow up of 43.5 months. The group used the same treatment paradigm as the Marseille group and indeed took part in a multi centre study with Marseille. After GKNS no patient was seizure free [48]. The first patient to be operated was treated surgically 39 months after GKNS. A considerable improvement in Engels score was achieved after surgery. Three of the patients suffered marked raised intracranial pressure after GKNS which resulted in a lowering of the prescription dose to 18 Gy. This is lower than often advised. Even so it was not low. The group conclude that they are not convinced that the question of GKNS for MTLE has been settled.

From the Cleveland Clinic five patients were reported who received 20 Gy to the appropriate treatment volume. However, the epilepsy was not controlled and two patients died from epilepsy related complications at 1 month and 13 months after treatment. Since no improvement had occurred the surviving three patients were operated at 18, 20 and 22 months after treatment [49].

The group from Sheffield published their experience with a small series of eight patients followed for 24–63 months. Only three patients in this period became seizure free even though seizure frequency did reduce in all patients [50]. The dosimetry was as described by Régis both in terms of location, volume and prescription dose. One of the patients requested a lobectomy though in fact it didn't really help all that much. The group regarded the success rate as less good than surgery and again were worried about the latent interval and the potential risks involved.

Hypothalamic Hamartomas and Gelastic Epilepsy

Hypothalamic hamartomas are malformations of redundant grey matter in the region of the hypothalamus. They grow at the same rate as the body. Some are associated with precious puberty which is mostly treated medically with LHRH analogues. These lesions also possess an intrinsic epileptogenicity. This is a very rare condition, perhaps as low as 0.1% of all patients with seizures. The seizures normally start in the neonatal period or early childhood with a peak incidence between 2 and 3 years of age. The condition can often evolve into a generalized epileptic encephalopathy with severe seizures and cognitive and behavioural disturbances in about two thirds of patients. The attacks are usually brief; lasting from 10 to 30 s and consisting of unmotivated mirthless laughter which may be silent or loud. Crying attacks may occur in a minority of patients. Children with hamartomas and precocious puberty but without seizures do not develop behavioural disturbances. The author would like to emphasise here that most paediatricians prefer a medical approach in the treatment of precocious puberty so that attention here is directed only towards the treatment of epilepsy.

The epilepsy tends to be resistant to AEDs. Surgery has been tried from a variety of approaches but today the preferred approach is either transcallosal or transventricular using an endoscope. The risk of the transcallosal approach is damage to both fornices with resulting short term memory deficit. The advantage of the endoscope is that it is applied through the foramen of Monro and only abuts on one fornix. However, to be successful it must be inserted on the same side as the attachment of the hamartoma to cerebral tissue. So while the results of these methods have improved previous efforts they are far from problem free [51].

GKNS has been tried in an effort to avoid the complications of surgery and in this it has proved remarkably successful [52–59]. To understand the possibilities for GKNS it is necessary to understand the classification of these lesions which is as follows together with the recommended treatment modality from the report concerned [56].

Type I	Located in hypothalamus may extend third ventricle	GKNS
Type II	Mainly in third ventricle with root in hypothalamus	Resection or GKNS
Type III	Floor of third ventricle	GKNS if small
Type IV	Sessile lesions below the floor of the third ventricle	Resection
Type V	Pedunculous under floor of third ventricle	Rarely epileptic resection
Type VI	Giant including all the above. Multimodality with surgery and GKNS	

This classification is an amalgam of previous classifications. The types are not however quantified in terms of size. It has been shown that relief of epilepsy is related to the prescription dose which in turn is related to lesion volume. In one of the earlier papers all the successful results were in cases where the prescription was more than 17 Gy. Thus, it is suitable for smaller lesions which permit a higher dose. The permitted dose is limited by the dose to the visual pathway which was 10 Gy. To achieve this in two patients the prescription dose was over 17 Gy but the lesion cover was sub-optimal. Even so the epilepsy was improved.

While the major work has been done by the Marseille group there have been other small series. The Marseille group had a mean dose of 16.75 Gy (range 13–26 Gy). The mean lesion diameter was 11.15 mm (range 5–26 mm). The group in Guadeljara achieved marked improvement in 2 of 3 cases in both epilepsy and behaviour using doses between 12.5 and 15 Gy [52]. The Graz group with 4 cases achieved Engels 2 in 3 and Engels 3 in one and social reintegration in all. Moreover, they also used a smaller prescription dose of 12–14 Gy to lesions with a range of diameters between 11 and 17 mm. Four patients were treated in Pittsburgh. Two attained Engels 2 status. The group in Yonsei University had disappointing results with no improvement in 4 cases. However, they treated larger lesions with a mean diameter of 21 mm (range 10–35 mm) with a low mean dose of 11.5 Gy (range 9–12.5 Gy.

The precise place for GKNS in the treatment of MTLE and the gelastic epilepsy associated with hypothalamic hamartomas would seem as yet to be incompletely defined. The biggest advantage with the method is its low operative morbidity. The biggest disadvantage is the latency of several months between treatment and effect. These are complex conditions and in common with most other complex conditions a variety of treatments are available. It is suggested that these should be used not in competition but in cooperation. This is another example of where a multidisciplinary team offering all the possible treatments should be responsible for the management. This notion implies the centralisation of these uncommon treatments to centres of excellence where all the necessary expertise is present, including neurologists, neurophysiologists, neuroradiologists and in the case of hamartomas paediatric neurologists. These lesions should not be treated on an ad hoc basis just because an institution has acquired a Gamma Knife.

Pain

Intracranial Pain Syndromes

Nerve Related Pain Syndromes

There are four intracranial pain conditions which may be or have been treated using GKNS. They are three cranial nerve neuralgias and cluster headaches. Trigeminal neuralgia is such complex topic it has been covered in its own chapter (Chap. 20). There are only case history reports on glossopharyngeal neuralgia and sphenopalatine neuralgia and no more will be said about them here. The treatment of cluster headache has been reported in three papers [25, 60, 61]. The desperation of the patients with this condition which has been said to be the worst pain known to man makes it reasonable to try any treatment with even a small chance of success. Unfortunately, all three papers were consistent in their findings in series of ten patients that GKNS does not help cluster headaches

Thalamic Pain

There have been attempts to relieve thalamic pain using GKNS in two different ways. The first derives from the original work of Leksell where thalamotomy was used to treat thalamic pain [62–64]. The pain is excruciating and gamma thalamotomy does help up to a point. The doses used varied between 130 and 180 Gy. The targets included the centrum medianum nucleus, parafascicular nucleus and the medial dorsal nucleus. In between 60 and 70% initially excellent or good pain relief: that is to say a useful effect [62–64]. One patient had useful but not total pain relief so that he needed no medication for up to 7 years after the treatment.[26]

Another way to treat thalamic pain is by means of gamma knife anterior hypophysectomy. There are three current references on the topic [65, 66]. The results are consistent. The technique used is gamma knife anterior hypophysectomy. There is some risk of temporary diabetes insipidus [65, 66]. Hormone replacement has also been necessary on occasion [66]. These are treatable complications. Effective pain relief is achieved in roughly 70% of patients but unfortunately in over half this relief fades away over about 6 months.

Extracranial Pain Syndromes

In the 1970s it was quite usual to perform anterior hypophysectomies for patients with breast or prostate cancer with metastases. It became clear that the method only worked on pain due to bone metastases. Attempts were made to replace the stress of a transsphenoidal operation under general anaesthetic to trans-nasal injection of toxic chemicals. Over time it became the general opinion that the complications of these various procedures outweighed their benefits and the method fell into desuetude.

It was thus interesting to note that so distinguished a colleague as Dr. Dieter Lüdecke in Hamburg revived the validity of the method in a case report published in 2008. Impressed by the degree of pain relief Lüdecke raises the question as to whether this procedure should be reconsidered. The author of this book recalls a patient with breast cancer with dreadful pain from a metastasis in the neck of her femur. During the lifting of the patient onto and off the operating table a pathological fracture occurred through the tumour. Even so, after the trans-ethmoidal anterior hypophysectomy performed by Mr. Huw Griffith of Frenchay Hospital Bristol, the patient no longer required morphine for her pains.

In this context it is interesting to see that attempts have been made with to perform the hypophysectomy using the Gamma Knife. In 15 patients reported in two papers [67, 68] all patients were pain free from operation to death. However, it must again be emphasised that the method is only useful for pain from skeletal metastases arising from breast or prostate cancer. It is hoped in accordance with the suggestion of Dr. Lüdecke that this most effective treatment be considered on a wider basis.

Psychosurgery

The problems surrounding this topic do not relate to the methodology of lesion making. They are more social, political, and religious in origin. Just as it is up to the neurologist to decide when a patient's epilepsy is treatment resistant so is it up to the psychiatrist to decide if surgical intervention is required for one of his/her patients. The subject has had a long and contentious history, and the improvements in medication for psychiatric diseases have much reduced the potential indications. Recently, a paper has been published concerning 3 cases with 60% control of medically refractory symptoms [69]. The paper suggests that GKNS treatment should be reconsidered. It remains to be seen if the milieu is ready to consider this possibility seriously. However, a very recent paper indicates that also in this field DBS is likely to become the preferred interventional treatment [70].

References

1. Laitinen LV. Brain targets in surgery for Parkinson's disease. Results of a survey of neurosurgeons. J Neurosurg 62(3): 349–351; 1985
2. Duma CM, Jacques DB, Kopyov OV, Mark RJ, Copcutt B, Farokhi HK. Gamma knife radiosurgery for thalamotomy in parkinsonian tremor: a five-year experience. J Neurosurg 88(6): 1044–1049; 1998

3. Friehs GM, Ojakangas CL, Schrottner O, Ott E, Pendl G. Radiosurgical lesioning of the caudate nucleus as a treatment for parkinsonism: a preliminary report. Neurol Res **19(1)**: 97–103; 1997

4. Ohye C, Shibazaki T, Hirato M, Inoue H, Andou Y. Gamma thalamotomy for parkinsonian and other kinds of tremor. Stereotact Funct Neurosurg **66(Suppl 1)**: 333–342; 1996

5. Ohye C, Shibazaki T, Ishihara J, Zhang J. Evaluation of gamma thalamotomy for parkinsonian and other tremors: survival of neurons adjacent to the thalamic lesion after gamma thalamotomy. J Neurosurg **93(Suppl 3)**: 120–127; 2000

6. Ohye C, Shibazaki T, Sato S. Gamma knife thalamotomy for movement disorders: evaluation of the thalamic lesion and clinical results. J Neurosurg **102(Suppl)**: 234–240; 2005

7. Ohye C, Shibazaki T, Zhang J, Andou Y. Thalamic lesions produced by gamma thalamotomy for movement disorders. J Neurosurg **97(5 Suppl)**: 600–606; 2002

8. Pan L, Dai JZ, Wang BJ, Xu WM, Zhou LF, Chen XR. Stereotactic gamma thalamotomy for the treatment of parkinsonism. Stereotact Funct Neurosurg **66(Suppl 1)**: 329–332; 1996

9. Rand RW, Jacques DB, Melbye RW, Copcutt BG, Fisher MR, Levenick MN. Gamma knife thalamotomy and pallidotomy in patients with movement disorders: preliminary results. Stereotact Funct Neurosurg **61(Suppl 1)**: 65–92; 1993

10. Young RF, Jacques S, Mark R, Kopyov O, Copcutt B, Posewitz A, Li F. Gamma knife thalamotomy for treatment of tremor: long-term results. J Neurosurg **93(Suppl 3)**: 128–135; 2000

11. Young RF, Shumway-Cook A, Vermeulen SS, Grimm P, Blasko J, Posewitz A, Burkhart WA, Goiney RC. Gamma knife radiosurgery as a lesioning technique in movement disorder surgery. J Neurosurg **89(2)**: 183–193; 1998

12. Young RF, Shumway-Cook A, Vermeulen SS, Grimm P, Blasko J, Posewitz A. Gamma knife radiosurgery as a lesioning technique in movement disorder surgery. Neurosurg Focus **2(3)**: e11; 1997

13. Friehs GM, Ojakangas CL, Pachatz P, Schrottner O, Ott E, Pendl G. Thalamotomy and caudatotomy with the gamma knife as a treatment for parkinsonism with a comment on lesion sizes. Stereotact Funct Neurosurg **64(Suppl 1)**: 209–221; 1995

14. Friedman JH, Epstein M, Sanes JN, Lieberman P, Cullen K, Lindquist C, Daamen M. Gamma knife pallidotomy in advanced Parkinson's disease. Ann Neurol **39(4)**: 535–538; 1996

15. Okun MS, Stover NP, Subramanian T, Gearing M, Wainer BH, Holder CA, Watts RL, Juncos JL, Freeman A, Evatt ML, Schuele SU, Vitek JL, DeLong MR. Complications of gamma knife surgery for Parkinson disease. Arch Neurol **58(12)**: 1995–2002; 2001

16. Young RF, Vermeulen S, Posewitz A, Shumway-Cook A. Pallidotomy with the gamma knife: a positive experience. Stereotact Funct Neurosurg **70(Suppl 1)**: 218–228; 1998

17. Jawahar A, Cardenas RJ, Zwieg RM, Willis BK, Nanda A. A case report of complete disappearance of essential tremor after gamma knife radiosurgery. J La State Med Soc **156(3)**: 140–142; 2004

18. Kida Y, Kobayashi T, Tanaka T, Mori Y, Hasegawa T, Kondoh T. Seizure control after radiosurgery on cerebral arteriovenous malformations. J Clin Neurosci **7(Suppl 1)**: 6–9; 2000

19. Niranjan A, Kondziolka D, Baser S, Heyman R, Lunsford LD. Functional outcomes after gamma knife thalamotomy for essential tremor and MS-related tremor. Neurology **55(3)**: 443–446; 2000

20. Siderowf A, Gollump SM, Stern MB, Baltuch GH, Riina HA. Emergence of complex, involuntary movements after gamma knife radiosurgery for essential tremor. Mov Disord **16(5)**: 965–967; 2001

21. Starr PA, Vitek JL, Bakay R. Ablative surgery and deep brain stimulation for Parkinson's disease. Neurosurgery **43(5)**: 989–1013; 1998

22. Maciunas RJ, Galloway RL Jr, Latimer JW. The application accuracy of stereotactic frames. Neurosurgery **35(4)**: 682–695; 1994

23. Oh S, Niranjan A, Weiner WJ. Movement disorder in (eds) Chin LS, Regine WF. Principles and Practice of Stereotactic Radiosurgery. Springer Science + Business Media LLC, New York: pp 541–548; 2008

24. Davies KG, Edwards A. Epilepsy: surgical perspective in (eds) Chin LS, Regine WF. Principles and Practice of Stereotactic Radiosurgery. Springer Science+Business Media LLC, New York: pp 541–548; 2008
25. Donnet A, Valade D, Régis J. Gamma knife treatment for refractory cluster headache: prospective open trial. J Neurol Neurosurg Psychiatry 76(2): 218–221; 2005
26. Keep MF, Mastrofrancesco L, Craig AD, Ashby LS. Gamma knife surgery targeting the centromedian nucleus of the thalamus for the palliative management of thalamic pain: durable response in stroke-induced thalamic pain syndrome. J Neurosurg 105(Suppl): 222–228; 2006
27. Kondziolka D, Ong JG, Lee JY, Moore RY, Flickinger JC, Lunsford LD. Gamma Knife thalamotomy for essential tremor. J Neurosurg 108: 111–117; 2008
28. Kurita H, Kawamoto S, Suzuki I, Sasaki T, Tago M, Terahara A, Kirino T. Control of epilepsy associated with cerebral arteriovenous malformations after radiosurgery. J Neurol Neurosurg Psychiatry 65(5): 648–655; 1998
29. Schauble B, Cascino GD, Pollock BE, Gorman DA, Weigand S, Cohen-Gadol AA, McClelland RL. Seizure outcomes after stereotactic radiosurgery for cerebral arteriovenous malformations. Neurology 63(4): 683–687; 2004
30. Sutcliffe JC, Forster DM, Walton L, Dias PS, Kemeny AA. Untoward clinical effects after stereotactic radiosurgery for intracranial arteriovenous malformations. Br J Neurosurg 6(3): 177–185; 1992
31. Steiner L, Lindquist C, Adler JR, Torner JC, Alves W, Steiner M. Clinical outcome of radiosurgery for cerebral arteriovenous malformations. J Neurosurg 77(1): 1–8; 1992
32. Whang CJ, Kim CJ. Short-term follow-up of stereotactic Gamma Knife radiosurgery in epilepsy. Stereotact Funct Neurosurg 64(Suppl 1): 202–208; 1995
33. Whang CJ, Kwon Y. Long-term follow-up of stereotactic Gamma Knife radiosurgery in epilepsy. Stereotact Funct Neurosurg 66(Suppl 1): 349–356; 1996
34. Schröttner O, Eder HG, Unger F, Feichtinger K, Pendl G. Radiosurgery in lesional epilepsy: brain tumors. Stereotact Funct Neurosurg 70(Suppl 1): 50–56; 1998
35. Barcia Salorio JL, Roldan P, Hernandez G, Lopez Gomez L. Radiosurgical treatment of epilepsy. Appl Neurophysiol 48(1–6): 400–403; 1985
36. Barcia-Salorio JL, Barcia JA, Hernandez G, Lopez-Gomez L. Radiosurgery of epilepsy. Long-term results. Acta Neurochir Suppl 62: 111–113; 1994
37. Lindquist C, Kihlstrom L, Hellstrand E. Functional neurosurgery – a future for the gamma knife? Stereotact Funct Neurosurg 57(1–2): 72–81; 1991
38. Régis J, Peragui JC, Rey M, Samson Y, Levrier O, Porcheron D, Régis H, Sedan R. First selective amygdalohippocampal radiosurgery for 'mesial temporal lobe epilepsy'. Stereotact Funct Neurosurg 64(Suppl 1): 193–201; 1995
39. Régis J, Bartolomei F, Rey M, Hayashi M, Chauvel P, Peragut JC. Gamma knife surgery for mesial temporal lobe epilepsy. J Neurosurg 93(Suppl 3): 141–146; 2000
40. Bartolomei F, Hayashi M, Tamura M, Rey M, Fischer C, Chauvel P, Régis J. Long-term efficacy of gamma knife radiosurgery in mesial temporal lobe epilepsy. Neurology 70: 1658–1663; 2008
41. Régis J, Bartolomei F, Hayashi M, Chauvel P. Gamma knife surgery, a neuromodulation therapy in epilepsy surgery! Acta Neurochir Suppl 84: 37–47; 2002
42. Régis J, Bartolomei F, Rey M, Genton P, Dravet C, Semah F, Gastaut JL, Chauvel P, Peragut JC. Gamma knife surgery for mesial temporal lobe epilepsy. Epilepsia 40(11): 1551–1556; 1999
43. Régis J, Rey M, Bartolomei F, Vladyka V, Liscak R, Schrottner O, Pendl G. Gamma knife surgery in mesial temporal lobe epilepsy: a prospective multicenter study. Epilepsia 45(5): 504–515; 2004
44. Rheims S, Fischer C, Ryvlin P, Isnard J, Guenot M, Tamura M, Régis J, Mauguiere F. Long-term outcome of gamma-knife surgery in temporal lobe epilepsy. Epilepsy Res 80(1): 23–29; 2008

45. Régis J, Kerkerian-Legoff L, Rey M, Vial M, Porcheron D, Nieoullon A, Peragut JC. First biochemical evidence of differential functional effects following gamma knife surgery. Stereotact Funct Neurosurg **66(Suppl 1)**: 29–38; 1996

46. Barbaro NM, Quigg M, Broshek DK, Ward MM, Lamborn KR, Laxer KD, Larson DA, Dillon W, Verhey L, Garcia P, Steiner L, Heck C, Kondziolka D, Beach R, Olivero W, Witt TC, Salanova V, Goodman R. A multicenter, prospective pilot study of gamma knife radiosurgery for mesial temporal lobe epilepsy: seizure response, adverse events, and verbal memory. Ann Neurol **65(2)**: 167–175; 2009

47. Spencer SS. Gamma knife radiosurgery for refractory medial temporal lobe epilepsy. Too little too late? Neurology **70(5)**: 1654–1655; 2008

48. Vojtech Z, Vladyka V, Kalina M, Nespor E, Seltenreichova K, Semnicka J, Liscak R. The use of radiosurgery for the treatment of mesial temporal lobe epilepsy and long-term results. Epilepsia **50(9)**: 2061–2071; 2009

49. Srikijvilaikul T, Najm I, Foldvary-Schaefer N, Lineweaver T, Suh JH, Bingaman WE. Failure of gamma knife radiosurgery for mesial temporal lobe epilepsy: report of five cases. Neurosurgery **54(6)**: 1395–1402; 2004

50. Hoggard N, Wilkinson ID, Griffiths PD, Vaughan P, Kemeny AA, Rowe JG. The clinical course after stereotactic radiosurgical amygdalohippocampectomy with neuroradiological correlates. Neurosurgery **62(2)**: 336–344; 2008

51. Feiz-ErfanEIZ I, Horn EM, Rekate HL, Spetzler RF, Ng Y-T, Rosenfeld JV, Kerrigan JF III. Surgical strategies for approaching hypothalamic hamartomas causing gelastic seizures in the pediatric population: transventricular compared with skull base approaches. J Neurosurg **103(4 Suppl)**: 325–332; 2005

52. Barajas MA, Ramirez-Guzman MG, Rodriguez-Vazquez C, Toledo-Buenrostro V, Cuevas-Solorzano A, Rodriguez-Hernandez G. Gamma knife surgery for hypothalamic hamartomas accompanied by medically intractable epilepsy and precocious puberty: experience in Mexico. J Neurosurg **102(Suppl)**: 53–55; 2005

53. Mathieu D, Kondziolka D, Niranjan A, Flickinger J, Lunsford LD. Gamma knife radiosurgery for refractory epilepsy caused by hypothalamic hamartomas. Stereotact Funct Neurosurg **84(2–3)**: 82–87; 2006

54. Régis J, Bartolomei F, de Toffol B, Genton P, Kobayashi T, Mori Y, Takakura K, Hori T, Inoue H, Schrottner O, Pendl G, Wolf A, Arita K, Chauvel P. Gamma knife surgery for epilepsy related to hypothalamic hamartomas. Neurosurgery **47(6)**: 1343–1351; 2000

55. Régis J, Hayashi M, Eupierre LP, Villeneuve N, Bartolomei F, Brue T, Chauvel P. Gamma knife surgery for epilepsy related to hypothalamic hamartomas. Acta Neurochir Suppl **91**: 33–50; 2004

56. Régis J, Scavarda D, Tamura M, Nagayi M, Villeneuve N, Bartolomei F, Brue T, Dafonseca D, Chauvel P. Epilepsy related to hypothalamic hamartomas: surgical management with special reference to gamma knife surgery. Childs Nerv Syst **22(8)**: 881–895; 2006

57. Régis J, Scavarda D, Tamura M, Villeneuve N, Bartolomei F, Brue T, Morange I, Dafonseca D, Chauvel P. Gamma knife surgery for epilepsy related to hypothalamic hamartomas. Semin Pediatr Neurol **14**: 73–79; 2007

58. Shim KW, Chang JH, Park YG, Kim HD, Choi JU, Kim DS. Treatment modality for intractable epilepsy in hypothalamic hamartomatous lesions. Neurosurgery **62(4)**: 847–856; 2008

59. Unger F, Schrottner O, Feichtinger M, Bone G, Haselsberger K, Sutter B. Stereotactic radiosurgery for hypothalamic hamartomas. Acta Neurochir Suppl **84**: 57–63; 2002

60. Donnet A, Tamura M, Valade D, Régis J. Trigeminal nerve radiosurgical treatment in intractable chronic cluster headache: unexpected high toxicity. Neurosurgery **59**: 1252–1257; 2006

61. McClelland S III, Tendulkar RD, Barnett GH, Neyman G, Suh JH. Long-term results of radiosurgery for refractory cluster headache. Neurosurgery **59**: 1258–1262; 2006

62. Young RF, Jacques DS, Rand RW, Copcutt BC, Vermeulen SS, Posewitz AE. Technique of stereotactic medial thalamotomy with the Leksell gamma knife for treatment of chronic pain. Neurol Res **17(1)**: 59–65; 1995

63. Young RF, Jacques DS, Rand RW, Copcutt BR. Medial thalamotomy with the Leksell Gamma Knife for treatment of chronic pain. Acta Neurochir Suppl **62**: 105–110; 1994

64. Young RF, Vermeulen SS, Grimm P, Posewitz AE, Jacques DB, Rand RW, Copcutt BG. Gamma knife thalamotomy for the treatment of persistent pain. Stereotact Funct Neurosurg **64(Suppl 1)**: 172–181; 1995

65. Hayashi M, Chernov MF, Taira T, Ochiai T, Nakaya K, Tamura N, Goto S, Yomo S, Kouyama N, Katayama Y, Kawakami Y, Izawa M, Muragaki Y, Nakamura R, Iseki H, Hori T, Takakura K. Outcome after pituitary radiosurgery for thalamic pain syndrome. Int J Radiat Oncol Biol Phys **69(3)**: 852–857; 2007

66. Hayashi M, Taira T, Ochiai T, Chernov M, Takasu Y, Izawa M, Kouyama N, Tomida M, Tokumaru O, Katayama Y, Kawakami Y, Hori T, Takakura K. Gamma knife surgery of the pituitary: new treatment for thalamic pain syndrome. J Neurosurg **102(Suppl)**: 38–41; 2005

67. Hayashi M, Taira T, Chernov M, Fukuoka S, Liscak R, Yu CP, Ho RT, Régis J, Katayama Y, Kawakami Y, Hori T. Gamma knife surgery for cancer pain-pituitary gland-stalk ablation: a multicenter prospective protocol since 2002. J Neurosurg **97(5 Suppl)**: 433–437; 2002

68. Hayashi M, Taira T, Chernov M, Izawa M, Liscak R, Yu CP, Ho RT, Katayama Y, Kouyama N, Kawakami Y, Hori T, Takakura K. Role of pituitary radiosurgery for the management of intractable pain and potential future applications. Stereotact Funct Neurosurg **81(1–4)**: 75–83; 2003

69. Lopes AC, Greenberg BD, Noren G, Canteras MM, Busatto GF, de Mathis ME, Taub A, D'Alcante CC, Hoexter MQ, Gouvea FS, Cecconi JP, Gentil AF, Ferrao YA, Fuentes D, de Castro CC, Leite CC, Salvajoli JV, Duran FL, Rasmussen S, Miguel EC. Role of pituitary radiosurgery for the management of intractable pain and potential future applications. J Neuropsychiatry Clin Neurosci **21(4)**: 381–392; 2009

70. Bear RE, Fitzgerald P, Rosenfeld JV, Bittar RG. Neurosurgery for obsessive-compulsive disorder: contemporary approaches. J Clin Neurosci **17(1)**: 1–5; 2010

Part VI
The Gamma Knife and Specific Diseases: Less Common Indications

Chapter 22
Rare Tumours and Other Lesions

Introduction

This is a short chapter included for the sake of completeness. There are two rare intraparenchymal tumours which have been treated with GKNS where there are published series to which one can refer. There are also a number of rare conditions which have been treated with the Gamma Knife and published as case histories. A list is found at the end of the chapter.

Hemangiopericytoma

One time considered to be a variant of meningiomas this tumour has been considered as a separate entity since 1954 [1]. This is due to its aggressive behaviour and tendency to recur locally and to metastasise inside and outside the cranium. The best description of the role of the Gamma Knife in the treatment of these tumours is summed up a paper from Steiner's group published in 2000. There it states "Gamma surgery is effective in palliating the patients by decreasing tumor volume and delaying recurrence" [2]. It would be an exaggeration to believe that GKNS has a greater role than this. The earliest preliminary paper of a series found marked shrinkage in patients where images were available. The follow up period varies from 4 to 17 months for the 11 tumours in the five cases treated. This is in marked contrast to the slow decrease in volume of a proportion of meningiomas. This kind of speedy volume reduction can be an index of the tumours aggression, since cell death may occur after a number of cell divisions and in an aggressive tumour the cells divide quickly resulting in faster initial shrinkage. It also carries with it the possibilities for relatively speedy recurrence of those tumour cells which were not killed by the radiation. This is mentioned because if a tumour thought to be a meningioma suffers a rapid shrinkage, the nature of the tumour may need to be considered and the frequency of follow up MR examinations increased at least for 2 or 3 years.

J.C. Ganz, *Gamma Knife Neurosurgery*,
DOI 10.1007/978-3-7091-0343-2_22, © Springer-Verlag/Wien 2011

Retreatment for these lesions is quite often needed [3, 4]. The aggressiveness of the tumour is of importance in terms of control [3, 5] as is the dose [5]. A high prescription dose is desired but in practice has varied between 10 and 20 Gy in the varying studies in relation to the tumours' locations and size [3–8]. There are three series of over 20 patients published within the last 2 years. The first from Pittsburgh indicates that dose and tumour aggression are crucial for a better result [5]. The mean follow up was 48.2 months. Eight out of 20 patients had died of metastases or local progression. All the patients had been operated and 13 had received fractionated external beam radiotherapy. This radiotherapy seemed to have no effect on survival, recurrence or tumour control. Similar findings have been recorded earlier by other workers [3]. Twenty one of 29 tumours were under control after a mean/median follow up of 23.3/37.9 months. The more recent work from Charlottesville had a mean follow up of 62 months for 21 patients. At the most recent follow up only 47.6% patients were still alive. This worse result may be related to the longer follow up or to a different distribution of aggressive tumours in this later material, since the mean prescription dose of 16.7 Gy was higher than the mean dose of 14.8 Gy in the Pittsburgh material [4]. Again, the use of prior radiotherapy did not seem to have an effect on the survival of the patients. Finally there is a material from Beijing. In this series with a mean follow up of 26 months the exclusively recurrent tumours received a mean prescription dose of 13.5 Gy. There were 58 tumours. The control rate for these 58 tumours was 89.7%. Nonetheless four patients died; one from local progression and the other three from distant metastases. Yet again in this series post operative fractionated external beam radiotherapy had no effect on either the recurrence rate or the latency to recurrence [8].

In view of the reported findings outlined above it seems fair to say that there is a case for using GKNS soon after surgery, since conventional radiotherapy does not seem to have a striking effect on tumour control. It is necessary to be aware of the grade of the tumour. Every effort should be made to maximise the tumour dose, which again would be simpler if the patient has not received prior radiotherapy. Nonetheless, the patient numbers and follow up remain too small and short to do more than suggest that perhaps GKNS could be the preferable first choice adjunctive treatment for this condition. Hopefully, more and better data in the future will clarify this issue.

Lymphoma

In general there is no place for focal intracranial interventions with intracerebral lymphomas, with the exception of biopsy. However, in recurrent cases the treatment could have value to relieve symptoms and palliate the progression of the illness. In one paper six patients without immunodeficiency disease had relapsing intracranial lymphomas which were treated with radiosurgery [9]. The symptoms in all patients were markedly improved or disappeared. However, all the patients suffered tumour recurrence between 3 and 13 months. The second paper reports the findings in 22 cases with primary central nervous system lymphoma [10]. Here the standard treatment is whole brain radiotherapy and methotrexate. Eighteen of the patients had undergone some form of microsurgery with or without conventional radiotherapy. Four patients had received no treatment. The lesions disappeared after GKNS. However, new lesions appeared in other locations and were treated with repeat GKNS in ten patients. The mean prescription dose used was 16.5 Gy to a mean tumour volume of 4.14 cm [3]. There were no local recurrences and quality of life was good during the mean follow up period of 19.4 months. Again there is not enough clinical material to form a policy for the treatment of either kind of lymphoma. However, these early results indicate that in carefully selected cases GKNS can deliver useful benefit not least to the patients quality of life.

Rare Conditions Where the Information Is Based on Case Reports

There are a number of other conditions that have been treated using GKNS. However, the reporting is limited to case reports so that it is not possible to comment on principles of treatment. The various conditions concerned are listed below.

Masson's Hemangioendothelioma
Meningeal Melanocytoma
Plasmacytoma
Subependymoma
Cerebral Alveolar Hydatid Disease
Langerhans Cell Histiocytosis
Rosai Dorfman Disease

References

1. Begg CF, Garrett R. Hemangiopericytoma occurring in the meninges. **Case report.** Cancer 7: 602–606; 1954
2. Payne BR, Prasad D, Steiner M, Steiner L. Gamma surgery for hemangiopericytomas. Acta Neurochir **142(5)**: 527–536; 2000
3. Ecker RD, Marsh WR, Pollock BE, Kurtkaya-Yapicier O, McClelland R, Scheithauer BW, Buckner JC. Hemangiopericytoma in the central nervous system: treatment, pathological features, and long-term follow up in 38 patients. J Neurosurg **98(6)**: 1182–1187; 2003
4. Olson C, Yen CP, Schlesinger D, Sheehan J. Radiosurgery for intracranial hemangiopericytomas: outcomes after initial and repeat Gamma Knife surgery. J Neurosurg **112(1)**: 133–139; 2010
5. Kano H, Niranjan A, Kondziolka D, Flickinger JC, Lunsford LD. Adjuvant stereotactic radiosurgery after resection of intracranial hemangiopericytomas. Int J Radiat Oncol Biol Phys **72(5)**: 1333–1339; 2008

6. Coffey RJ, Cascino TL, Shaw EG. Radiosurgical treatment of recurrent hemangiopericytomas of the meninges: preliminary results. J Neurosurg **78(6)**: 903–908; 1993

7. Sheehan J, Kondziolka D, Flickinger J, Lunsford LD. Radiosurgery for treatment of recurrent intracranial hemangiopericytomas. Neurosurgery **51(4)**: 905–910; 2002

8. Sun S, Liu A, Wang C. Gamma knife radiosurgery for recurrent and residual meningeal hemangiopericytomas. Stereotact Funct Neurosurg **87(2)**: 114–119; 2009

9. Matsumoto Y, Horiike S, Fujimoto Y, Shimizu D, Kudo-Nakata Y, Kimura S, Sato M, Nomura K, Kaneko H, Kobayashi Y, Shimazaki C, Taniwaki M. Effectiveness and limitation of gamma knife radiosurgery for relapsed central nervous system lymphoma: a retrospective analysis in one institution. Int J Hematol **85**: 333–337; 2007

10. Kenai H, Yamashita M, Nakamura T, Asano T, Momii Y, Nagatomi H. Gamma knife surgery for primary central nervous system lymphoma: usefulness as palliative local tumor control. J Neurosurg **105(Suppl)**: 133–138; 2006

Chapter 23
Orbital Indications

Introduction

When this author was a student in London in 1966 he was introduced to a quotation regarding intraocular melanomas. Interestingly enough in 1997 a Dr. Gordon wrote a letter to the New England Journal of Medicine with the identical quote "Look for the person with a glass eye and a big liver" [1]. In London the words "Look for" were replaced with "Beware of". Dr. Gordon tells how he spent nearly 4 decades seeking the answer to this "mystery". The London teachers were kinder. They made the comment at the bedside of a patient with the diagnosis, which is intraocular melanoma or uveal melanoma. The point being made was that despite removing the eye which contained the tumour the patient could still die later from tumour metastases.

Uveal Melanomas Background Information

Death in this condition is usually the result of liver metastases. In a study called the Collaborative Ocular Melanoma Study (COMS) the tumours were divided into small (up to 3 mm elevation) medium (3–8 mm thick) and large more than 8–10 mm thick. Small tumours were not treated until they grew to medium size. Then they were randomised into plaque brachytherapy or enucleation [2]. The large tumours were randomised into two groups. All were enucleated but one group received pre-surgical radiotherapy and one group did not. The pre-enucleation radiation made little difference. In another study based on COMS there was a 5-year mortality of 16% for small tumours, 32% for medium tumours and 50% for big tumours [3]. Both series comment that larger and more anterior tumours are more dangerous. Yet another recent series is more pessimistic suggesting that the mortality is 50% after only 3 years [4]. The longest follow up study to date is known as the Helsinki study which followed patients up to a maximum of 35 years.

J.C. Ganz, *Gamma Knife Neurosurgery*,
DOI 10.1007/978-3-7091-0343-2_23, © Springer-Verlag/Wien 2011

The 4-year tumour related mortality was 31%, the 15-year tumour related mortality was 45% and the 35-year tumour mortality was 52%, indicating how vital long term follow up is [5]. Assessing the results of treatment is made more difficult by the variability of the clinical course of this tumour [2]. In addition to the influence of size and location there are variations in the cells of the tumour [2, 6]. Very simply the predominant cells may be spindle cells, epithelioid cells or mixed. The presence of epithelioid cells is associated with more aggressive behaviour [6].

Thus it is important to recognise that for shorter term follow up, results can only be reliably reported in relation to tumour control and not to mortality. One of the odd features of this tumours is its well known ability to prove deadly from systemic metastases, years after an enucleation of an affected eye; metastases usually in the liver. Where the metastases reside in the interval is not known.

Radiosurgery has not been generally adopted by the ophthalmological community as a new contributor to the treatment of this condition. Thus, the available information concerns in COMS terms small to medium tumours treated in a few centres manned by enthusiasts. The mortality of these smaller tumours is not so clear cut. COMS also showed that the anterior tumours had a worse prognosis. A requirement for GKNS treatment of these tumours is an ophthalmologist who believes in the technique and its possibilities because it is this specialist who will select patients, follow them up and who will fix the eye on the day of treatment.

It is worth underlining that to place the results of GKNS in this condition in the context of other studies mentioned above the minimum follow up should be at least 3 years.

Treatment Technique

The idea of radiosurgery is to obviate the need for enucleation and increase the chance of retaining vision. It has proven to be a difficult path to travel. There have been successes but also problems. To begin with the patient has to have the eye fixed before imaging. This is done using a retrobulbar injection of marcaine. The duration of the effect of the injection is such that the procedure must be completed within roughly 4 h from fixation to finished treatment. The position of the patient during treatment can be uncomfortable because of the eccentric location of the tumour, though with the introduction of "Perfexion" this must be less of a problem.

The treatment is undertaken with MR images which give the best visualisation of the tumour. The most useful images are a 3D gradient echo T1 series with and without contrast and an axial T2 series. Again because of its eccentric location and small size special care is needed to check the geometric accuracy of the MR machine used for this purpose. The most extensive published material to date on this topic comes from Prague [7]. These workers checked the positions in the dose plan against physical measurements using polymer gel with MR images. There is good concordance for lesions that are 15–20 mm from the surface. For lesions closer to the surface the concordance is less good with inaccuracies of up to

15–20% in localisation leading to reduced dose delivery. The Prague group compensate for this by attaching a tissue equivalent mass of material over the eye to be treated. The precise details of how this is done are not specified. Nor is it clear if the this inaccuracy will apply with Gamma Knife "Perfexion" with its different design.

Case Selection

There is no definite rule for the selection of cases but the current literature does offer guidelines. The purpose of GKNS is to provide tumour control, limit metastases and avoid the need for enucleation. If possible it would be preferable if vision could be preserved. It is known that tumour aggression [4, 7] tumour volume [8–11], and anterior location with involvement of the ciliary body [7, 12, 13] are negative factors for local control. In addition pre-treatment systemic metastases is a negative factor for survival [7]. Distal metastases after treatment are the major cause of death in uveal melanomas, in particular liver metastases [8, 9, 11, 12, 14, 15]. There is no clear evidence as to what factors pre-dispose to post-treatment metastasis although in one paper it was suggested it could be related to tumour height [8]

Table 22.1 Tumour height and width in reported series

Reference	Case no.	Tumour height mm (range)	Tumour width mm (range)
Haas et al. [9]	32	5.16 (2.12–11.5)	11.1 (4.9–21.4)
Langmann et al. [13]	60	6.7 (3–12)	12.2 (3–22)
Langmann et al. [16]	66	≤10	≤16
Marchini et al. [17]	12	(3.5–13)	(8–16)
Marchini G et al. [18]	36	(3.5–14)	(8–21)
Modorati et al. [19]	78	6.1 (4.7–8.8)	
Mueller et al. [10]	35	9.1 (3.1–13.9)	13.1 (6.5–25)
Rennie et al. [14]	14	6.3 (3.5–11.8)	12.9 (10.9–17)
Simonova et al. [15]	75	8.5 (4–15)	
Woodburn et al. [20]	11	(2.9–7)	(6–13)

It can be seen from Table 22.1 that there a wide variety of sizes treated embracing all three of the COMS size definitions from small through medium to large. The tendency today is try to avoid tumours involving the ciliary body and to shape the dose where possible to protect the optic nerve. It is also conventional to enclose a 2 mm boundary outside the visible tumour to ensure improved local control [7].

Results in Terms of Local Control

Local tumour control varied from 84 to 100% [7–11, 13–21]. Precise causes of loss of local control vary. The matter of dosimetry shall be taken up lower down. However, there is the question of the price the patient must pay in terms of complications. It is part of the nature of uveal melanomas that once they have spread below the Bruch membrane they spread in the subretinal space giving a characteristic mushroom like appearance and also provides a mechanism for the known associated retinal detachment [7, 9–12, 19].

There are other radiation techniques in use, proton therapy and brachytherapy with either iodine-125, iridium-192 or ruthenium-106. GKNS in common with these techniques is aimed at avoiding enucleation of the eye. To make this viable the method must achieve adequate local control of the tumour as indicated above. It must also be free of serious complications, particularly those which affect quality of life.

Experience has shown that GKNS is associated with a number of fairly frequent complications. The development of complications is affected by the location and size of the tumour together with the presence of other illnesses such as hypertension and diabetes [7]. Complications are classified as early (within 90 days of treatment) and late (after 90 days). The early complications tend to be transient while the late complications tend to persist. The Prague material has perhaps the most comprehensive analysis of the incidence of complications and the parameters which affected them [7]. They found that toxicity to cornea and optic nerve was reduced if the dose to these structures was kept below 10 Gy. The limit dose for the lens was 7.5 Gy and for the iris 15 Gy. The most severe complications were retinopathy (15%), optic neuropathy (9%) lens damage (26%) and glaucoma (18%). Eleven percent of eyes had to be enucleated because of secondary glaucoma. Vision deteriorated in 34% of patients due to tumour progression in 3%, optic neuropathy in 8%, retinopathy in 9%, neovascular glaucoma in 14%. It may be noted that the mean time for the development of glaucoma was 18 months. In this material from Prague the effects of GKNS recorded in the literature are tabulated in comparison with other radiation techniques. The method scores reasonably well in terms of tumour control but has a relatively high incidence of retinopathy and enucleation.

Complications

Some years ago the author was present at a meeting where the eminent Dutch neuro-radiobiologist Dr. Albert van der Kogel asked the question why are such high doses used in the treatment of uveal melanoma? In his view there was little chance of a better control of tumour cells with prescription doses exceeding 25 Gy. (A van der Kogel personal communication). The initial high doses were based on experiment work done by Rand on melanomas in the eyes of rabbits where doses of 60–90 Gy to the 90% isodose were recommended [22]. In the great majority of papers the prescription doses have varied between 30 through 50 up to 80 Gy [8, 9, 12–21]. Two papers report treatment using prescription doses of 25 Gy [10] or 20–25 Gy [11].

The first of these series reported 25 patients with a relatively short follow up specified as more than 12 months [10]. There was 97% tumour control. There were two enucleations one due to treatment failure and one due to glaucoma. In the second report there were only 14 patients followed for a mean period of 32 months. There was 93% tumour control. Retinopathy with neovascularisation and vitreous haemorrhage occurred in 2 cases (14%). One patient had neovascular glaucoma and another with closed angle glaucoma required enucleation. Nine patients (64%) suffered worsening of vision.

Conclusion

Despite much work by distinguished and dedicated colleagues, the results of GKNS for uveal melanoma are in some ways disappointing. Certainly the local control rate is good but it is not noticeably better than other radiation techniques. There remains a significantly high rate of complications which reduce the chance of retaining vision. In the two papers where the dose was reduced, one had too short a follow up to be certain of the incidence of late complications and the other shows little benefit in terms of complications from a lower dose. On the other hand the tumour control rate with the lower doses were as good as in series with a higher dose, indicating that maybe Dr. van der Kogel is right and a lower dose would be more appropriate.

In view of the variability in the nature of these tumours, their rarity and the risk of GKNS induced complications it seems advisable to recommend that while attempts to improve GKNS for this condition should continue, the technique's use for this indication should be limited to specialist centres with the necessary expertise and experience. It should not be considered a routine indication for every Gamma Knife user to attempt. It will be interesting to see if the application of Gamma Knife Perfexion will permit an improvement in the results and complications from the treatment of these melanomas.

Finally, at the time of writing there is no follow-up material long enough to permit an analysis of the effect of GKNS on late metastases from these tumours.

Choroidal Haemangioma

This is a benign retinal tumour which exists in localised and diffuse forms. The diffuse form is usually a component of the Sturge Weber syndrome. The localised form may be observed unless by growth or secondary effects it may threaten vision. Laser photocoagulation is used to control growth but the failure rate is between 20 and 30% [23]. Radiotherapy has also been used but these tumours are small objects for conventional radiotherapy. GKNS provides a possible solution. In three patients treated in Seoul in Korea, two circumscribed tumours had GKNS as the primary treatment and one diffuse tumour had GKNS after failed photocoagulation. 10 Gy was the prescription dose and the maximum dose to the optic nerve was never more than 8 Gy and to the lens never more than 2.4 Gy. Control of tumour growth and a dramatic improvement in vision was recorded in all three patients. The current follow up of these patients is short but nonetheless this would appear to be an interesting new indication for GKNS.

Glaucoma

The group in Prague noted that during their treatment of other intra-ocular conditions a number of patients who had co-incidentally secondary painful glaucoma experienced a reduction in intra-ocular pressure following GKNS. This led to first a pilot project [24] and then a more formal study [25]. In this study there was a mixture of patients some with secondary glaucoma and some with primary open angle glaucoma. The treatment method developed from tentative partial ciliary body radiation into its current form where the entire ciliary body is the target volume and a median prescription dose of 15 Gy is used. 77% of patients experience disappearance of pain accompanied by a fall in intra-ocular pressure. Only one patient in the original pilot study required enucleation after the treatment. The effects on vision are not recorded.

Complications were not serious. Transient lacrimation related to the surgical fixation of the eye occurred in 61% of patients. Cataract was a problem in some patients requiring operative intervention in two patients. Compared with other treatments this would appear to be promising and useful and it is a little surprising that it has not been taken up more widely.

Optic Nerve Gliomas and Optic Nerve Sheath Meningiomas

These tumours are dealt with in the chapters on meningiomas (Chap. 14) and gliomas (Chap. 16).

Rare Conditions Where the Information is Based on Case Reports

There are a number of other conditions that have been treated using GKNS. However, the reporting is limited to case reports so that it is not possible to comment on principles of treatment. The various conditions concerned are listed below.

Rhabdomyosarcoma
Retinoblastoma
Endocrine Ophthalmopathy
Neovascular Macular Degeneration

References

1. Gordon RM. Solution to a medical mystery. N Engl J Med **336(19)**: 1393–1394; 1997
2. Kincaid MC. Uveal melanoma. Cancer Control **5(4)**: 299–309; 1998
3. Margo CE. The collaborative ocular melanoma study: an overview. Cancer Control **11(5)**: 304–309; 2004
4. Sandinha T, Farquharson M, McKay I, Roberts F. Correlation of heterogeneity for chromosome 3 copy number with cell type in choroidal melanoma of mixed-cell type. Invest Ophthalmol Vis Sci **47(12)**: 5177–5180; 2006
5. Kujala E, Mäkitie T, Kivelä T. Very long-term prognosis of patients with malignant uveal melanoma. Invest Ophthalmol Vis Sci **44(11)**: 4651–4659; 2003
6. El-Shabrawi Y, Ardjomand N, Radner H, Ardjomand N. MMP-9 is predominantly expressed in epithelioid and not spindle cell uveal melanoma. J Pathol **194(2)**: 201–206; 2001
7. Simonova G, Liscak R, Novotny J Jr. Ocular and orbital lesions. in (eds) Chin LS, Regine WF. Principles and Practice of Stereotactic Radiosurgery. Springer Science + Business Media LLC, New York: pp 593–610; 2008
8. Fakiris AJ, Lo SS, Henderson MA, Witt TC, Worth RM, Danis RP, Des Rosiers PM, Timmerman RD. Gamma-knife-based stereotactic radiosurgery for uveal melanoma. Stereotact Funct Neurosurg **85(2–3)**: 106–112; 2007
9. Haas A, Pinter O, Papaefthymiou G, Weger M, Berghold A, Schrottner O, Mullner K, Pendl G, Langmann G. Incidence of radiation retinopathy after high-dosage single-fraction gamma knife radiosurgery for choroidal melanoma. Ophthalmology **109(5)**: 909–913; 2002
10. Mueller AJ, Talies S, Schaller UC, Horstmann G, Wowra B, Kampik A. Stereotactic radiosurgery of large uveal melanomas with the gamma-knife. Ophthalmology **107(7)**: 1381–1387; 2000
11. Schirmer CM, Chan M, Mignano J, Duker J, Melhus CS, Williams LB, Wu JK, Yao KC. Dose de-escalation with gamma knife radiosurgery in the treatment of choroidal melanoma. Int J Radiat Oncol Biol Phys **75(1)**: 170–176; 2009
12. Cohen VM, Carter MJ, Kemeny A, Radatz M, Rennie IG. Metastasis-free survival following treatment for uveal melanoma with either stereotactic radiosurgery or enucleation. Acta Ophthalmol Scand **81(4)**: 383–388; 2003
13. Langmann G, Pendl G, Klaus Mullne R, Papaefthymiou G, Guss H. Gamma knife radiosurgery for uveal melanomas: an 8-year experience. J Neurosurg **93(Suppl 3)**: 184–188; 2000
14. Rennie I, Forster D, Kemeny A, Walton L, Kunkler I. The use of single fraction Leksell stereotactic radiosurgery in the treatment of uveal melanoma. Acta Ophthalmol Scand **74(6)**: 558–562; 1996
15. Simonova G, Novotny J Jr, Liscak R, Pilbauer J. Leksell gamma knife treatment of uveal melanoma. J Neurosurg **97(5 Suppl)**: 635–639; 2002
16. Langmann G, Pendl G, Mullner K, Feichtinger KH, Papaefthymiouaf G. High-compared with low-dose radiosurgery for uveal melanomas. J Neurosurg **97(5 Suppl)**: 640–643; 2002
17. Marchini G, Babighian S, Tomazzoli L, Gerosa MA, Nicolato A, Bricolo A, Piovan E, Zampieri PG, Alessandrini F, Benati A. Stereotactic radiosurgery of uveal melanomas: preliminary results with gamma knife treatment. Stereotact Funct Neurosurg **64(Suppl 1)**: 72–79; 1995
18. Marchini G, Gerosa M, Piovan E, Pasoli A, Babighian S, Rigotti M, Rossato M, Bonomi L. Gamma knife stereotactic radiosurgery for uveal melanoma: clinical results after 2 years. Stereotact Funct Neurosurg **66(Suppl 1)**: 208–213; 1996
19. Modorati G, Miserocchi E, Galli L, Picozzi P, Rama P. Gamma knife radiosurgery for uveal melanoma: 12 years of experience. Br J Ophthalmol **93(1)**: 40–44; 2009
20. Woodburn R, Danis R, Timmerman R, Witt T, Ciulla T, Worth R, Bank M, Coffman S. Preliminary experience in the treatment of choroidal melanoma with gamma knife radiosurgery. J Neurosurg **93(Suppl 3)**: 177–179; 2000

21. Song WK, Yang WI, Byeon SH, Koh HJ, Kwon OW, Lee SC. Clinicopathologic report of uveal melanoma with persistent exudative retinal detachment after gamma knife radiosurgery. Ophthalmologica **224(1)**: 16–21; 2009

22. Rand RW, Khonsary A, Brown WJ, Winter J, Snow HD. Leksell stereotactic radiosurgery in the treatment of eye melanoma. Neurol Res **9(2)**: 142–146; 1987

23. Kong DS, Lee JI, Kang SW. Gamma knife radiosurgery for choroidal hemangioma. Am J Ophthalmol **144(2)**: 319–322; 2007

24. Vladyka V, Liscak R, Subrt O, Vymazal J, Pilbauer J, Hejdukova I, Nemec P. Initial experience with gamma knife radiosurgery for advanced glaucoma. J Neurosurg **93(Suppl 3)**: 180–183; 2000

25. Vladyka V, Liscak R, Simonova G, Pilbauer J, Hejdukova I, Novacek L. Progress in glaucoma treatment research: a nonrandomized prospective study of 102 patients with advanced refractory glaucoma treated by Leksell gamma knife irradiation. J Neurosurg **102(Suppl)**: 214–219; 2005

Part VII
Conclusions

Chapter 24
Conclusion and Possible Future Trends

Introduction

Gamma Knife radiosurgery was introduced at the end of the 1960s to treat functional disorders of the brain and is used now, for the most part, to treat tumours and malformations. It was initially designed to treat very small volumes. It is unlikely that it will be able to treat really large targets but it is also possible that it may be safely used with targets which are somewhat larger than those currently accepted as appropriate. However, this implies that the dosimetry is similar to that reported in this book.

It is also true that the techniques of focused radiation treatments have now expanded from the head, where they were first used to the rest of the body and to organs unrelated to the Central Nervous System. This means that radiosurgery will increasingly be managed by tumour oncologists, using technology which is different from the Gamma Knife. The sub millimetre accuracy necessary for intracranial treatments are neither possible nor necessary outside the cranium. The movements of the circulation and respiration make such accuracy impossible. The author is happy to have been involved in the use and development of a technology which slowly but surely has developed into something with a range of use far beyond what was originally envisaged.

However, it might be an error to forget the original concept. That is why this book is called Gamma Knife Neurosurgery rather than Gamma Knife Surgery.

The Responsible Physician

In the context of this book this could be considered an outmoded concept since no individual physician can possess all the necessary knowledge and experience to take single handed responsibility for the treatment of the conditions described in this book.

The Therapeutic Team

This perhaps should be the basic unit involved in the treatment of the conditions under consideration. Members of such a team should include expertise from a mixture of the specialities which refer and those who treat the patients and those who follow up the patients after treatment. The author is aware that this point has been laboured during the course of this book, but that is because it is perceived to be so important.

Team Members with Treatment Expertise Would Have to Include

Neurosurgeons
Neuro-radiologists
Medical Physicists
Oncologists
Nurses

Team Members Who Refer and Follow Up Might Include

Neuroosurgeons
Oncologists
Neurologists
Ophthalmologists
Otolaryngologists
Endocrinologists

Yet every management team must have a chairman or leader and it seems logical that this task should fall to the neurosurgeon. The diseases to be treated fall within his/her area of expertise. Only the neurosurgeon can offer all three therapeutic options, surgery, radiosurgery or wait and see. Moreover, he/she is the only member of the treatment team with adequate experience in the clinical assessment of the neurological symptoms and signs and the effects of treatment on them. In this he/she is guided by the other members of the team. The radiologist is vital to ensure the use of optimal technique for visualisation of the target. The oncologist is needed for the purpose of advising on radiobiology, dose and volume limitations and in the case of malignant tumours such as metastases, the integration of GKNS into to a total treatment program directed for the benefit of the patient as a whole. The physicist is responsible for the technical working of the Gamma Knife, the accuracy of its dose planning and the accuracy of the images imported into the dose planning system. The value of the nurses needs no special explanation since no hospital treatment can work effectively without their participation and particularly their humanity.

Functions of the Team

The initial function is to assess referred patients. The reaction to a referral will lead to either acceptance for treatment, refusal or a request for further additional treatment or investigation before a decision can be reached. However, once the team has accepted a patient for treatment it is to be hoped that every patient's lesion will be planned where necessary for multi modality treatment from the start. This would replace the current practice where the microsurgeon does his best and radiosurgery is required when safe radical surgery has not been feasible. With multi-discipline planning, the surgeon could with modern stealth technology remove what is safe and accessible and leave the rest for GKNS. The patient would be informed that this approach provided the optimal benefit in terms of disease control and safety from complications.

It cannot be emphasised too much that microsurgery and radiosurgery are not competing techniques but complimentary methodologies each fulfilling the other.

Personal Radiosensitivity: A Concluding Remark

While efforts to improve the mechanical and imaging accuracy of radiosurgery are ongoing, there is little likelihood that there will be dramatic improvements in these parameters in the foreseeable future. Indeed, it is perhaps unlikely that any such improvement could have anything but a marginal effect on the quality of treatment.

There is however an area of knowledge which would benefit greatly from investment in research. This is individual radiosensitivity. Anyone who has worked with therapeutic radiation will become aware that different people have different sensitivity to the same radiation dose. What is needed is a simple clinical test which could be applied prior to treatment. This would in time enable more sophisticated tailoring of the radiation dose to the particular patient's requirements. However, to date this matter, because of its complexity and technical difficulty in practice, has received relatively little attention. It is believed that a simple test as outlined above could materially improve the quality of any radiation treatment. It is hoped that investment and ingenuity will find a way sooner rather than later.

Appendix A: A Simple Unassisted Frame Application

Introduction

Most readers of this book will already know a method for frame application. However, it happens that for a variety of mainly administrative reasons the Gamma Knife user can find him/herself in the situation where a frame has to be applied and there is no qualified assistance.

What follows is a very simple guide as to how a frame may be applied with confidence without assistance.

The process is divided into several steps.

Frame Application

The process is shown in the accompanying figures and legends (Figs. A.1–A.7).

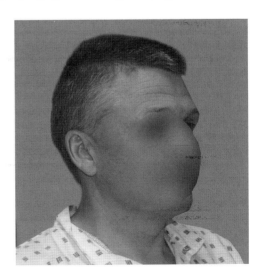

Fig. A.1 Stable position waiting to start

Fig. A.2 Note stable
position. MRI box in place.
Height of frame controlled by
number of compresses. In a
high lesion the top horizontal
line of the box should be
above the top of the head. In
the current case the target is
low sitting

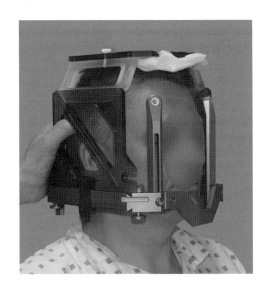

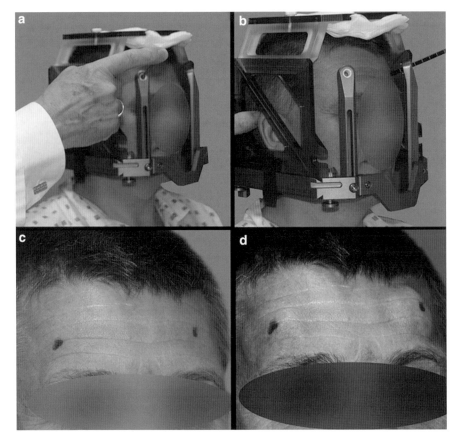

Fig. A.4 The anterior screws are in place. The surgeon's left hand is stabilising the frame from behind

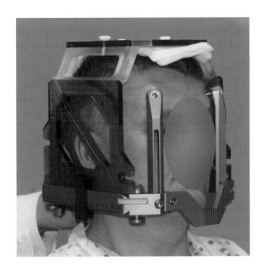

Fig. A.5 The safe posterior grip used while the local anaesthetic is injected at the back and the frame is held for 2–3 min until the regions are without sensation. Mostly the injection is through the holes in the posts. In cases where the distance from the post to the head is unusually long inserting a pin and screwing it in far enough that the location of its tip may be seen in relation to the head, can be helpful in placing the local anaesthetic in the right place

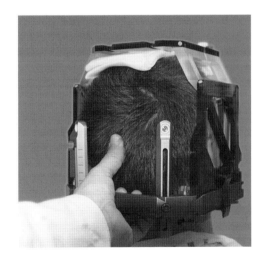

←

Fig. A.3 (**a**) and (**b**) show the ruler used to make ink marks (**c**) forehead with ink marks in place (**d**) local anaesthetic applied. Note that the anterior pins should avoid the thin part of the temporal bone and that if lateral the local anaesthetic should be allowed to spread posteriorly to ensure maxillary branches are anaesthetised as well as ophthalmic branches. Wait 2–3 min for the local anaesthetic to work. We use 1% xylocaine + adrenaline

Fig. A.6 The plastic box which ensures that there is no portion of the head or frame which will collide with Gamma Knife Perfexion. However, this is an approximation. With lesions which are at the occipital or frontal poles and for patients with metastases it is wise to measure the length of the posts and pins at the time of frame application, since this is a more accurate measurement than the plastic box

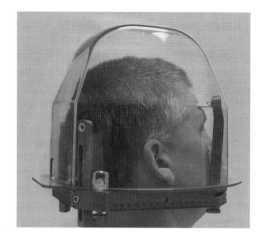

Fig. A.7 The plastic 'bubble' is fixed to the frame and measurements are made as indicated to insert into the dose planning software. This enables the software to calculate how much of a beam passes through air and how much passes through tissue. As a result the dose at the target can be calculated more accurately

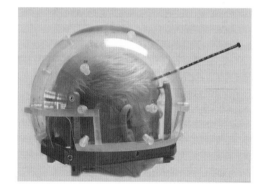

Completion

At this stage the patient is ready to be taken to the MR or CT laboratory for stereotactic imaging.

Index

Printing: Ten Brink, Meppel, The Netherlands
Binding: Stürtz, Würzburg, Germany